# OBSTETRIC and GYNECOLOGIC CARE

## in Physical Therapy

Linda J. O'Connor, BS, PT
Rebecca J. Gourley, BS, PT

SLACK Incorporated, 6900 Grove Rd., Thorofare, N.J. 08086

Printed in the United States of America

Library of Congress Catalog Card Number: 89-043071

ISBN: 1-55642-139-7

Published by:  SLACK Incorporated
6900 Grove Road
Thorofare, NJ 08086

Last digit is print number:  10  9  8  7  6  5  4  3  2

# Acknowledgments

The authors wish to thank Jane Frahm, Z. Annette Iglarsh, and Linda M. Pipp for their participation in interviews; Barbara Savi for her assistance in manuscript preparation; David P. Simmons, M.D., for his support and help with library privileges; Melanie Wallace for acting as our model; and the Section on Obstetrics and Gynecology of the American Physical Therapy Association for providing background material on the development of practice.

# Dedications

To my husband John for his evenings spent alone; to my three children—John, Scott, and Lisa— for letting me use the computer; and to the many physical therapists and physical therapy students who expressed the need and desire to perpetuate a new field of practice—LJO

To Jared and David for their love, patience, support, and confidence that allowed me the freedom to undertake and complete this project; and to the memory of Steve Rose whose zest for life, enthusiasm for physical therapy, and drive to pursue a vision, live on as an inspiration for all in physical therapy—RJG

# Table of Contents

# Preface

Pregnancy is not a pathologic condition, and a pregnant woman does not become a physical therapy client simply because she is pregnant. However, pregnancy does impose normal physiologic changes. The pregnant woman's ability to adapt to these changes will determine her need for services. Physical therapists have discovered that not every pregnant woman must suffer from posturally-induced backache, numb hands and arms, aching legs, pelvic joint pain, or the long-term effects of disease, injury, or traumatic event. Indeed, the effects of childbirth and of some gynecologic conditions can cause disorders years later. Many of the symptoms of these disorders, however, can be relieved to some extent and even prevented by therapeutic instruction during the childbearing years.

The flexible nature of physical therapy allows the practitioner to develop intimate, one-to-one relationships with patients. This potential relationship and an understanding of kinesiology, physiology, and family dynamics, make physical therapists uniquely qualified to build upon an already solid knowledge base and modify techniques for the pregnant woman. But, when considering the health of the fetus, in addition to the altered effects of standard therapy techniques during pregnancy, evaluation and treatment become complicated.

How, then, does a physical therapist learn about changes that occur during pregnancy and the implications these changes may have for future health? Physical therapy curricula, in general, lack adequate instruction in obstetrics and gynecology. Those who later become involved in the field must acquire that specialized knowledge through extensive reading, on-the-job training, and more recently, through continuing educations courses offered regionally by the Section on Obstetrics and Gynecology of the American Physical Therapy Association. Most of the other literature and educational courses, though, are presented from a physician's or nurse's viewpoint and lack that critical link to physical therapy. Physical therapists have written books on perinatal exercise and childbirth techniques, but so far, none have presented a comprehensive overview of the field for the physical therapy student or clinician with no background in obstetrics and gynecology. As even the specialized field of obstetric and gynecologic physical therapy branches into subspecialties (early pregnancy education, perinatal exercise, supportive care for labor and delivery, pain management post-Cesarean, remediation of musculoskeletal disorders of pregnancy and the postpartum, development of programs for high-risk pregnancy patients, and treatment of gynecologic conditions), the need for a single basic reference becomes crucial for practitioners.

This volume attempts to answer that need by providing current literature reviews, examination of controversial evaluation and treatment methods, and exposure to current practices. For physical therapy students and perennial students, many of the chapters include self-assessment reviews. At the end of the book are appendices for suggested readings and product information related to this field of practice. Through an awareness of the many facets of obstetric and gynecologic practice, physical therapists can expand their services for the female client and improve their value to the medical community.

# The Evolution of the Role of Physical Therapy in Obstetrics and Gynecology

# ONE

# Overview of Obstetrics and Gynecology

## *History of Obstetrics and Gynecology*

Why should a physical therapist be interested in the development of obstetrics and gynecology? Many would be hard-pressed to give a satisfactory answer. This topic is addressed in this text for the simple reason that obstetrics is a field that tends to go in circles—what goes around, comes around. For instance, people tend to think that "natural childbirth" is something of an oddity—a rare occurrence in this age of technology. But less known is that there was an outcry against medical intervention during a woman's labor and delivery as early as the 14th century. This outcry subsided and general acceptance reigned until this century. Therefore, it seems that the physical therapist well-versed in the development of this field may be able to provide clients with insightful advice. In this case, hindsight may indeed prove more valuable than foresight.

Obstetric care was chiefly provided by women until the role of men as physicians and healers also relegated the responsibility for women to males. However, it is believed that the early male "mid-wives" were ridiculed and embarrassed by physicians and patients alike.[1] Yet, the role of men as physicians confirmed their role in the care of women. More recent, however, is the acceptance by some (not all) physicians that gynecologic problems can cause a variety of symptoms previously categorized as psychosomatic or even hysterical. Hence, it should be obvious that certain events in history have brought the field of obstetrics and gynecology to its present state. Cianfrani, in his review of this topic, suggests that the progress of the field was minimal until around 1809 when McDowell performed the first documented gynecologic surgery. He further marks progress by the development of anesthesia, bacteriology, antibiotics, and endocrinology. Cianfrani identifies 20 stages of progress, ranging from the invention of the speculum to the application of endocrine physiology to the menstrual cycle. Rather than explore these 20 stages, this overview will concentrate on the relatively few events that are of interest to the physical therapist practicing in this field.

## *Famous Practitioners*

When studying obstetric history, several names constantly appear in the literature—Peter Chamberlen, William Smellie, William Hunter, and Joseph DeLee are but a few of the physicians who added to the current state of practice.

Although the story of the Chamberlens reads like a soap opera, it is enough to know that they attended the medical needs of the royal family in England. They also are remembered for their use of forceps, and possibly the invention of that instrument in the late 1500s.

Smellie was a noted British physician and pelvic anatomist, as was Hunter; both active practitioners of the mid-1800s. Smellie authored *Anatomic Tables* and Hunter authored *The Anatomy of the Human Gravid Uterus*. Hunter, unlike Smellie who used forceps but hid them in large pockets in his lab coat, touted nonintervention. "In his obstetric practice Hunter allowed nature to take its course whenever possible. He rarely used forceps. In fact, he was wont to publicly exhibit his own rusty pair during obstetric lectures as proof of this fact."[2] DeLee is credited with the establishment of the Chicago Lying-In Hospital, now part of the University of Chicago. He was also the inventor of a variety of obstetric equipment, the first to use motion pictures to instruct colleagues in new techniques, a proponent of episiotomy and low cervical Cesarean delivery, plus the author of *The Principles and Practice of Obstetrics* in 1929.

## *Tools of the Trade*

Invention of x-ray, the microscope, the speculum, sounds, and for-ceps are viewed by some historians as the miracles of gynecologic and obstetric practice.

X-ray assisted diagnosis and treatment, and Leeuwenhoek's micro-scope opened the door for medical and chemical research. The invention of the microscope, in particular, is most likely responsible for gynecologic anatomic and physiologic discoveries, including the follicles of de Graaf and the existence of sperm. These discoveries, in turn, led to an understanding of conception, gestation, and events surrounding childbirth.

Leeuwenhoek's 16th century introduction of the microscope en-abled a number of anatomists and physiologists to unfold the mys-teries associated with reproduction. Although dissection revealed many anatomic answers, it wasn't until the microscope was invented that researchers were able to confirm the existence of sperm and ova in the 17th century. De Graaf identified the ovarian follicle, and the way was paved for discoveries of tubal pregnancies, the difference between secretions of disease and of normal discharge, and the identification of fibroids and ovarian cysts. Sperm was discovered quite a bit earlier than the ovum, however. It was proposed origi-nally that the father alone gave rise to the fetus; the uterus was merely the incubator.[1] The invention of the speculum, used to dilate the vagina and explore the vagina and uterine cervix, dates back to at least the second century, A.D., and perhaps earlier than that. It is believed that an early speculum, dating to 1300 B.C., was possibly made from a hollow plant tube, similar to bamboo. Remains from Pompeii revealed evidence of at least two types of specula. Modern specula are based on the same principles introduced by the ancient Hebrews but tend to be easier for both patient and physician to use. The introduction of metal specula came later, in the 1500s.[1] The speculum fell in and out of favor until the 1800s when it started to gain popularity with physicians performing gynecologic surgery.

Sounds for dilating the urethra and cervix became popular in the 1600s, although it is believed primitive types of sounds were used by the ancient Egyptians as far back as 3500 B.C. It is also believed, however, that the early sounds were used strictly for applying medi-cations and for probing wounds rather than as a tool for explora-tion. Now, with the advent of fiberoptic tools for exploration, appli-cation of various treatments through narrow passageways inside the body is again part of the medical regimen. Perhaps the single most controversial tool introduced into the field was forceps. Not that the forceps themselves were the problem; rather it was the idea of assisted delivery. In this area in particular, the practitioner that keeps an eye on historical events will recognize that the idea of nonintervention during delivery may be associated with the earliest uses of forceps. Prior to their introduction, the only assisted deliveries occurred as embryotomies (*i.e.,* the extraction of a dead fetus from the womb via dismemberment). The instruments used for this were a fillet, a hook, a lever, and finally the forceps.

The fillet was a loop, usually of either muslin, linen, leather, or whalebone, used to lasso the fetal presenting part. Often, however, it was difficult to apply the fillet to the fetus, and blunt hooks were used in conjunction with the fillet. The hook, however, tended to injure soft tissues more easily, and appears to have been primarily reserved for embryotomy.

The lever, also called vectis or tractor, was perhaps the forerunner of the modern forceps. This tool was curved and had a blade for cephalic presentations. It was used for gynecologic procedures, such as pessary extraction, as well as for obstetric maneuvers. Although there is some disagreement as to who invented this tool, its use is documented in writings of the 18th century from Holland. Because of problems with slippage and injuring maternal tissues, this tool was abandoned, but paved the path for the forceps—two levers in combination. "The embryotomy group of instruments, those formidable instruments, long the stock in trade of physicians, continued as such for many years before the forceps were accepted and Cesarean section attained its great stature; yet even to this day these instruments of destruction are included in the armamentarium of some maternity hospitals for occasional use, if anyone around knows how."[1]

The credit for the first documented delivery of a live child goes to Peter Chamberlen, the Elder, but disagreement exists as to whether he invented the forceps. One reason for the confusion is that use of the forceps was so controversial that it was often applied as a secret method. Even the patient was blindfolded when it was used, according to some sources. Considerable modification of the forceps has occurred since its appearance in the late 1500s, but the principle of two forces joined to apply traction and leverage continues intact. What has fluctuated over the years is the attitude towards forceps' use. Many believed forceps held the same risk of injury to the mother or fetus as the lever. And in many cases, this fear was justified, as unskilled practitioners did indeed injure mothers and newborns (see Figure 1-1).

Among the prominent physicians that opposed indiscriminate use of forceps were William Hunter and Thomas Denman. The forceps, however, was the first instrument that could assist delivery

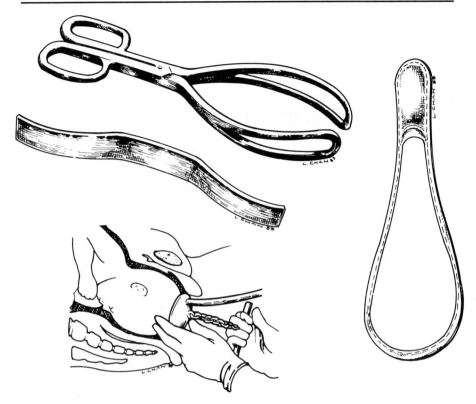

Figure 1-1: Obstetric instruments through the ages: (from top left, clockwise) early forceps, fillet or loop, vacuum extractor, lever.

of a live child. There was no way to discourage use of such a tool that could potentially save a fetus entrapped within the pelvis.

As this life-saving instrument gained favor, design modifications appeared, and actually continue to this day. Alterations of the blade curvature (compensation curve), inclination of the handles, closed or open shank blade, and type of lock between handles, are a few of the changes made for specialized deliveries. Certain obstetric maneuvers also required forceps, like Kjelland's for rotations, Tarnier's or Hodge's forceps for particular presentations, axis-traction forceps for applying external force, and Simpson's forceps, still in use today.

Forceps were welcomed into the obstetric armamentarium, and many women in danger of losing their own life, or that of their baby during childbirth, believed that any complications potentially imposed by the use of forceps certainly outweighed the risks. For the first two centuries or so, obstetricians' use of forceps received little criticism. In the early 1800s, however, public sentiment shifted back in favor of the wisdom of nature, and obstetricians followed suit. Obstetric practice continued with less emphasis on instrumentation until the late 19th century, when technology was viewed as progress. Forceps led the way for technological advancement in obstetrics—

an idea that also emphasized the need for delivery in the hospital. "In the early decades of the 20th century, the concept of prophylactic forceps' fit in well with the idea of delivery as a surgical, scientific procedure best conducted in a hospital setting.

Routine instrumentation was finally run aground in recent years when a new backlash against instrumental assistance developed. What is unclear is whether the pendulum will swing back and whether instrumental delivery will again become popular."[2] The idea of a vacuum extractor, used to extract the fetal head via suction, is credited to Simpson of forceps-fame in 1849. Based on the notion of creating negative pressure through cupping, vacuum extraction held promise for deliveries in which forceps could not be applied. Technical and technological difficulties, however, led to the disappearance of the vacuum extractor until Malmstrom developed the forerunner for variants that exist today (see Figure 1-1).

The only alternative to forceps or the vacuum extractor was, and is, the Cesarean section. This procedure dates back to 1500 A.D. when a physician, Jacob Nufer, desperately attempted to save his wife. Other Cesarean sections are documented in the 16th century, but these were performed without anesthesia and largely only when the mother's life was in jeopardy. Despite the concerns of modern consumers of obstetric care that Cesarean sections may be performed at the convenience of the caregiver, and not because the mother or fetus needs the procedure, this operation has saved many a life. The advent of anesthesia made this life-saving procedure easier for both physician and patient.

Anesthesia helped not only surgery but forceps application as well. Yet, it was not really popular until notable persons began to demand relief from the pain of labor, once it was known that such relief existed. In fact, Queen Victoria is reported to have asked for chloroform for her eighth delivery in 1853. "Following a discussion with her doctors concerning the proposed and controversial use of this anesthetic, the queen remarked, Gentlemen, We are having the baby and We are having the chloroform...."[2] In an obstetric nursing textbook from 1929, Carolyn C. Van Blarcom, RN, states, "In the early days, the idea of using anesthesia during labor was greeted with a storm of protest, both from the clergy and the laity, because of their belief that the relief of women in childbirth was contrary to the teachings of the Bible, as set forth in God's curse on Eve, when He said, In sorrow thou shalt bring forth children."[3] Even at that time there was objection to the use of anesthesia for spontaneous, uncomplicated deliveries.

Some physicians objected to chloroform on the grounds that the mother's pain guided the birth attendant about the progress of the labor. Simpson argued that the contraction of the uterus was the vital element for labor, not the pain. Van Blarcom adds, "Those of us who are accustomed to seeing anesthetics used to relieve patients of the worst of their pain, during labor, find it hard to realize that until comparatively recent years women went through this suffering without mitigation."[3]

Chloroform was often administered only for delivery, not during labor, and strictly as an agent to decrease "the danger of perineal tears, as the accoucheur has better control of the delivery when the patient lies quietly than when she tossed violently about the bed . . . ." There also existed some wariness that too much anesthetic might prolong labor and adversely affect the fetus. Today, this wariness still exists, but more is known about types of anesthesia and analgesia and their effects on the fetus and mother. These effects will be discussed in more detail in the chapters on labor and delivery.

## OB/GYN Physical Therapy: Development of Practice

Although the practice of obstetric physical therapy is relatively new in the United States, the idea of physical therapists having something to offer the pregnant patient is more firmly entrenched in countries such as England, South Africa, Australia, and Canada. This does not imply, however, that referrals are more frequent, nor that physician acceptance and awareness of physical therapy skills is any better. When Elizabeth Noble, Australian physical therapist, came to the United States, she was disappointed to learn that little, if any, physical therapy practice was conducted in this field. About the closest physical therapists were to treating the obstetric patient was through instructing childbirth education classes; a practice spearheaded by physical therapist, Elisabeth Bing, in New York in the 1960s. Bing's *Moving Through Pregnancy* was the first American book to apply the concepts of body mechanics training to the pregnant woman. Other foreign books preceded hers: *Relaxation and Exercise for Childbirth,* by Helen Heardman (see Appendix), *Physiotherapy in Obstetrics* (out of print) by Maria Ebner, and *Preparation for Childbirth,* by Mabel Lum Fitzhugh (see Appendix).

In the '70s came Noble's *Essential Exercises for the Childbearing Year,* a book that meshed nicely with Americans' burgeoning interest in health and exercise. Noble coincidentally founded the OB/GYN Special Interest Section of the American Physical Therapy Association (APTA) in 1976 and drafted a document of the potential state of practice for physical therapists interested in this field. With much foresight, and based on her experience in her homeland, this document, the Position Paper for the Establishment of the OB/GYN Section, continues to be a valuable guideline for practitioners and for those therapists wishing to convince department administrations of the need for such a service.[4]

To further trace the development of the field in the United States, the best record is probably found in back issues of the *Bulletin of the Section of the American Physical Therapy Association*. Perhaps some quotations from assorted issues will help the historian trace the growth of this still developing role:

"Over 30 physical therapists responded to the paragraph in the APTA's August 1976, issue of *Progress Report* concerning a special group in obstetrics and gynecology. There must be many more PTs involved or interested; probably they are not members of the APTA because in the past this association has had nothing to offer specialists in OB/GYN."

"Unlike other countries, American physical therapists traditionally have not been trained in OB/GYN as undergraduates, employed by women's hospitals or otherwise involved in this field apart from recent participation in childbirth education.... This leaves glaring deficiencies in early prenatal education, which would stress the role of body mechanics, postural and other physical adjustments throughout the childbearing year, exercise, and other preventive measures."[5]

"Four out of the six major independent childbirth organizations in the USA were actually founded by physical therapists."[6]

"As physical therapists we have much to offer in the field of childbirth education, and it should not be the sole domain of the RN-CNM (Registered Nurse-Certified Nurse-Midwife). We've got to get together for the sake of the public's education. The man on the street' image of a physical therapist is hazy to begin·with. He's confused about what we're doing in respiratory care and burn tanks, and now obstetrics-gynecology.

"Unfortunately if the public in unclear about physical therapy, the professional sector is not much better. How does one obtain referrals to childbirth class or postpartum care if the physician thinks of physical therapists as the ladies in the gym?'"[7]

"Exposure to the OB/GYN area is noticeably sparse in the American physical therapy school curriculum. This seems a logical place to begin to generate interest."[8] "Obstetrical physical therapy...is not a practice in which therapists must train as childbirth educators, but it is a field where therapists practice as therapists."[9]

"I am constantly asked how a physical therapist can get involved with obstetrical patients. For those of you who are hospital-based, Cesarean rehabilitation is an excellent starting place. Our ability to improve the quality of care in this patient population is remarkable. For many of you, the opportunity is there. All it takes is a little initiative to get started!"[10] And with a little initiative, the role of the physical therapist in treating obstetric and gynecologic problems of the female patient became better understood and welcomed by women who were suffering needlessly. Yet, this role is far from being totally accepted by the medical profession and even within the field of physical therapy itself. In a survey of curricula in physical therapy in the United States, data revealed that less than half of the schools offered instruction in treatment of obstetric and gynecologic ailments.[11] Hopefully, future surveys will lend support to this expanding role. Besides Bing and Noble, therapists who have assisted in the promotion of the field include those who belong to the Section of Obstetrics and Gynecology of the American Physical Therapy Association, which offers a quarterly journal and continuing education programs at regional and national APTA meetings (see Appendix). Additionally, there are many physical therapists who do not belong to the section, but are also practicing as childbirth educators or as instructors of prenatal and postnatal exercise.[12] Finally, there are therapists who do none of the above, but are practicing as independent consultants in OB/GYN physical therapy, as employees of obstetricians and gynecologists, or as staff or administrative therapists in hospitals or clinic departments developing services for perinatal clients. The current role of the therapist will be discussed more fully in the next chapter.

## *References*

1. Cianfrani T: A Short History of Obstetrics and Gynecology. Springfield, Charles C Thomas, 1960.
2. O'Grady J: Modern Instrumental Delivery. Baltimore, Williams & Wilkins, 1988.
3. Van Blarcom C: Obstetrical Nursing (2nd ed). New York, MacMillan, 1928.
4. Noble E: Position paper. Bull Sect Obstet Gynecol, APTA 8(1):6-10, 1984.
5. Noble E: Special Interest Group in Obstetrics & Gynecology Newsletter 1(1):1, 1976.
6. Noble E: Bull Sect Obstet Gynecol, APTA 1(4):1, 1977.
7. Frahm J: Bull Sect Obstet Gynecol, APTA 2(3):10, 1978.
8. Frahm J: Bull Sect Obstet Gynecol, APTA 3 (3&4):1, 1979.
9. Iglarsh ZA: Bull Sect Obstet Gynecol, APTA 6(4):18, 1982.
10. Kotarinos R: Bull Sect Obstet Gynecol, APTA 8(4):5, 1984.
11. Hulme J, Nieman K, Miller K: Obstetrics in the physical therapy curriculum. Phys Ther 65(1):51-53, 1985.
12. Wallis K, Curtis PR, Kondela-Cebulski P: The physical therapist

in obstetrics practice: Results of an initial survey of section members. Bull Sect Obstet Gynecol, APTA 11(1):5-8, 1987.

# Two

# Current Role of the Physical Therapist in OB/GYN

## *Current Role*

The role of the obstetric and gynecologic physical therapist in the United States has expanded greatly over the last 15 years. Initially, physical therapists were viewed by other maternal health providers as childbirth educators, edging in on an area traditionally thought of as part of nursing. OB/GYN practice, however, is a natural area of interest for physical therapists because of the intimate relationship of muscle physiology, mechanics, and exercise to the changes of pregnancy. Noble's three objectives for the Special Interest Section on Obstetrics and Gynecology of the American Physical Therapy Association (APTA) still serve practitioners well as the role of OB/GYN therapists expands: (1) to promote the role of physical therapists in OB/GYN, (2) to facilitate training of physical therapists wishing to specialize in OB/GYN, and (3) to foster research and study.[1]

Today, physical therapists interested in this specialty evaluate, treat, counsel, and monitor obstetric and gynecologic patients. Areas of interest within the field now include treatment of gynecologic dysfunction and changes associated with pregnancy (physiological, biomechanical, and emotional); instruction in prenatal, childbirth education, and exercise classes for prenatal, postpartum, and post-Cesarean clients. As recognition grows, so does the need for education. More colleges offer OB/GYN classes as options for a more in-depth view of this specialty. Northwestern University, for example, has been open to individual design of a Master's degree program in physical therapy with a specialty in OB/GYN. In addition, the Section on Obstetrics and Gynecology of the APTA is exploring requirements for clinical competency exams leading to certification as a specialist in this field. With further education, experience, and understanding of the OB/GYN patient, physical therapists will gain access to clients in need of services.[2,3]

In 1977, the Section on Obstetrics and Gynecology of the APTA prepared a position paper on the scope of practice within this specialty area. Because one of the most commonly asked questions by newcomers to the field is, what does an OB/GYN physical therapist do, this position paper has been reprinted below to answer that question and to provide experienced practitioners with reminders about options in practice that may have been forgotten.

## *Position Paper, Section on Obstetrics and Gynecology of the American Physical Therapy Association*

(Adapted with permission of the Section on Obstetrics and Gynecology, APTA)

### The Scope of Practice of Physical Therapy in Obstetrics and Gynecology

1. Physical and psychological preparation for childbirth
2. Education for early pregnancy and postpartum in exercise, body mechanics, and other health and comfort measures
3. Training the labor partner, and/or assisting the parturient with: breathing patterns, relaxation techniques, massage, changes of body position, administration of heat or cold, and pain management skills
4. Evaluation and treatment of musculature involved in childbearing
5. Treatment of orthopedic problems related to pregnancy and postpartum
6. Exercise regimes for maternity patients confined to bed and rest prenatally

7. Post-Cesarean section rehabilitation
8. Post-gynecologic surgery rehabilitation
9. Electrotherapy for pelvic disorders
10. Institution of OB/GYN curriculum in undergraduate and graduate physical therapy schools
11. In-service education to: labor, delivery, and postpartum staff; obstetric and gynecology clinics; nursing and allied health professions; schools; childbirth education conferences; and media programs for the general public.

**Areas of Overlap with Other Disciplines**    Primarily: registered nurses, certified nurse-midwives, lay midwives, and certified childbirth educators of lay or varied professional backgrounds.

Other areas of overlap include: dancers; yoga instructors; health educators; teachers; psychologists; physical education teachers; respiratory and occupational therapists; Masters of public health; medical doctors; chiropractors; osteopaths; naturopaths; acupressure, acupuncture, and biofeedback specialists; hypnotists; and social workers.

### The Role of the Physical Therapist in Obstetrics and Gynecology

The physical therapist practicing in the specific area of OB/GYN demonstrates expertise in the roles of educator, clinical practitioner, consultant, researcher, and administrator. The required functions and skills will be examined in the following pages:

### The Scope of Knowledge for Physical Therapy Practice in OB/GYN

Basic Sciences:     anatomy, physiology, kinesiology, embryology, histology, genetics

Clinical Sciences:  obstetrics, gynecology, neonatology, pharmacology, anesthesiology, nutrition

Social Sciences:    psychology, sociology, statistics, methodology, communications, group dynamics, history and theories of childbirth education

### The Function of the Physical Therapist as an Educator in OB/GYN

1. To provide education to the obstetric patient and her partner for health, comfort, and the accommodation of body changes during the childbearing year
2. To provide education to prepare the couple for labor, delivery and postpartum
3. To provide instructional programs and continuing education

for physical therapists, other medical personnel, and the public

**Skills Needed to be an Educator in OB/GYN**   As an educator in the specific area of OB/GYN, the physical therapist must be knowledgeable in:

1. Fetal development and psychology
2. Physical, hormonal, psychological, and sexual maternal changes associated with the childbearing year (three quarters, pregnancy; one quarter, postpartum)
3. Nutritional requirements for pregnancy and lactation
4. The obstetric process and parameters of normal labor
5. Complications and interventions; especially Cesarean section
6. Hospital procedures and patients' rights
7. Medication and anesthesia
8. Educational preparation for parenthood:
   a. Appearance and care of normal newborn
   b. Neonatal complications
   c. Parent-infant bonding
   d. Physiology of lactation and breastfeeding
   e. Postpartum adjustments
   f. Milestones of child development
9. Instructional programs and continuing education:
   a. Curricula and clinical affiliations for physical therapy students at the undergraduate and graduate level, and physical therapy assistants
   b. Continuing education for practicing physical therapists
   c. Educational programs for allied disciplines
   d. In-service education to OB/GYN units in hospitals and clinics
   e. Community education programs and public relations

## The Function of the Physical Therapist as a Clinical Practitioner in OB/GYN

1. To conduct a musculoskeletal evaluation of the obstetric patient
2. To conduct a cardiovascular evaluation and institute a program of conditioning
3. To demonstrate knowledge of comfort measures and preventive body mechanics
4. To instruct in therapeutic exercise appropriate to each phase of the childbearing year
5. To provide training in relaxation and breathing
6. To demonstrate techniques for pain management
7. To provide psychosocial and psychosexual support

8. To provide electrotherapy, ultrasound, hydrotherapy, and ultraviolet light treatments when prescribed
9. To provide chest physical therapy to mother or newborn when prescribed
10. To provide orthotic devices for the obstetric patient or newborn when prescribed
11. To assist and coach the parturient during labor
12. To advise the mother on breastfeeding, care of the episiotomy, and positioning for postpartum

**Skills Needed to be a Clinical Practitioner in OB/GYN**    The physical therapist practicing in the specific area of OB/GYN shall demonstrate expertise in the following:
1. Musculoskeletal evaluation
   a. Posture and gross muscle testing
   b. Specific evaluation of the abdominal wall (especially diastasis recti) and the pelvic floor (Kegel's perineometer) c. Assement of pelvic and spinal joint and nerve dysfunction, especially pubic symphysis and sacroiliac, sciatic nerve, and thoracic outlet syndrome
2. Cardiovascular evaluation and conditioning
   a. Edema evaluation
   b. Exercises and positioning to improve circulation
   c. Supine hypotension
   d. Training effects of exercise programs
   e. Vasodilation effects of connective tissue massage, acupressure
3. Biomechanics, preventive body mechanics
   a. Bed mobility and transfers
   b. Posture, gait, lifting, stooping
   c. Activities of daily living, modification of household and hospital equipment
4. Comfort measures
   a. Positioning and mobilization
   b. Orthotic devices and mechanical aids
   c. Work efficiency
5. Therapeutic exercise
   a. Active and progressive exercises adapted for each phase of the childbearing year
6. Psychosocial and psychosexual support
   a. Culture pressure and old wives' tales
   b. Physical and hormonal changes
   c. Alternative positions and methods for sexual satisfaction
   d. Consumer impact on health care providers
   e. Options in maternity care

7. Relaxation training
   a. Passive relaxation—yoga and meditation techniques
   b. Progressive relaxation—Jacobsen
   c. Touch relaxation—Kitzinger
   d. Biofeedback
8. Breathing management
   a. Diaphragmatic breathing
   b. Coordination of respiration with exercises
   c. Avoidance of Valsalva maneuver and hyperventilation
   d. Psychoprophylactic breathing patterns for labor (Lamaze)
   e. Controlled exhalation for expulsive effort in second stage
9. Techniques for pain management
   a. Conditioned response (Pavlov)
   b. Use of focal point—visual, auditory, and tactile stimuli
   c. Practice and repetition of psychoprophylactic techniques
   d. Administration of heat and cold
   e. Transcutaneous Electrical Nerve Stimulation (TENS), biofeedback
10. Massage
    a. Effleurage
    b. Kneading and deep frictions
    c. Counterpressure
    d. Connective tissue massage and acupressure (especially in gynecologic disorders)
    e. Reflexology and zone therapy
    f. Perineal massage
11. Chest physical therapy
    a. Postural drainage, percussion, and vibrations
    b. Instruction in breathing exercises, expectoration of sputum
    c. Suctioning
    d. Effects of anesthesia
12. Use of modalities in GYN conditions
    a. Short-wave diathermy, high-voltage galvanic stimulation for pelvic inflammatory conditions
    b. Faradic stimulation for pelvic floor weakness
    c. Iontophoresis, ultrasound (postpartum), ultraviolet light
    d. Hydrotherapy
    e. TENS, biofeedback
13. Labor coaching
    a. Assistance with relaxation and breathing
    b. Administration of comfort measures and pain management
    c. Meet with obstetric staff

14. Care of the neonate
    a. Respiratory care (hyaline membrane disease, respiratory distress syndrome, aspiration of meconium, pneumonia)
    b. Infant stimulation, oral stimulation
    c. Neurologic evaluation and behavioral assessment

## The Function of the Physical Therapist as a Consultant in OB/GYN

1. To develop a more physiologic approach to the present conduct of labor and use of hospital equipment
2. To expand existing services to provide clinical and educational programs for the entire childbearing years
3. To provide consultation to OB and GYN units with regard to physical therapeutic skills previously listed
4. To advise childbirth education groups on those aspects of their programs which relate to physical therapy skills
5. To be a resource person for physical therapy, medical, and allied health profession schools
6. To provide consultation for government and insurance agencies

### Skills Needed to be a Consultant in OB/GYN

1. Documentation and communications skills
2. Broad knowledge of other related disciplines
3. Public relations

## The Function of the Physical Therapist as a Researcher in OB/GYN

1. To determine the efficacy of current practices, such as:
   a. Exercise regimes in pregnancy and postpartum
   b. Positions for labor and delivery
   c. Breathing techniques and methods of expulsion in second stage
2. To study national and cross-cultural approaches to the conduct of labor and delivery
3. To determine the effects of obstetric intervention on maternal and neonatal outcome, parent-infant bonding, and child development
4. To investigate the benefits of exercise modalities and massage (acupressure) in gynecologic conditions

### Skills Needed to be a Researcher in OB/GYN

1. Statistics and methodology
2. Documentation
3. Grantsmanship

**The Function of the Physical Therapist as an Administrator in OB/GYN**

1. To meet with OB/GYN units in order to provide physical therapy services
2. To establish physical therapy departments in women's hospitals
3. To develop childbearing year programs and to coordinate, where necessary, early pregnancy and postpartum classes with established prepared childbirth programs
4. To schedule inpatient and outpatient obstetric and gynecology treatments
5. To provide quality assurance and peer review
6. To develop teaching resources, library, visual aids
7. To meet with other departments involved in the care of the OB or GYN patient
8. To coordinate fiscal management

**Skills Needed to be an Administrator in OB/GYN**

1. Definition of objectives
2. Documentation and communication
3. Promotion of physical therapy input in multidisciplinary team
4. Evaluation of staff, knowledge of peer review techniques
5. Evaluation of instructional programs for professionals and patients
6. Facilitation of consumer feedback
7. Interviewing and personnel management
8. Budgeting
   ©Section on Obstetrics and Gynecology of the American Physical Therapy Association, 1977

## *State of Practice*

Z. Annette Iglarsh, P.T., Ph.D., former chairman of the APTA section (1979-1983), believes that the current status of physical therapists in this specialty has not progressed as it should. Iglarsh thinks that hospital-based programs, if given a chance and reimbursement, may take off. For this reason, she believes specialists should direct their attention to the care of high-risk obstetric and gynecologic patients. Iglarsh is concerned that the specialty has not kept pace with the rest of the profession. Because OB/GYN is predominantly a female-oriented domain, and general private practice has been successful because it is largely male-spirited, women have the laborious task of working all that much harder to promote the OB/GYN specialty. Media focus on exercise and health has resulted in sociological flutters of interest in prenatal and postnatal exercise, but, in general, the physical therapist must heavily market these services to the OB/GYN department.

Iglarsh remembers her early days of trying to get into an obstetric department in 1976. By bribing the evening shift nurses with donuts and promises to do some of the less enjoyable chores around the ward, she was allowed to attend deliveries from 2:00 a.m. to 6:00 a.m. She recalls her frustration when she assisted a young teenager with no support person, and the attending physician wondered why she was helping and asked, "What difference will it make?"[4] Iglarsh contends that there are still many women in America who blindly accept routine anesthesia for labor and delivery and who need information about alternative pain relief. It is not that we need a new introduction, she states, it's that we need to be "rerecognized"; and that will take a great deal of additional hard work to get the message out in a more diverse nature. It is also not enough that physical therapists in this specialty help make women feel better, she points out, but that a monetary reward must be connected to the service. Insurance companies need to know that women may experience fewer complications and may return to work faster after assistance from an OB/GYN specialist. The attitudes of other medical professionals need to shift, as well. "Physical therapy is a necessity, not a nicety."[4]

The current shortage of physical therapists, in general, is reflective of a drop off of those active in the profession over the past several years. Iglarsh urges the profession, and especially OB/GYN specialists, to explore, develop, and undertake the methods necessary for making this a profession, not just a job where people can drop out.

Jane Frahm, P.T., charter member and Program Chairperson of the APTA section, has been formally recognized as an OB/GYN specialist at Hutzel Hospital, in Detroit, Michigan. A new position was created and titled, Coordinator of Obstetrics and Gynecology for Rehabilitation Services. Hopefully, this is an indication of an increasing awareness of the OB/GYN specialty.

Frahm sees the role of the OB/GYN therapist evolving into one of innovative patient education. She sees hospitals looking for new programs—and establishing them. The general public, for example, is not aware that conditions such as pelvic floor dysfunction or high-risk pregnancy are diagnosable problems, let alone that therapy exists to alleviate their symptoms. She believes education must be a major ongoing commitment for the benefit of the medical and lay communities, and, therefore, has been instrumental in developing multidisciplinary protocols for high-risk and diabetic patients. A high-risk patient in danger of premature labor due to an incompetent cervix may be on bed rest for 5 days to 5 weeks. Without physical therapy education, such a patient adopts poor body mechanics, like sitting up in jackknife positions or holding her breath when sitting on a bedpan, and thereby increases intraabdominal pressure and pressure on the cervix. Sometimes, then, merely prescribing bed rest is not enough.

Frahm has found that education of the medical staff leads to a greater understanding of OB/GYN specialists and less incongruity in requests for services. Because the specialty is small, Frahm believes there should be more sharing of ideas and inspiration among physical therapists in the field. Frahm hopes that private and hospital OB/GYN specialists will gain greater recognition and greater access to patients as consciousness is raised in the medical community.[5]

Linda Pipp, P.T., has been involved with prenatal programs for over 15 years at Providence Hospital in Southfield, Michigan, and instructs physical therapy students at Wayne State and Oakland Universities in the role of the OB/GYN physical therapist. She has seen the specialty grow from one of overtrained prenatal exercise instructors to one that includes (1) prenatal care (comfort, body mechanics, pain control, musculoskeletal assessment and treatment, posture, relaxation); (2) labor and delivery intervention; (3) postpartum care (exercise, body mechanics, posture, musculoskeletal assessment and treatment); (4) high-risk pregnancy care; and (5) gynecologic care (pre- and post-surgical). Each expanded role, she believes, was a natural progression of the previous one. With the increased interest in wellness and fitness for the childbearing year, women are even preparing their bodies before pregnancy. Pipp also sees our role as that of educators. As more schools incorporate OB/GYN into their curricula, the greater the exposure for entry-level physical therapists, and perhaps, the greater the interest.[6]

Based on these interviews with practicing specialists and on the scope of practice identified in the APTA position paper, it is apparent that the initial role of OB/GYN physical therapists as childbirth educators has grown to include roles as clinical practitioners, consultants, researchers, and as physical therapy educators and administrators. As clinical specialists, physical therapists can treat patients with gynecologic disorders, pre- and post-surgery; perform musculoskeletal evaluations and treatment of obstetric patients; act as labor support persons; and teach therapeutic exercise for prenatal, postpartum, high-risk, and post-Cesarean clients. As consultants, physical therapists can expand hospital-based and private practice programs, as well as act as resource persons for the public and medical communities, insurance companies, and the government. As researchers, physical therapists have their work ahead of them, since the specialty is relatively new and little documentation exists in this field. Physical therapists have started, however, to explore the effects of exercise, modalities, and current practices; the benefits of cross-cultural approaches to labor and delivery; and the long-term effects of obstetric intervention on both the fetus and the mother. Lastly, as administrators and educators for physical therapy students, patients, and medical personnel, physical therapists have the opportunity to promote services, knowledge, and experience to increase access to patients. Physical therapists in these roles have the chance to promote not only the OB/GYN specialty, but the profession as a whole as part of the multidisciplinary team approach to patient care.

## *References*

1. Noble E: Prepared childbirth: Facts and fallacies. Bull Sect Obstet Gynecol, APTA 8(1):11-15, 1984.
2. Noble E: Reminiscence: Then and now. Bull Sect Obstet Gynecol, APTA 11(2):7-8, 1987.
3. O'Connor L: The first ten years. Bull Sect Obstet Gynecol, APTA 11(2):8-9, 1987.
4. Iglarsh ZA: Telephone interview with R Gourley, March 1989.
5. Frahm J: Telephone interview with R Gourley, April 1989.
6. Pipp LM: Telephone interview with R Gourley, April 1989.

# Foundation for Specialization in OB/GYN

THREE

# Functional Anatomy of the Female Patient

### *Historical Perspectives*

The women who appear in the paintings by Leonardo da Vinci seem so lifelike, one can almost palpate the muscles. This realistic representation, however, was no accident. To achieve this realism, da Vinci became one of the early students of human anatomy, and certainly one of the first to record his work so intricately.[1] Prior to da Vinci's illustrations of human anatomy, physicians had a limited awareness of human muscle and bone function, learning what they could from surface anatomy and from animal dissection, and extrapolating that information to the human. Yet, once human dissection became scientifically acceptable, a taboo persisted on the study of female anatomy.[2]

Prior to the Renaissance, the only anatomic illustrations of the female depicted her pregnant, nude, and in a squatting position. The uterus was either bicornuate, multichambered, or shaped like an inverted light bulb. An inner lining encased a fetus, fully-formed from conception, and merely growing in size until delivery. During the Renaissance, da Vinci's artistic obsession with detail provided both artists and physicians with a new understanding of human development and human anatomy, complete with pictorial observations from various angles, including cross- sectional. But many of da Vinci's illustrations were lost until the twentieth century, and hence, a variety of anatomists' names have been attached to female anatomic structures.[3] Bartholin, Montgomery, Douglas, Cooper, Mackenrodt, Fallopius, and de Graaf are but a few of the anatomists who have been immortalized through their discoveries. Perhaps the only human parts untouched by eponyms are the bones. But, because the physical therapist must examine obstetric and many gynecologic patients solely on the basis of observation and palpation, this discussion of anatomy will be oriented from the exterior to the interior. Presuming that readers are familiar with basic anatomy common to both genders, this chapter will highlight normal female anatomy from an obstetric viewpoint, focusing on the female during pregnancy and on changes that occur anatomically from adolescence to senescence.

## *Hormonal Factors Affecting Anatomic Relations*

When reviewing female anatomy, it is vital that the therapist keep in mind the pervasive influence of relaxin and its effect on connective tissue. Although relaxin is a peptide hormone produced by the corpus luteum and generally associated only with pregnancy and the postpartum, research is contradictory regarding the existence of small amounts of relaxin in nonpregnant and menstruating females and in the male seminal fluid.[4-6] Although recent studies suggest relaxin may only affect cervical and uterine tissues, other studies offer evidence that relaxin may be responsible for relaxation of the connective tissue, including ligaments, fasciae, and symphyses. It is believed that relaxin affects tissues in the pregnant woman immediately after conception, peaks at 3 months, and then either remains at a constant level or drops 20% to a stable level for the remainder of the pregnancy.[7] Some believe there is also an increase prior to delivery,[8] although other studies suggest no rise prior to delivery, but significant rise during labor. Joint laxity associated with relaxin has been recorded in peripheral joints up to 3 to 5 months postpartum.[9] There is also evidence, however, that relaxin levels are higher in some women than in others, and even higher in women with multifetal pregnancies. Pelvic pain has been linked to women with higher relaxin levels than average, although this association is not firmly substantiated.[10] There is also evidence that relaxin may inhibit uterine contractions and maintain the integrity of the cervix during pregnancy.[11]

## The Female Chest Wall and Mammary Gland

The influence of relaxin upon ligamentous structures, connective tissue within the breast, and underlying fascia, combined with the increased weight of the breasts during pregnancy and lactation, may cause stress on the chest musculature and upper spine. Thoracic kyphosis associated with lumbar lordosis is a frequent postural change seen in pregnant women. The breast lies superficially to a layer of fascia overlying the pectoralis major, serratus anterior, external abdominal oblique, and the anterior wall of the rectus abdominis sheath, ending in the axillary tail near the axillary lymph nodes. The mammary glands or breasts consist of glandular tissue, fibrous tissue, adipose tissue, blood vessels, lymph vessels, and nerves. The fibrous tissue connects 15 to 20 lobes, formed by lobules of alveoli joined by areolar tissue, blood vessels, and lactiferous ducts that drain into lactiferous sinuses.[12] The ducts contain elastic tissue and narrow as they enter the papilla or nipple, encircled by the pigmented areola and areolar glands. The upper fascia is supported by suspensory ligaments (Cooper's). In addition to strain of chest musculature and postural stress, the pull exerted by pendulous breasts and edema of the upper extremities may result in nerve compression, either at the brachial plexus, or more distally in the median nerve at the wrist[13] (see Figure 3-1).

## The Female Abdomen and Abdominopelvic Relations

### Abdominal and abdominopelvic muscles

As a brief review of landmarks important to the obstetric physical therapist, the abdominal muscles may be viewed as belonging to two groups, one posterior and one anterolateral. The posterior group is comprised of the quadratus lumborum. The anterior group, which is probably the most stressed during pregnancy, boasts two longitudinal muscles, the rectus and pyramidalis; and three layers of muscles (the external abdominal oblique, internal abdominal oblique, and transversus abdominis) with alternating fiber directions, which extend their aponeuroses to ensheathe the longitudinal muscles. The iliopsoas, although it originates at the lumbar vertebrae and inserts on the lesser trochanter of the femur, serves as a landmark for nerves exiting the lumbar plexus. This muscle group also crosses the sacroiliac joint and runs under the inguinal ligament[12] (see Figure 3-2).

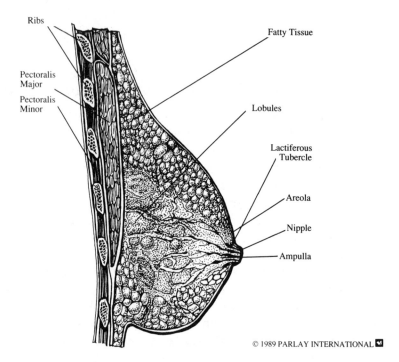

Figure 3-1: Sagittal section, female breast

## Abdominal fascia

As part of relaxin's potential influence on the connective tissue, the fasciae of the trunk and pelvis may be affected as well. The transversalis fascia covers the quadratus lumborum and psoas muscles and spreads to the lumbar spine and anterior longitudinal ligament. Iliacus fascia extends from the transversalis fascia, attaches to the inguinal ligament, crosses the superior pubic ramus, and blends into the fascia lata.[13]

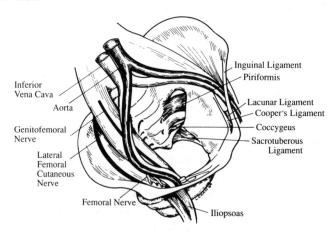

Figure 3-2: Abdominopelvic relationships

## Abdominal wall

As pregnancy advances, the influence of relaxin and the pressure exerted by the growing fetus create new relationships for thoracic and abdominal contents. In some cases, women experience pain or postural discomfort because of normal changes in the abdominal wall during pregnancy. As the fetus enlarges, the abdominal wall must stretch to accommodate. And as the recti and oblique muscles stretch, some weakening is expected. Yet, this is the time when the abdominal muscles must perhaps work harder than ever before to maintain an upright posture, despite the forces of gravity bearing down on the uterus. On top of this paradoxical situation, relaxin may have an additional influence on the linea alba and a diastasis of the recti may occur.[14] Should diastasis occur, the pregnant woman's ability to provide support without assistance for the enlarging uterus is tenuous at best. Diastasis can occur in varying degrees, and there have been severe cases in which the uterus is partially covered anteriorly only by peritoneum, fascia, and skin.[15] Faced with these potential problems, the physical therapist should be well versed in abdominal wall anatomy to identify the extent of abdominal weakness and fascial involvement.

## Abdominopelvic ligaments

The external abdominal oblique and internal abdominal oblique aponeuroses form the inguinal ligament and lacunar ligament and give rise to the fascia lata. The inguinal (Poupart's) ligament stretches from the anterior superior iliac spine to the pubic tubercle. Fibers passing to the pectineal line create the lacunar ligament. From the combined aponeuroses of the internal abdominal oblique muscle and the transversus abdominis muscle rises the conjoint tendon, extending from the inguinal ligament to the pectineal line of the pubis. Also attached to the pectineal line is the reflected inguinal ligament (triangular fascia). One other ligament, the iliolumbar, extends from the vertebral column to the pelvis and blends with the thoracolumbar fascia. Sudden stretching of this latter ligament is believed to cause both acute and persistent pain in pregnant women.

## Influence of postural changes on nerve supply

As fetal weight causes an increased lumbar lordosis, the pelvis may tilt anteriorly, and the iliopsoas muscles, with a common insertion, may be stressed. Since part of the lumbar plexus (see Table 3-1) lies within the psoas muscle, strain in this region may cause additional symptoms, particularly irritation of sensory nerves. The ilioinguinal, iliohypogastric, lateral femoral cutaneous, and femoral nerves exit laterally from the psoas, and the genitofemoral nerve travels

**Table 3-1. Sensory Innervation of the Lumbar Plexus**

| | |
|---|---|
| Iliohypogastric (L1): | symphysis pubis and lateral iliac crest |
| Ilioinguinal (L1): | medial thigh, mons pubis, labia major |
| Lateral femoral cutaneous (L2, L3): | anterior thigh |
| Femoral (L2, L3, L4): | anterior thigh |
| Genitofemoral (L1, L2): | anterior vulva and anterior thigh |
| Obturator (L2, L3, L4): | medial thigh |

through the belly. The obturator nerve exits medially and passes through the obturator foramen (see Figure 3-2).[12]

As the fetus enlarges, the pressure of the uterus and dependent edema may result in neuropathies or neural compressions, especially of the lateral femoral cutaneous and femoral nerves and its branches as they pass beneath the inguinal ligament (see Figure 3-2). In addition, the possibility of spinal laxity may create conditions favorable for compressions of spinal or peripheral nerves exiting at the spine, although the incidence of disc herniations is no greater during pregnancy than in the normal population.[16]

### Diaphragm and rib cage

Laxity around the spine may result in more mobile rib articulations, and the lower ribs do flare laterally. The subcostal angle widens, the transverse diameter of the rib cage increases about 2 cm, and its circumference expands approximately 6 cm.[17]

With this expansion comes an altered relation to the diaphragm, which radiates from the ribs, costal cartilages, sternum, and lumbar vertebrae to the central tendon. In the nonpregnant state, the diaphragm may reach as high as the fifth rib on the right and the fifth interspace on the left during expiration.[12] During pregnancy, the diaphragm rises approximately 4 cm in position, and excursion is thought to be greater than during nonpregnant states. Additional compensatory changes in pulmonary function are not necessarily structurally related and will be addressed in Chapter 4.

Anatomically, although undocumented, it is conceivable that the origins of the diaphragm and the influence of relaxin may cause other structures to be influenced by positional changes. The diaphragm has a sternal, costal, and lumbar portion. The costal origins interdigitate with the transversus abdominis muscle to a slight degree, and the lumbar segments attach to aponeuroses over the psoas and quadratus lumborum muscles. Further, it is possible that the diaphragmatic crura may add stress to the anterior longitudinal ligament in the lumbar area, especially at L1 and L2 into which both crura attach. The lumbocostal fascial arches also give rise to portions of the diaphragm. Finally, the diaphragm may be responsible for affecting those structures which pass through it, namely the esophagus, the vena cava, hemiazygos vein, lymphatic channels, and splanchnic nerves. The aorta does not pass directly through the diaphragm, although the diaphragm forms a hiatus posteriorly for its passage.[12]

## Abdominopelvic blood vessels and internal organs

The potential diaphragmatic influence upon the major blood vessels has been largely ignored by maternal health researchers, but the aorta and the vena cava may be occluded by the enlarging uterus in certain women when the supine position is assumed for a prolonged period during late pregnancy (supine hypotensive syndrome or aortocaval occlusion). The heart normally becomes slightly rotated, enlarged, elevated, and displaced to the left from the fundal pressure. Other organs with altered anatomy during pregnancy include a distended gallbladder and enlarged pituitary and thyroid.[15]

Of greater interest to researchers has been the partial occlusion of the inferior vena cava and the pelvic veins by the enlarging uterus, not only when the woman lies supine for prolonged periods, but also when she is standing for prolonged periods. This compression not only can reduce venous return, but also may increase venous pressure and contribute to dependent edema in the lower extremities. The inferior vena cava exits the abdomen via the central tendon of the diaphragm at the level of T8. It lies directly anterior to the lower lumbar vertebrae, the anterior longitudinal ligament, the right-sided psoas muscles, and lumbar sympathetic trunk among other structures, and its occlusion may directly impact the inferior tributaries. These tributaries include the common iliac veins, the lumbar veins, the ovarian veins, and their tributaries, reviewed in Table 3-2.[18-20]

## *The Female Perineum and Pelvis*

### The bony pelvis

When teaching childbirth classes, the analogies of the abdominal wall as a corset and the pelvis as a basin may become rather mundane for the instructor, but one cannot argue with the sheer descriptive power of these terms. Forming a continuous cavity with the abdomen, the pelvis serves to support the trunk and provide a site for attachment of the lower extremity. Yet, the female pelvis serves another vital function, that is, to protect the reproductive organs and, during the early months of pregnancy, the developing fetus. Bounded by the sacrum and coccyx posteriorly, and by the innominates laterally and anteriorly, the bony structure meets at the symphysis pubis and at two sacroiliac joints (see Figure 3-3).

**Table 3-2. Venous Return Potentially Affected by Uterine/Fetal Pressure**

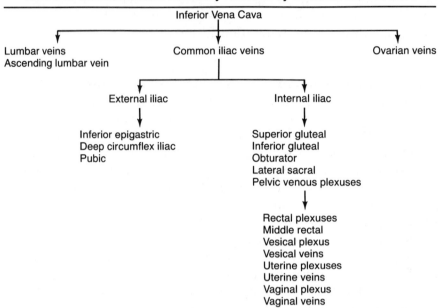

The ilium, ischium, and pubis meet to form the acetabulum and fuse during adolescence to form the coxal or innominate bones. The iliac crest borders the top of the ilium, extending from the anterior superior iliac spine to the posterior superior iliac spine. Muscles attach to a path along the crest between the inner and outer lip of the crest. The anterior and posterior inferior iliac spines are also useful landmarks. The ischium offers a weightbearing surface in sitting position and forms the greater and lesser sciatic notches.

Joining with the ilium and ischium is the pubis with superior and inferior rami. The inferior or descending rami form in the normal, average female a 90 to 100 degree angle for passage of the fetal head (pubic arch is 70-75 degrees in males)[21] (see Figure 3-4). Ligaments and fibrocartilage join the two pubic portions together at the symphysis pubis. The pubic crest may be palpable as it rises to form the pubic tubercle, which extends laterally to the pectineal line, finally joining the arcuate line and ending at the terminal line. The superior and inferior rami fuse with the ischial ramus and the body of the ischium to form the obturator foramen, through which passes vessels and nerves to the lower extremity.

The sacral promontory projects most deeply into the pelvic cavity, and provides a site for measurement of pelvic size. Normal value for a straight line drawn from the promontory to the sacral apex is 10 cm, and 12 cm along the ventral surface of the sacrum.[22] The anterior of the sacrum hosts four paired foramina, through which pass

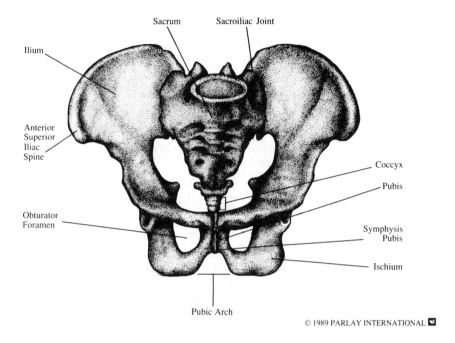

Sacrum

Sacroiliac Joint

Ilium

Anterior
Superior
Iliac
Spine

Obturator
Foramen

Coccyx

Pubis

Symphysis
Pubis

Ischium

Pubic Arch

Figure 3-3: Bony pelvis

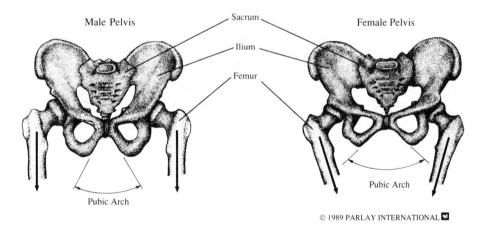

Male Pelvis

Sacrum

Ilium

Femur

Female Pelvis

Pubic Arch

Pubic Arch

Figure 3-4: Comparison of female and male pelves

the anterior divisions of the sacral nerves and tributaries from the lateral sacral vessels. The posterior of the sacrum also permits passage of the posterior primary divisions of the sacral nerves. Inferior to the median sacral crest at about S4 or S5 is a sacral hiatus that points the way to the sacral canal. The sacral canal is of importance to the obstetric anesthesiologist in that it allows access to the epidural space for caudal conduction anesthesia[18] (see Figure 3-5). The lateral portion of the sacrum articulates with the innominate bone. Superiorly is a facet for articulation with L5 and inferiorly, a facet for coccygeal articulation.

The four coccygeal vertebrae are usually fused into one bone, as are the five vertebrae of the sacrum. However, the vertebral canal does not continue into the coccyx.

## Ossification

When treating females of childbearing age, it should be remembered that biologic reproduction can start much earlier than socially accepted dictum. Emphasis has been focused on the mother over 35 years of age because of the risk to fetal health, but maternal health is a greater problem to the adolescent mother. The physical therapist treating the pregnant adolescent should keep in mind that bony ossification may not be complete until adulthood. The bones of the innominate fuse at different times. At 7 or 8 years of age the inferior

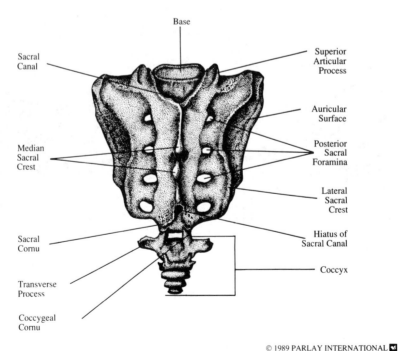

Figure 3-5: Landmarks of the sacrum

rami of the pubis fuses with the ischium, but ossification at the acetabulum occurs later. A Y-shaped cartilage is still present in the acetabulum where the three bones join. The fusion of the ilium and pubis occurs at about 18 years, followed by the joining of the ilium and ischium, and finally the pubis and ischium by 24 to 25 years. The sacrum and coccyx, however, may not ossify until 25 to 30 years, and the coccyx may totally fuse with the sacrum even later in life.[20]

Those bony landmarks of the pelvis, which are of special significance to the obstetric or gynecologic examiner, are summarized in Table 3-3.

## Pelvic ligaments and articulations

The two sacroiliac joints and the symphysis pubis are the only articulations of the pelvis. The sacroiliac joints are synovial, with the articular surface of the sacral surface covered by fibrocartilage, and the ilial surface covered by hyaline cartilage. The symphysis pubis is a cartilaginous joint with an interpubic disc of fibrocartilage. Hyaline cartilage on the bony surfaces meets the disc, which varies in shape and thickness. Relaxin is thought to soften the fibrocartilage. The ligaments, described in Table 3-4, provide support to the pelvis, despite the effects of relaxin. They may be viewed in five groups: abdominopelvic ligaments (iliolumbar, inguinal, lacunar); sacroiliac ligaments (anterior sacroiliac, posterior sacroiliac, and interosseus);

**Table 3-3. Bony Landmarks of the Pelvis Palpable During Pelvic Examination**

| | |
|---|---|
| Ischial spine | determines level of fetal descent into true pelvis and shortest diameter of cavity |
| Pubic arch | forms bony framework for vulva and perineum |
| Pubic tubercle | provides medial attachment site for the inguinal ligament |
| Obturator foramen | allows passage of obturator nerve and vessels |
| Ischial tuberosity | marks inferior boundary of pelvis |
| Sacral promontory | provides measurement site with sacral tip for dimension of pelvic outlet |

**Table 3-4. Abdominopelvic Ligaments**

| | |
|---|---|
| Iliolumbar | connects pelvis with vertebral column |
| Inguinal | forms lower border of external abdominal oblique aponeurosis, fuses with iliopsoas fascia and fascia lata |
| Lacunar | forms medial boundary of femoral ring |
| Anterior sacroiliac | runs from ventral sacrum to ilium |
| Posterior sacroiliac | connects dorsal sacrum to PSIS (posterior superior iliac spine) |
| Interosseus sacroiliac | connects sacral and ilial tuberosities |
| Sacrotuberous | provides passage for coccygeal plexus |
| Sacrospinous | separates lesser and greater sciatic foramina |
| Anterior sacrococcygeal | runs from ventral sacrum to coccyx |
| Posterior sacrococcygeal | completes distal sacral canal |
| Lateral sacrococcygeal | completes foramen for S5 |
| Interarticular | joins sacral and coccygeal cornua |
| Superior pubic | joins superior pubis to pubic tubercle |
| Arcuate pubic | spans inferior pubic archway |
| Pectineal | extends along pubic bone |

sacroischial ligaments (sacrotuberous, sacrospinous); sacrococcygeal ligaments (anterior sacrococcygeal, posterior sacrococcygeal, lateral sacrococcygeal, and interarticular); and pubic ligaments (superior pubic, arcuate pubic, pectineal).

Although anatomists describe these ligaments from a structural viewpoint, the clinician may find it more helpful to analyze ligamentous support functionally as it relates to presenting symptoms or to the pelvic biomechanics (see Figure 3-6).

## Biomechanics of the female pelvis

The pelvis has been compared to a ring, appearing as a curved beam in the frontal plane, and as an irregular, angular lever in the sagittal plane.[23] In the frontal plane, the iliolumbar ligament, the lumbosacral ligamentous support, the posterior back muscles, and the lateral abdominal muscles maintain stability. When the body is in motion, the ligaments and muscles must control rotatory and translatory movements. Sacroiliac stress increases on lateral motion. If there is anomaly or sacralization of the fifth lumbar vertebra, range of motion may be limited, and impingement creating a lever force on the sacrum may occur. The sacroiliac joint receives weight stress, resulting in both vertical and horizontal components entering the femoral head and neck and entering the symphysis pubis. Shear (horizontal force) is resolved by ligamentous support. Pressure (vertical force) transmits to the femoral head. In the sagittal plane, the line of gravity appears to fall behind the hip joint and anterior to the sacroiliac joint. Gravity acting upon the pelvis will force the posterior pelvic ring into a downward rotation about the hip axes. If the

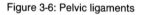

Figure 3-6: Pelvic ligaments

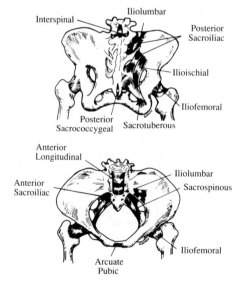

posterior pelvis is forced downward, the anterior will be forced upward. However, the hip flexors and iliofemoral ligament resist the anterior upward force. The more horizontal the pelvic inclination, the greater the downward force and the greater the lever arm between the lumbosacral junction and the sacroiliac joint. It is believed that, because of the relation of the lumbosacral joint and the sacroiliac joint, rotatory force will first be transmitted to the lumbosacral; and only to the sacroiliac after force passes into the lumbosacral joint and into the sacrum.[24]

As the sacrum joins the ilia, the lumbosacral articulation bears the force of the upper body weight. This force is dispersed in two directions. One component attempts to drive the sacrum caudally and dorsally between the ilia, and one attempts to rotate the cephalic sacrum caudally and ventrally into the pelvic cavity.[20] The ligaments, then, may be identified as preventing the rotational forces imposed upon the sacrum. The interosseus sacroiliac, posterior sacroiliac, and the iliolumbar ligaments are positioned to resist the caudal and dorsal drive upon the sacrum, whereas the sacrotuberous, and the sacrospinous ligaments resist ventral rotation of the sacral promontory.[19]

The pubic ligaments assist the disc and maintain the integrity of the joint by superior pubic ligament and by the arcuate, which supports the pubic arch inferiorly.[22] It is believed that relaxin softens the ligaments as well as the fibrocartilage; yet this softening does not appear to impair the strength of the joint during childbirth. The natural force of the body weight to push the ilia together may add rotatory and compressive forces to the symphysis. In sitting, the pubic arch resists spreading forces. The symphysis pubis is able to withstand the force of the fetal head moving beneath it; hence, it appears that most problems of symphysial separation during pregnancy are related to trauma or faulty pelvic mechanism. If strain of the symphysis pubis occurs, torsion may appear in the sacroiliac joints, and pelvic ring instability may result. Normal separation of the symphysis has been measured at 1 to 5 mm, increasing approximately 0.5 to 7 mm more during pregnancy, and decreasing by 2 mm on an average within the first week postpartum.[25] Labor does not seem to widen the diastasis. There has been no documentation regarding the amount of separation and association with pelvic pain.

There appears to be a normal accentuation of the lumbar lordosis during pregnancy, possibly attributable to the stress of added fetal weight anteriorly and to the effects of relaxin, which may cause supporting spinal ligaments, such as the longitudinal ligaments, to allow greater spinal joint laxity. Exactly how much accentuation is normal is unknown. There is little documentation to support observations made by physical therapists that, as the center of gravity shifts upward and anteriorly with increasing fetal weight, the lumbar spine shifts forward. There have also been claims that there are compensatory increases in the dorsal curve and cervical curve as well.[26]

It is conceivable that as pregnancy advances, the increase in lumbar lordosis and influence of relaxin add additional stresses on the sacral ventral rotatory force. Resisting rotation is the middle segment of the sacrum, in which the sacral convexities interlock with the ilial concavities. During delivery, as the fetus descends into the ventral sacrum, this interlocking mechanism of the middle segment, reinforced by the sacrospinous and sacrotuberous ligaments, prevents sacral dislocation.[15] It is believed that during defecation and parturition the coccyx rotates backward at the sacrococcygeal joint.[20]

Because of the relaxation of the pelvic articulations and biomechanical forces, pain in the pelvic region may be related to the relaxation of ligamentous attachments to the ischial tuberosity, ischial spine, lateral border of the sacrum and coccyx, posterior iliac spines, pubic bones, or the obturator internus fascia.

## Pelvic axes, position, diameters, and shape

When viewed as a whole, the pelvis may be obstetrically divided into a true pelvis and a false pelvis. The linea terminalis separates the true and false pelvis, with the false pelvis lying superiorly to the linea and the true pelvis lying inferiorly. The major or false pelvis actually harbors the lower portion of the abdominal cavity. The true or lesser pelvis lies below a plane created by the linea terminalis and the sacral promontory; this also identifies the pelvic inlet. The inlet is directed posteriorly and intersects the vertical axis at approximately 30 degrees.[21] The pelvic outlet, however, because of its anatomic structure (the sacrum posteriorly and the pubis anteriorly) lies in an almost horizontal plane.

The cavity of the true pelvis has been compared to a bent cylinder, the top portion directed down and back and the lower portion pointed down and forward.[21] The true pelvis is posteriorly bound by the anterior sacrum, inner ischium, sacrosciatic notch, and sacrosciatic ligaments. Anteriorly, the true pelvis if formed by the pubis, the ascending superior ischial ramus, and the obturator foramen. It has been estimated that the planes of the walls of the true pelvis converge at the knees.[21]

The irregularity of the pelvis compared to the long bones led anatomists to develop a system of diameters for ease in describing pelvic anomalies. Four planes (pelvic inlet, pelvic outlet, greatest pelvic dimension, and least pelvic dimension) are divided into various diameters and shapes for obstetrical reference. These are summarized in Table 3-5. The inlet diameter of importance is the obstetric conjugate, which is estimated by manually measuring the diagonal conjugate and subtracting a value between 1.5 to 2.0 cm from that distance, depending on the tilt and length of the symphysis pubis. The plane of greatest dimensions, as the name implies, is not of major importance to the obstetric attendant, because this part from S2-S3 to the pubis is the most spacious for the fetal head. If any of these other diameters are reduced, however, and cause delay of fetal descent during labor, the pelvis is considered contracted.[15]

Although the pelvic shapes have been carefully delineated, the intermediate type, a combination of shapes, is the usual occurrence. The shapes are based on the line drawn through the transverse diameter to form a posterior and anterior pelvic inlet. The intermediate shapes are described by the posterior division as the pelvic type or hindpelvis; the anterior as the tendency or forepelvis. The gynecoid occurs in over half of all women.[15]

## Abnormal pelvis

The abnormal pelvis presents, in some cases, a life-threatening situation for the fetus. Contraction of pelvic diameters may occur at the inlet, outlet, midpelvis (greater and lesser dimensions), or in any

### Table 3-5. Diameters and Shapes of the Female Pelvis

**Pelvic inlet**
Anteroposterior
    *obstetric conjugate*—narrowest width-promontory to pubis; 10cm
    *true conjugate*—cephalad pubis to promontory
    *diagonal conjugate*—caudal pubis to promontory
Transverse—greatest distance between opposite sides of linea terminalis; intersects a/p 4 cm anterior to promontory
Right Oblique—right sacroiliac synchondrosis to left iliopectineal eminence; about 13 cm
Left Oblique—left sacroiliac synchondrosis to right iliopectineal eminence; about 13 cm
**Least pelvic dimensions**
Interspinous—10 cm; smallest of pelvis
Anteroposterior—at ischial spines; 11.5 cm
Posterior sagittal—sacrum to intersect with interspinous; 4.5 cm
**Greatest pelvic dimensions**
Anteroposterior—12.5 cm
Transverse—12.5 cm
Right and left oblique—unmeasurable
**Pelvic outlet**
Anteroposterior—lower pubis to sacral tip; 11.5 cm
Transverse—between ischial tuberosities; 10.0 cm
Posterior sagittal—sacral tip to intersect transverse; 7.5 cm
**Shapes**
Gynecoid—round and wide
Android—small, narrow, and wedge-like
Anthropoid—oval, narrow, pointed
Platypelloid—shallow and wide
Intermediate—combination of types

combination of the above areas. A contracted inlet can prevent passage of the fetal head, by altering the presentation of the fetus from occiput leading to face or shoulder leading or prolapsed cord or extremities. Cervical dilatation may be reduced because of premature membrane rupture and diminished fetal head pressure. Overstretching or rupture of the lower uterine segment may occur, and there may be a predisposition to fistula from impaired circulation. Midpelvis contractions appear more commonly and may result in arrest of fetal descent. Outlet contraction may contribute to perineal tearing as the fetal head is directed away from the pubic arch. When all or multiple parts of the pelvis are contracted, labor is jeopardized by mechanical resistance and diminished uterine contractions.[15] Other pelvic abnormalities which may interfere with labor include kyphotic or scoliotic pelvis (lumbosacral kyphosis may obstruct inlet), postfracture pelvis (malunion or callus formation reduce birth canal), and the coxalgic pelvis (from abnormal development of lower extremity). Tumors arising from the pelvic walls may also obstruct the pelvic cavity.[15]

### Contents of the pelvic cavity

Comparing the pelvic cavity to a bowl, Crafts and Kreiger[21] identify the bottom of this bowl as the pelvic floor. Above the floor lies the pelvic cavity proper, and below the floor is the external genitalia. Inside the pelvic cavity is the rectum, which lies anterior to the sacral promontory. The uterus and its peritoneal attachments come between the rectum and the urinary bladder, creating the rectouterine (Douglas) and vesicouterine pouches, respectively. The rectouterine pouch is a continuation of the vagina. The uterine (Fallopian) tubes, ovaries, subserous and parietal fascia, ureters, uterine ligaments, sacral, pudendal and coccygeal plexuses, piriformis muscle, coccygeal muscle, obturator internus muscle, and levator ani muscles also lie within the cavity (see Figure 3-7).

The vagina parallels the pelvic inlet and at its superior end encloses the uterine cervix. This relationship causes the vaginal walls to be unequal in length; about 7.5 cm anteriorly and 9.0 cm posteriorly.[21] Anterior, lateral, and posterior fornices surround the cervix. The anterior wall of the vagina relates half to the urinary fundus and half to the urethra. The posterior wall relates in thirds to the rectouterine pouch, rectum, and the perineal body. Vaginal plexuses are situated between the vagina and the pelvic diaphragm. The vaginal tissue is mucosal, erectile and muscular.

The uterine tubes are about 10 cm long and are divided into isthmus, ampulla, and infundibulum. The isthmus branches off the

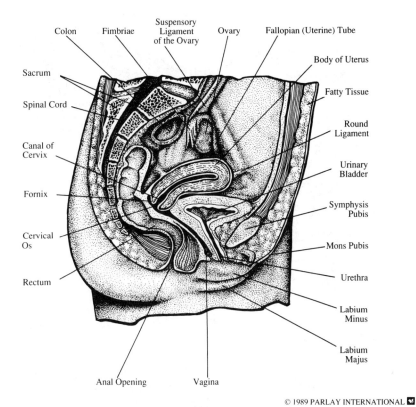

Figure 3-7: Contents of the female pelvic cavity

Labels on figure:
Colon, Fimbriae, Suspensory Ligament of the Ovary, Ovary, Fallopian (Uterine) Tube, Body of Uterus, Sacrum, Fatty Tissue, Spinal Cord, Round Ligament, Canal of Cervix, Urinary Bladder, Fornix, Symphysis Pubis, Cervical Os, Mons Pubis, Rectum, Urethra, Labium Minus, Labium Majus, Anal Opening, Vagina

uterus, the ampulla extends and caps the ovary, and the infundibulum spreads its fimbriae projections over the ovary.

The ovaries rest against the lateral pelvic walls sheltered by the broad ligament, the ureter, and the external iliac vessels. In standing, the ovary is oriented vertically. The suspensory ligament of the ovary extends past the iliac vessels and the psoas muscles. This is differentiated from the ovarian ligament which connects it to the uterus (see Figure 3-8).

The uterus has been compared to an inverted pear the size of a fist. In a nonpregnant state, the uterus is about 7.5 cm long, 5.0 cm wide, and 2.5 cm in thickness. The fundus (top) and body (middle) of the uterus lie over the urinary bladder in an almost horizontal plane, bending (anteflexed) at a 100 to 110 degree angle at the cervix (neck) to meet the vagina. Because of its relation to the urinary bladder, the position and the uterine angle can change with urine volume. The fundus is that portion above the area where the uterine tubes exit the uterus. The body has the greatest amount of broad ligament associated with it, and gives rise to the isthmus, just above the cervix. The cervix is considered the lower 2 cm and it meets the vagina obliquely. The uterus is supported by the pelvic floor and by

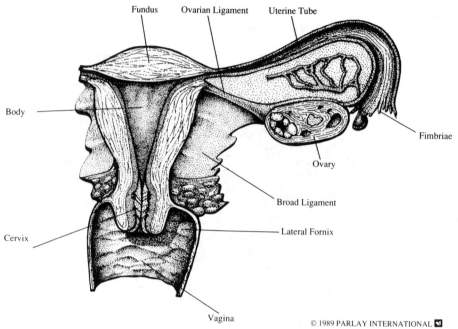

Fundus
Ovarian Ligament
Uterine Tube
Body
Fimbriae
Ovary
Broad Ligament
Cervix
Lateral Fornix
Vagina

Figure 3-8: Uterine support structures

the surrounding viscera. Anatomists believe that the pelvic floor is essential for support, and that the broad, round, and uterosacral ligaments merely maintain position within the cavity.[15,20-21,23]

The pelvic contents are partially covered by peritoneum and partially embedded in dense connective tissue called the endopelvic fascia. The placement of the uterus creates two peritoneal pouches on either side, but broad ligaments of the uterus reach from the uterus, ensheathing the uterine tubes and the ovaries laterally to the pelvic walls (see Figure 3-9). The round ligament of the uterus and the ovarian ligament attach to the side of the uterus below the uterine tube.

The round ligaments keep the fundus forward and spread anterolaterally from the uterine tubes to the labium majora. The uterosacral ligaments maintain a backward and upward position of the cervix and attach to deep fascia and sacral periosteum. These ligaments are augmented by smooth rectouterine muscle. Cardinal ligaments, once thought to be prime supporters for the uterus, are now believed to be connective tissue covering around the uterine blood vessels. The uterosacral ligaments and the cardinal ligaments also carry visceral nerve fibers, both sympathetic and parasympathetic efferent fibers, as well as afferent or sensory fibers to thoracic, lumbar, and sacral spinal cord levels.[12]

The urinary bladder lies between the pubis, the vagina, the cervix, and the pelvic diaphragm. The trigone of the bladder rests on the anterior middle third of the vagina. The bladder is attached to and

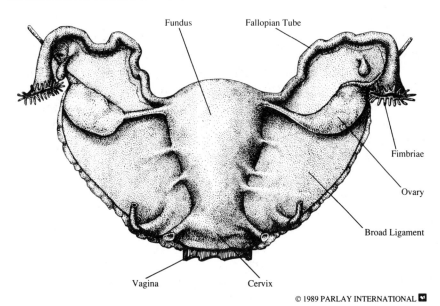

Figure 3-9: Broad ligament

supported by the endopelvic fascia, but remains separate from the vagina. Pubovesical ligaments provide additional support. Nerves reach the bladder through the vesicovaginal ligament, cardinal ligament, and lateral vesical ligament.[18]

The urethra is supported by the anterior vaginal wall, by the urogenital diaphragm, and by pubourethral ligaments (from endopelvic fascia). The support of the diaphragm assists in providing urethral resistance. Skene's or paraurethral glands and ducts lie within the urethral wall, and empty into the vestibule.

The rectum lies close to the vagina until the two openings are separated by the perineal body. The puborectalis and the external sphincter ani are responsible for fecal continence. The role of the internal sphincter in fecal continence is not clear.[20] The vascularity and position of the anal opening make it subject to both internal and external varicosities.

## Muscles of the pelvis and perineum

The anatomist researching pelvic muscles is faced with considerable confusion regarding terminology associated with the various structures of the female pelvis and genitalia. The terms pelvic floor, pelvic diaphragm, urogenital diaphragm, urogenital triangle, anal triangle, perineum, vulva, and pudendum are frequently used interchangeably—and often incorrectly. In addition to confusion about the perineum and the pelvis, there are muscles that technically belong to the lower extremity, but originate in the pelvis, and are therefore part of its anatomy. The iliopsoas has been discussed in the abdominopelvic muscle section, but it should be remembered that the tendon inserts on the lesser trochanter, and the iliacus covers the medial surface of the false pelvis. The piriformis, which hosts the sacral and pudendal plexuses, originates from the lateral sacrum, exits the pelvis through the greater sciatic foramen, and inserts into the greater trochanter of the femur. The obturator internus muscle originates from the innominate and obturator membrane, passes through the lesser sciatic foramen, and inserts also into the greater trochanter. Thick fascia covers the obturator internus and gives rise to the levator ani muscle.[20]

Pelvic floor is probably the most general and abused term, but should probably be used only when referring to the pelvic diaphragm. Arising from the posterior superior pubic rami, the inner ischial spines, and the obturator fascia, the fibers of the pelvic diaphragm insert into a raphe between the vaginal and rectal openings (perineal body) and below the rectal opening (anococcygeal raphe), at midline around the vaginal and rectal openings to form sphincters, and into the coccyx. As separate entities, the pelvic diaphragm is composed of the coccygeus and levator ani muscles. The coccygeus muscle arises from the ischial spine and inserts into the lateral coccyx. Anterior to the coccygeus muscle is the levator ani, which is divided by anatomists into three or four parts. A portion (pubovaginalis) blends with the vagina and is sometimes considered separate from the rest of the parts of the levator ani muscle. The puborectalis, pubococcygeus, and the iliococcygeus are the more commonly known divisions of the levator ani muscle. Fibers from the puborectalis merge with the rectum and blend with the corresponding muscle opposite, along with the pubococcygeus and iliococcygeus muscles as they insert into the coccyx. The combination of these muscles creates a sling mechanism to support the internal organs and the openings transsecting the pelvic diaphragm (see Figure 3-10).

The urogenital diaphragm is a second muscular layer external to the pelvic diaphragm that adds support to the region transsected by the openings of the urethra and vagina. It spans across the ischiopubic rami and is sandwiched between two fascial sheets that fuse near the pubis to form the transverse ligament of the pelvis. The muscular portion forms a triangle from the urethral sphincter and the deep transverse perineal muscles; however, this area is different than that called the urogenital triangle of the perineum.[18] The deep transverse perineal muscle arises from the ischial ramus, passes medially and posteriorly to the vagina. It forms a tendinous raphe with contributions from the external sphincter ani and the puborectalis, blending into the vaginal wall. The female sphincter urethrae muscle is an arch of fibers that end in the urethral and vaginal walls.[12]

The urogenital triangle, on the other hand, is the anterior portion

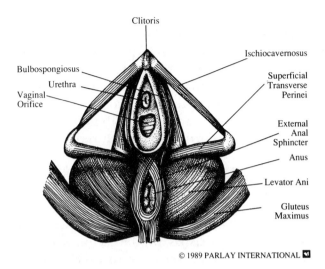

© 1989 PARLAY INTERNATIONAL

Figure 3-10: Superficial muscles of the pelvic floor that define the urogenital and anal triangles

of the perineum. The posterior portion, divided by a line drawn between the ischial tuberosities, is the anal triangle. The anal triangle of the perineum is bounded by the sacrotuberous ligaments, the gluteus maximus, and the urogenital triangle, and contains the anus, external sphincter ani muscle, and the ischiorectal fossae. The perineum, then, is inferior to the pelvic diaphragm and the urogenital diaphragm. The urogenital triangle may be further divided into the superficial and deep perineal spaces. The deep perineal space hosts the urethra and the lower vagina. The superficial structures of the urogenital triangle of the perineum are also known as the external genitalia, the vulva, or the pudendum. This area includes the mons pubis, labia majora, labia minora, clitoris, vestibular bulb, bulbocavernosus (bulbospongiosus) muscles, greater vestibular glands (Bartholin's), ischiocavernosus muscles, superficial transverse perineum muscles and, in some texts, the urogenital diaphragm.[12] For this discussion, the perineum will be considered separately from the muscular diaphragms. The urogenital triangle, though, has several layers of its own, primarily fascial. The skin and fatty layer lie superior to the superficial space. The superficial space contains a membranous layer of fascia and a muscular layer. The perineal membrane which stretches across the inferior pubic rami, a muscular layer, and the deep fascia superior to that deep muscular layer make up the deep space. According to Danforth, the latter three layers are the urogenital diaphragm. It is no wonder that confusion exists. For the therapist in practice, though, an awareness of the fascial involvement in this area is probably all that is necessary for effective evaluation and treatment.

The labia majora blend anteriorly as the mons pubis and taper posteriorly at the anus. The inner skin is smooth, contains sebaceous glands, and bounds the areolar and fatty tissue of the labial fold. The labia meet at the anterior and posterior labial commissures. Hair and pigment mark the external labia. The labia minora are smooth, cutaneous folds, extending posteriorly from the clitoris for about 4 cm. Between the labia minora is the vestibule of the vagina, which hosts the external urethral orifice, the paraurethral (Skene's) glands, the vagina, and the ducts of the greater vestibular glands. The greater vestibular glands and the vestibular bulbs lie near the vagina. The labium minora form the prepuce and frenulum of the clitoris. Two crura form the clitoris, which angles, by a suspensory ligament to the symphysis pubis, towards the perineum. The clitoris is composed of erectile tissue, assisted by the ischiocavernosus muscles, and is covered by epithelium sensitive to touch. Arising from the ischial tuberosities passing medially to the central tendinous body of the perineum (perineal body), the superficial transverse perineum muscles stabilize the perineum for other muscle contraction. The external genital area is innervated by the pudendal nerve, vesical plexuses, and vaginal nerves. Lymphatics are rich in this area, which is covered by the superficial perineal fascia (Colles'), a space external to the superficial fascia of the urogenital diaphragm.[12]

Three nerves contribute to the cutaneous nerve supply to the vulva and perineum. The iliohypogastric, ilioinguinal, and genital branch of the genitofemoral innervate the anterior vulva. The pudendal nerve and branches innervate the clitoris, vestibule, labia, and perineum; and the perineal branch of the posterior femoral cutaneous nerve innervates the lateral perineum, posterior vulva and perianal region.

### Muscles and nerves of the lower extremity affected by pregnancy

The relation of several muscles that enter the pelvis but act on the lower extremity may be altered as the body adapts to pregnancy or the postpartum. These include those listed in Table 3-6. Much of the sensory innervation of the pelvic and genital region arises from nerves passing through the pelvis also. These are listed in Table 3-7.

## *Changes in Anatomic Structure Associated with Aging*

The breast changes considerably at puberty and during lactation. Consisting primarily of ducts in childhood, after puberty the ducts, stimulated by estrogen, develop potential alveoli. Premenstrually, the glandular tissue increases, vascular engorgement occurs, and the lumen of the ducts enlarges. During pregnancy, stimulation from estrogen and progesterone from the placenta causes the alveoli to

**Table 3-6. Muscles of the Pelvis and Lower Extremity Originating in or on the Pelvis**

| | | |
|---|---|---|
| Quadratus lumborum | Gemelli | Obturator internus and |
| Piriformis | Glutei | externus |
| Quadratus femoris | Hamstrings | Adductor group |
| Tensor fasciae latae | | Rectus femoris |

open and secrete milk, the adipose tissue increases, circulating blood increases, and the areola darkens and enlarges. Lactation lasts on an average about 5 or 6 months, but can last longer if estrogen and progesterone continue to interact with hypophysial hormones, prolactin, and growth hormone. There are many variations in lactation function. After lactation, milk is absorbed, alveoli shrink, and the glandular tissue rests. The glandular tissue atrophies after menopause and the ducts degenerate, as does the connective tissue support.

The sacroiliac joint cavities acquire fibrous or fibrocartilaginous adhesions, and synostosis may occur. About the tenth year of life, the interpubic disc develops a cavity in the upper and back of the joint.

The uterus enlarges, swells, and changes color during menstruation. During pregnancy, the uterine fibers hypertrophy and new fibers develop. The uterine walls grow thinner as pregnancy advances. After childbirth, the uterus involutes, but the cavity remains larger than prior to pregnancy, and it is believed that the muscular layers are thicker. The aged uterus is atrophied and portions are more defined.[20-22]

**Table 3-7. Sensory Nerves of the Pelvis and Lower Extremity Passing Through the Pelvis**

| | |
|---|---|
| **Sacral plexus (L4-S3)** | |
| Sciatic: | thigh and leg |
| Posterior femoral cutaneous: | vulva and perineum |
| **Pudendal plexus (S2-4)** | |
| Pudendal: | external sphincter ani, urogenital diaphragm, transverse perineal, bulbocavernosus, ischiocavernosus, urethra, skin of vulva, mucosa of vestibule, clitoris and prepuce |
| Pelvic splanchnics: | bladder, uterus, vagina, distal colon, rectum, external genitalia, erectile tissue, levator ani, coccygeus |
| **Coccygeal plexus (S4)** | |
| Anococcygeal: | skin over coccyx |
| **Visceral Afferent System** | |
| Pathways of abdominal and pelvic pain transmitted through pelvic plexus, superior hypogastric plexus, sympathetic trunks and pelvic splanchnic nerves | |

## Self-Assessment Review

1. Research is inconclusive regarding the action, levels, and effect of _____ on connective tissue in the pregnant woman.
2. _____ pain may occur in women with higher relaxin levels.
3. Weight gain and anatomic changes in breast structure may result in development of _____.
4. During pregnancy, the anterior abdominal wall _____.
5. The lumbar plexus is intimately related to the _____ muscle.
6. The circumference and transverse diameter of the _____ expands during pregnancy.
7. In pregnancy, the _____ may become enlarged, rotated, elevated, and displaced to the left.
8. The enlarged uterus may compress two major blood vessels: _____, _____.
9. When treating adolescents, it is important to remember that _____ may not occur fully until 25 to 30 years of age.
10. Name three important bony landmarks of the pelvis: _____, _____, _____.
11. Name the five ligamentous groups of the pelvis: _____, _____, _____, _____, and _____.
12. The ligaments resist _____ forces on the pelvis.
13. The pelvis has been divided into planes and diameters to _____.
14. The pelvic floor can also be referred to as the _____.
15. The _____ and _____ are muscular diaphragms of the inferior pelvis.

## References

1. O'Malley CD, Saunders JB: Leonardo on the Human Body. New York, Dover Publications, 1983.
2. Knight B: Discovering the Human Body. London, Imprint Books, 1980.
3. Chewning EB: Anatomy Illustrated. New York, Simon & Schuster, 1979.
4. Quagliarello J, Steinetz BG, Weiss G: Relaxin secretion in early pregnancy. Obstet Gynecol 53(1):62-63, 1979.
5. Yki-Jarvinen H, Wahlstrom T, Seppala M: Immunohistochemical localisation of relaxin in the genital tract of non-pregnant

women. In Bigazzi M, Greenwood FC, Gasparri F (eds): Biology of Relaxin and its Role in the Human. Amsterdam, Excerpta Medica, 1983.

6. Porter DG: The roles of relaxin in different species. In Bigazzi M, Greenwood FC, Gasparri F (eds): Biology of Relaxin and its Role in the Human. Amsterdam, Holland, Excerpta Medica, 1983.

7. MacLennan AH, Nicolson R, Green RC: Serum relaxin in pregnancy. Lancet :241-243, Aug 2, 1986.

8. Weiss G: The secretion and role of relaxin in pregnant women. In Bigazzi M, Greenwood FC, Gasparri F (eds): Biology of Relaxin and its Role in the Human. Amsterdam, Excerpta Medica, 1983.

9. Calguneri M, Bird HA, Wright V: Changes in joint laxity occurring during pregnancy. Ann Rheum Dis 41:126-128, 1982.

10. MacLennan AH, et al: Serum relaxin and pelvic pain of pregnancy. Lancet :243-245, Aug 2, 1986.

11. Norstrom A, et al: Inhibitory action of relaxin on human cervical smooth muscle. J Clin Endocrinol Metab 59(3):379-382, 1984.

12. Woodburne RT: Essentials of Human Anatomy. New York, Oxford University Press, 1973.

13. Massey EW, Cefalo RC: Neuropathies of pregnancy. Obstet Gynecol Surv 34(7):489-492, 1979.

14. Conant Van Blarcom C: Obstetrical Nursing. New York, MacMillan, 1929.

15. Pritchard JA, MacDonald PC, Gant NF: Williams Obstetrics. Norwalk, Appleton-Century-Crofts, 1985.

16. LaBan MM, Perrin JCS, Latimer FR: Pregnancy and the herniated lumbar disc. Arch Phys Med Rehabil 64:319-321, 1983.

17. Artal R, Wiswell RA: Exercise in Pregnancy. Baltimore, Williams & Wilkins, 1986.

18. Burnett LS: Anatomy. In Jones HW, Wentz AC, Burnett SL (eds): Novak's Textbook of Gynecology. Baltimore, Williams & Wilkins, 1988.

19. Basmajian JV: Grant's Method of Anatomy. Baltimore, Williams & Wilkins, 1971.

20. Goss CM (ed): Gray's Anatomy of the Human Body. Philadelphia, Lea & Febiger, 1970.

21. Crafts RC, Krieger HP: Gross anatomy of the female reproductive tract, pituitary, and hypothalamus. In Danforth DN, Scott JR (eds): Obstetrics and Gynecology. Philadelphia, JB Lippincott, 1986.

22. Warwick R, Williams PL (eds): Gray's Anatomy. Philadelphia, WB Saunders, 1973.
23. Steindler A: Kinesiology of the Human Body. Springfield, Charles C Thomas, 1970.
24. Steindler A: Mechanics of Normal and Pathological Locomotion in Man. Springfield, Charles C Thomas, 1935.
25. Heyman J, Lundqvist A: The symphysis pubis in pregnancy and parturition. Acta Obstet Gynecol Scand 12:191-225, 1932.
26. Siffert RS, Pruzansky ME, Levy RN: Orthopaedic complications. In Cherry SH, Berkowitz RL, Kase NG (eds): Rovinsky and Guttmacher's Medical, Surgical, and Gynecologic Complications of Pregnancy. Baltimore, Williams & Wilkins, 1985.

# FOUR

# Physiology

Physiologic changes during the life of the human female are numerous, occurring in every system of the body. Most changes, however, occur during and immediately following pregnancy. Altered function in the reproductive, renal, neurologic, cardiovascular, gastrointestinal, respiratory, endocrine, and dermatologic systems will be discussed, as well as general changes that occur when the pregnant woman exercises and as the normal female ages.

## *Reproductive Changes*

Uterine growth is brought about by hypertrophy of muscle cells, an increase in the total amount of elastic connective tissue, and an increase in the size and number of blood vessels to supply the rapidly growing tissues with oxygen and nutritive substances. Most of the uterine weight is gained by the 20th week of pregnancy. The myometrial walls become thicker at this time, only to become thinner in the latter half of pregnancy to allow for the growth of the fetus. Interestingly, in late pregnancy and during labor, myometrial contractions cause thickening of the upper uterine segment as the lower segment expands. This expansion of the lower segment allows for dilation of the cervix and easier passage of the infant. Uterine blood flow at term averages 500 ml/min as opposed to 50 ml/min in the nonpregnant state.[1]

The uterus undergoes irregular, usually painless, contractions, (Braxton-Hicks) throughout early pregnancy. Braxton-Hicks contractions, sometimes felt during the second trimester, increase after 30 weeks. Hypertrophied glands and softening of the tip of the cervix (Goodell's sign) are evident soon after conception; increased vascularity with congestion of the cervix, by the sixth week. Mucus secretion is increased and thickened, resulting in the formation of the large mucus plug at the opening of the cervix. This plug serves as a barrier to protect the fetus from bacterial or mechanical disruption. The round ligaments, which help stabilize the uterus and hold it close to the abdominal wall in nonpregnant states, become elongated and hypertrophied.

The fallopian tubes become elongated, edematous, and somewhat hyperemic, and the ovaries become enlarged and elongated because of their increased vascularity. The ovary containing the corpus luteum (the endocrine body that produces progesterone at the site of the ruptured follicle) is markedly longer and reaches its maximum development during the third month. Due to pituitary inhibition, ovulation is discontinued during pregnancy.[2]

The vaginal changes in pregnancy are marked. As vascularity increases, the vagina becomes congested and cyanotic (Chadwick's sign).[1] This is another of the objective signs of pregnancy. Secretions in the vagina have a highly acidic $pH$ of 3.3 to 5.5, because of the increased glycogen content of the epithelium. To prepare for delivery, the vagina's connective tissue decreases, the mucosa thickens, and the muscular wall hypertrophies. As a result, the space is lengthened and, with the acquired elasticity, the vagina can accommodate the fetal head without rupture. The vulva also increases because of edema and increased vascularity. Some multiparous women, say they feel as if they are "sitting on something," because of an increased edema reaction.[1,2,3]

## Renal

The renal system, too, must expand its function and capacity as the demand on it increases. Increased urination is a common, early complaint in pregnancy related to increased renal function. Effective renal plasma blood flow increases 60% to 80%, along with a 50% increase in the glomerular filtration rate.[4] In addition, as the uterus enlarges, the ureter may be obstructed at the level of the pelvic brim, causing bladder compression.[4] This hydroureter usually occurs more frequently on the right side. Although blood flow in the nonpregnant woman is maximal when she is supine, the assumption of this position by a pregnant woman may compromise vena cava renal blood flow because the uterus compresses the great vessels. For this reason, left-side lying is recommended in pregnancy.[4,5]

## *Neurologic*

There is no neurologic disorder that occurs solely during pregnancy. There are diseases of the peripheral and central nervous systems that occur more frequently in pregnancy or in the puerperium, and pregnancy may cause a recurrence of a preexisting neurologic disorder. These diseases and disorders will be discussed at length in Chapter 10.

## *Cardiovascular*

Extraordinary changes in hemodynamics occur during pregnancy as a result of increased metabolic needs for tissue growth, increase in the vascular network, and increased steroid hormone production.

Blood volume increases about 40% above nonpregnant values. The variation may be as much as 50% and fluctuates with maternal parity and body size. The largest increase in blood volume takes place during the first 20 to 30 weeks of pregnancy. There is an increase in both blood plasma and red cell mass (see Figure 4-1). The blood plasma volume, however, increases unequally, leading to hemodilution and possibly physiologic anemia. Supplemental iron alleviates this problem. Blood volume of women with twins increases more than that of women with a singleton gestation.

Cardiac output increases as early as the 12th week of pregnancy and peaks at 28 to 32 weeks to 30% to 50% above nonpregnant values (see Figure 4-2). Maternal position may have a great influence on cardiac output, especially if the inferior vena cava is compressed by the expanding uterus (see Figure 4-3). This reduced cardiac output in the supine position is termed "the vena cava syndrome" and disappears almost immediately when the woman is placed in a side-lying position (see Figure 4-4). The increased cardiac output in early pregnancy is attributed to increased stroke volume, which rises 20% to 40% at midpregnancy; however, after 28 to 32 weeks, the stroke volume declines until term, and increased cardiac output is related to tachycardia.

Heart rate increases throughout pregnancy. At term, it reaches a peak of about 10 to 15 beats/minute above nonpregnant values when

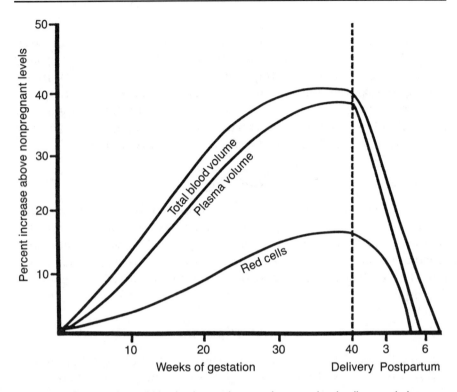

Figure 4-1: Changes in total blood volume, plasma volume, and red cell mass during pregnancy and puerperium (From Wilson JR, Carrington ER, Ledger WJ: Obstetrics and Gynecology (7th ed), St. Louis, Missouri: CV Mosby Co. 1983, p 235).

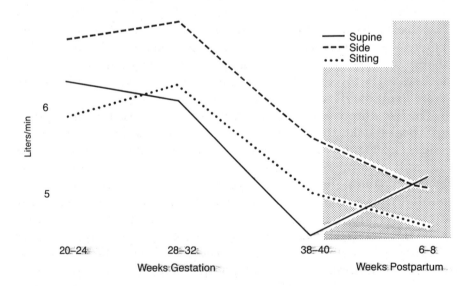

Figure 4-2: Cardiac output at different stanges of pregnancy and puerperium according to patient's position. (From Veland K, et al: American Journal of Obstetrics and Gynecology, 104: 856, 1969).

*Hemodynamic Parameters Throughout Pregnancy*

| Parameter | Patient Position | 1st Trimester | 2nd Trimester | 3rd Trimester | Postpartum |
|---|---|---|---|---|---|
| Heart rate | L | 77 ± 2 | 85 ± 2 | 88 ± 2 | 69 ± 2 |
| (beats/min) | S | 76 ± 2 | 84 ± 2 | 92 ± 2 | 70 ± 2 |
| Stroke volume | L | 75 ± 2 | 86 ± 4 | 97 ± 5 | 79 ± 3 |
| (ml/min) | S | 82 ± 5 | 85 ± 4 | 87 ± 5 | 79 ± 3 |
| Cardiac output | L | 3.53 ± 0.21 | 4.32 ± 0.22 | 4.85 ± 0.27 | 3.30 ± 0.17 |
| 1/min/m² | S | 3.76 ± 0.24 | 4.19 ± 0.21 | 4.54 ± 0.28 | 3.33 ± 0.21 |
| Left ventricular ejection time | L | 302 ± 2 | 290 ± 5 | 281 ± 4 | 310 ± 5 |
| (msec) | S | 301 ± 3 | 286 ± 4 | 260 ± 4 | 307 ± 5 |
| Systolic blood pressure | L | 98 ± 2 | 91 ± 2 | 95 ± 2 | 97 ± 2 |
| (mm Hg) | S | 106 ± 2 | 102 ± 2 | 106 ± 2 | 110 ± 2 |
| Diastolic blood pressure | L | 53 ± 2 | 49 ± 2 | 50 ± 2 | 57 ± 2 |
| (mm Hg) | S | 57 ± 2 | 60 ± 1 | 65 ± 2 | 65 ± 1 |

*L*, lateral; *S*, supine.

Figure 4-3: Hemodynamic parameters throughout pregnancy (Key TC, Resnik R: Maternal Changes in Pregnancy in Obstetrics and Gynecology 5th edition, Danforth DN, Scott JR (eds) Philadelphia, Pennsylvania, J.B. Lippincott, 1986; adapted from Katz R, Karliner JS, Resnik R: Effects of natural volume overload state (pregnancy) on left ventricular performance in human subjects. Circulation 58: 434, 1978, by permission of the American Heart Association, Inc.).

measured in a lateral position. Arterial blood pressure decreases near the end of the first trimester and throughout pregnancy, because of the substantial fall in systemic vascular resistance of about 2 to 3 mm Hg systolic and 5 to 10 mm Hg diastolic.[1]

## *Gastrointestinal*

Changes in gastrointestinal function arise from hormonal changes, as well as from structural adaptations to the fetus. Nausea, vomiting, appetite preference, constipation, heartburn, hemorrhoids, and mi-

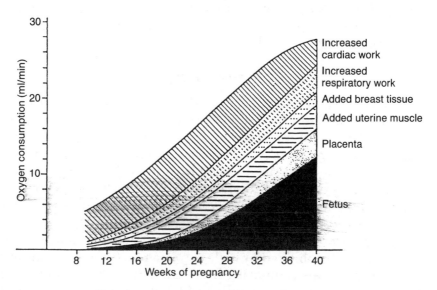

Figure 4-4: Components of increased oxygen consumption in pregnancy (from Hytten FE, Leitch I: The Physiology of Human Pregnancy. Oxford, Blackwell, 1964).

nor abdominal pains are common in pregnancy. Various degrees of nausea and vomiting, called "morning sickness," are experienced by 50% of women during the first trimester. Gastric disturbance can range from a mild, transient morning type, to a continual, severe type that threatens the life of the mother (hyperemesis gravidarum). Symptoms usually begin 2 weeks after the first missed period and abate by the 10th to 12th week, finally disappearing around the 14th week. However, some women experience nausea on and off during the entire pregnancy.

Nausea is more likely to occur first thing in the morning or before meals when the stomach is empty. There are several theories why nausea and vomiting occur, although the actual cause is unknown. It is believed that human chorionic gonadotropin (hCG) is secreted in large quantities by the placenta and may be a contributing cause. Another theory is that the rapid development of the trophoblastic cells that invade the uterine mucosa and develop into the placenta give off degenerative products that may produce the nausea and vomiting.[12]

It has recently been shown that many women have improved physiological adaptation to lactose digestion during pregnancy. Women who have an intolerance to lactose eliminate milk as a source of lactose, and calcium as well. There is, however, some evidence that those who are lactose-intolerant in early pregnancy improve enough to digest milk during the third trimester. This change may be the result of a progesterone-induced decrease in intestinal motility. Slower peristalsis allows for increased contact time with the layers of the intestine for lactose digestion.[6] The influences of pregnancy on the gastrointestinal system are listed below by location, changes, and etiology. (Table 4-1)

## Breast Changes

Breast changes are often one of the earliest signs of pregnancy. Typically, there will be a tingly feeling and increased sensitivity. Breast enlargement is usually noted by the eighth week. The venous supply to the breasts increases as they enlarge. The areola deepens in color, and there are small, palpable papules. These hypertrophied sebaceous glands are called glands of Montgomery. After the tenth week, colostrum, a clear substance, can be expressed. It is the forerunner of the milk that comes 2 to 3 days after delivery and is thought to prepare the infant's intestinal system for mother's milk. Full lactation is inhibited by high estrogen-progesterone levels prior to delivery. Estrogen stimulates production by the ducts, and progesterone increases the proliferation of lobule-alveolar tissue. This development is essentially completed by midpregnancy. After delivery,

**Table 4-1. Gastrointestinal Changes in Pregnancy**

| Location | Change | Etiology |
|---|---|---|
| Mouth | Gum hypertrophy, increased caries, ptyalism. | Unknown. |
| Esophagus | Decreased lower esophageal sphincter tone, increase of nonperistaltic contraction in distal esophagus; heartburn. | Possibly progesterone; pressure reduced in lower esophageal sphincter. |
| Appetite, thirst | Increased food cravings and aversions, occasionally pica (craving unnatural foods or substances). | Unknown. |
| Digestion | Nausea and vomiting, improvement in lactose digestion. | Possibly estrogens, hCG*, possibly progesterone, decreased intestinal motility. |
| Stomach | Decreased motility, tone, and acid secretion; increased incidence of hiatal hernia. | Possibly progesterone; mechanical effects of expanding uterus. |
| Small, large intestine | Possibly decreased motility. | Possibly progesterone. |
| Liver | Cholestasis, pruritus gravidarum (generalized itching). | Liver cell response to estrogen. |
| Appendix | Displaced upward as pregnancy develops. | Mechanical effects of expanding uterus. |
| Gallbladder | Decreased emptying time, possible buildup of cholesterol; gallstones. | Possibly progesterone. |
| Colon/anus | Constipation, hemorrhoids. | Decreased tone in rectal sphincter; pressure of expanding uterus; possibly progesterone; slower passage of food results in hard, dry feces difficult to expel. |

*hCG-human chorionic gonadotropin
Adapted from Manual of Obstetrics, Niswander, 1987. [3]

the suckling of the infant stimulates the secretion of prolactin by the anterior pituitary gland, which then stimulates the production and secretion of milk.[1,2,7]

## *Weight Gain*

Historically, physicians' opinions fluctuate about weight gain in pregnancy. In the mid-1950s, women were often restricted to a 15-pound gain, and some physicians even advised diet pills. Now it is known that weight gain not only affects fetal well-being but also alters the infant's ability to thrive after birth. Currently physicians believe the average woman with a singleton pregnancy should gain an average of 25-26 pounds, distributed as follows:

| | |
|---|---|
| Fetus | 7.5 lb. |
| Placenta | 1.5 lb. |
| Amniotic fluid | 2.0 lb. |
| Increased uterine muscle mass | 2.5 lb. |

| | |
|---|---|
| Increased blood volume | 3.5 lb. |
| Increased breast tissue | 2.0 lb. |
| Increased interstitial fluid | 2.0-3.0 lb. |
| Additional fat storage | 4.0 lb. |

Therefore, the uterus and its contents account for approximately 13.5 pounds, and maternal gains, about 11.5-12.5 pounds on the average. Maternal weight gain ranges from 20 to 40 pounds for a single birth and up to 50 or 60 pounds for a multiple birth. The general recommendation for weight gain during the first trimester is 2 to 4 pounds; and in the second and third, an average of slightly less than 1 pound per week. Extra fluid, protein, and fat are deposited as emergency stores in case the nursing mother is unable to get proper nutrition. The recommended daily allowance for women between the ages of 23 and 53 is about 2000 calories/day. During pregnancy, a mother should add 300 calories, and during lactation an extra 500 calories (above the 2000 calories/day base).

## *Metabolic Changes*

Profound metabolic changes occur during pregnancy. Metabolism of proteins, carbohydrates, fats, minerals, oxygen, and fluids is altered. Increased protein metabolism can be attributed to the demands of increased tissue growth (*e.g.*, in the uterus and breasts). The majority of protein is stored, causing a positive nitrogen balance early in gestation and increasing through the third trimester when fetal demands are the greatest. Carbohydrate metabolism also changes. Insulin is elevated because of the plasma expansion, and there is a reduction in the blood glucose for a given insulin load. Stress, therefore, is placed on the islet cells. These factors may be responsible for unmasking a latent deficiency in islet cell secretion.

The renal threshold for glucose may range from 100 to 150 mg/dl, a drop from the prepregnancy value (150-200 mg/dl) due to the increased glomerular filtration rate that occurs in pregnancy. The theory is that renal tubular reabsorption of glucose may not increase as the glomerular filtration rate does and may account for the many cases of glycosuria and the accompanying low blood sugar fasting levels found in pregnant women. This may also be the first evidence of diabetes, and a glucose tolerance test is needed to differentiate physiologic from diabetic glycosuria of pregnancy.

Sodium, potassium, and calcium are stored for maternal use, with large amounts of the sodium stored in amniotic fluid, placenta, and tissues. The largest portion of sodium (33%) is stored in the fetus. Potassium (48%) is also stored in the fetus, as well as in the breasts, uterus, and placenta. The fetus also harbors 90% of the stored calcium. The total value of maternal serum calcium diminishes during pregnancy, but serum ionized calcium is increased until delivery. At that time, the newborn's magnesium, phosphorus, and total and ionized calcium are greatly increased over the mother's normal level. Iron is not stored during pregnancy, and approximately 1000 mg must be supplied on a daily basis to meet the increased demands of the mother and fetus. Half is utilized by the fetus, placenta, and maternal red cell mass. Of the other half, approximately 450 mg remain in the maternal store and 150 mg are lost at delivery. Fat metabolism changes in concert with that of protein and carbohydrates. These changes include an increase in maternal fat stored and a related increase in insulin resistance. Wilson states, "The elevated level of the free fatty acid exerts an anti-insulin effect by interfering with peripheral use of glucose." There is evidence that progesterone may reset a fat thermostat in the hypothalamus.[8] This mechanism serves to store energy for the mother and fetus during periods of starvation or extreme physical exertion.[7]

In late pregnancy, swelling normally occurs in the eyelids, face, hands, and ankles. Fifty percent may develop eyelid edema and 70%, edema of the lower extremities (not associated with preeclampsia or eclampsia). The edema is usually present in the morning, decreases with activity, and is believed to be caused by sodium and water retention and by increased capillary permeability resulting from the additional circulating placental, ovarian, and adrenocortical hormones.[8]

## *Respiratory*

Respiratory physiology changes during pregnancy because of uterine enlargement, hormonal changes, increased cardiac output and increased blood volume. Normally, maternal plasma bicarbonate and total base values are reduced during pregnancy; the blood $p$H, however, remains unchanged. It has been suggested that because pregnant women hyperventilate, a respiratory alkalosis is caused by lowering the $PCO_2$ of the blood. There is an accompanying increase of sodium to compensate for the alkalosis, with little change in blood $p$H.

Oxygen consumption increases by 14%, half going to the fetus and placenta, and the other half supplying the needs of added uterine muscle and breast tissue. Accordingly, respirations and cardiac function increase. Increased levels of progesterone lead to hyperventilation, resulting in a decreased concentration of carbon dioxide in the alveoli. This reduced tension favors diffusion of carbon dioxide from fetal to maternal circulation. Pulmonary function is

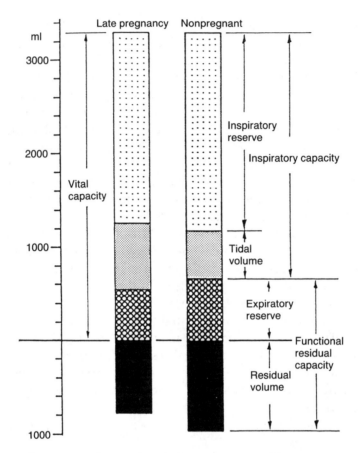

Figure 4-5: Components of lung volume in late pregnancy and in nonpregnant state (from Hytten FE, Leitch I: The Physiology of Human Pregnancy. Blackwell, Oxford, 1964).

not impaired, because the respiratory system accommodates these changes (see Figure 4-5).

There is a progressive elevation of the diaphragm caused by the enlargement of the uterus, and total excursion is reduced. The central part of the diaphragm appears flattened. As a result, breathing becomes more costal than abdominal. Dyspnea is a common complaint but appears unrelated to the encroachment of the uterus on the diaphragm in the first and second trimester. Because of an increase in respiratory tidal volume during normal respiration, there is a 26% increase in respiratory minute volume (see Figure 4-5), referred to as the "hyperventilation of pregnancy."

## Endocrine

During pregnancy, the major sources of hormone production are the adrenal, thyroid, parathyroid, anterior pituitary glands, and the placenta. After delivery, hormone secretions return to preexisting levels. The adrenal glands enlarge throughout the course of pregnancy because of hyperplasia at the adrenal cortex, and the thyroid is enlarged more than 50% in all pregnant women.[1] The enlargement of the thyroid is caused by new follicle formation, increased vascularity, and cell formation. The thyroid has a profound effect on the basal metabolism rate, which increases 10% to 30% by the 16th week. The basal metabolic rate measures total oxygen consumption, increased by the demands of the growing fetal and maternal tissues. The parathyroid glands are responsible for the calcium level and undergo hypertrophy as fetal calcium demands increase. The hypertrophy results in calcium absorption from the mother's bones to maintain normal calcium-iron concentration in maternal extracellular fluids for the fetus. The maternal pituitary gland enlarges during pregnancy from the effects of estrogen. The anterior lobe increases 20% to 40% due to the prolactin-containing "pregnancy cells." The posterior lobe does not hypertrophy. Presumably, the secretion of oxytocin and vasopressin (antidiuretic hormones) is increased. After delivery, the sudden loss of estrogen and progesterone secretion by the placenta allows for marked prolactin production by the pituitary. This stimulates production of fat and lactose by the mammary glands resulting in secretion of milk instead of colostrum.

The ovaries secrete relaxin from the corpus luteum which is the endocrine body developed at the site of the ruptured ovarian follicle.[10] In addition to its other functions of respiration, nutrition, and excretion for the fetus, the placenta acts as an endocrine gland. The primary purposes of this endocrine function are to maintain the pregnancy and support the fetus until gestation. By itself, the placenta is an incomplete endocrine organ. It is through the constant interaction of the fetus, placenta, and maternal system that steroid hormone levels increase. (See Table 4-2).

## *Dermatologic*

There are many skin changes that occur during pregnancy, including increased pigmentation, abdominal wall tissue modification, cutaneous vascular markings, skin tags, sweating, itching, hair growth or loss, and nail alteration.

An increase in pigmentation around the eyes and over the cheekbones sometimes occurs and is called chloasma, or "mask of pregnancy." It usually disappears at the end of pregnancy but may last for several weeks. Increased pigmentation also appears around the breast areola and on the linea alba, which becomes a brownish-black streak down the middle of the abdomen. These markings may not necessarily regress after delivery, but most often do.

As the uterus enlarges in some patients, the stretching and ten-

### Table 4-2. Hormones and their Functions in Pregnancy

| Hormone | A. Where Produced B. When Occurs | Function |
|---|---|---|
| hCG Human chorionic gonadotropin | A. Placenta, by the trophoblastic tissues of the early fertilized ovum into the fluids of the mother. B. Soon after fertilization. | Augments, maintains endometrial bed; causes persistence of corpus luteum to secrete larger quantities of progesterone and estrogen, prevents menstruation. |
| HPL Human placental lactogen, also known as human chorionic somatomammotropin (hCS) | A. By trophoblastic tissue, placenta, third week after ovulation in the trophoblast. B. 5th week, progressing with pregnancy. | Plays a major role in development of mother's breast prior to birth of baby; inhibits action of insulin to cause glucose transport through cell membranes; promotes cell growth and provides increased circulation of free fatty acids for energy for maternal metabolism and fetal nutrition; inhibition of glucose uptake and gluconeogenesis in mother; anti-insulin action raises levels of insulin, which favors protein synthesis and ensures mobilizable source of amino acids for transport to the fetus. |
| HCT Human chorionic thyrotropin | A. Produced by the placenta. B. Evident in early pregnancy and rises until term. | Increases secretion of thyroid hormones to stimulate incorporation of inorganic phosphates into thyroid to be neutralized by antipituitary TSH (pituitary thyrotropin). |
| HCACTH (HCCG) Human chorionic adrenocorticotropin | A. Pituitary-like hormone produced by placenta. B. Evident by 10th week of gestation. | Placental steroidogenesis. |
| Estrogen | A. Produced by ovarian follicle, placenta and adrenal cortex. B. Appears mid-pregnancy. | Levels used to assess fetal and placental functions; necessary for a viable placenta, healthy fetus; intact fetal circulation. |
| Progesterone | A. Formed by maternal adrenals, corpus luteum, placental syncytial cells, and fetal adrenals. B. Corpus luteum in early gestation; placenta in late pregnancy; polypeptide protein secreted by corpus luteum, evident by missed period. | Development, maintenance of endometrial bed; relaxation of pelvic ligaments and connective tissue, softening of the cervix, inhibition of uterine motility. |
| Prolactin | A. Produced by anterior lobe of pituitary gland. B. Produced immediately after birth of baby.[10,11,12] | Stimulates milk production. |

sion in the abdominal wall often causes changes in the collagen elastic fibers of the deep layers of the skin. These can also occur in the breasts and along the thighs. They are purplish irregular lines called "striae gravidarum," or stretch marks. There is some evidence that elevated levels of adrenal steroids may be responsible for this thinning of fibers. The striae are often a purplish color due to the increased venous distension beneath the skin. After delivery, the color fades to white, but the lines do not disappear.[1,2]

Cutaneous vascular changes, such as spider nevi, appear in two thirds of Caucasians and 10% of all black women. These small red elevations, with radiating branches from a central body, may appear on the face, upper chest, and arms. Telangiectasia are capillary dilations around the ankles and sometimes the thighs. They are related to varices but are not painful. There is no risk to the fetus, and they subside to an extent, but not completely, after delivery. Reddening of the palms (palmar erythema) is commonly encountered in two thirds of Caucasian and one third of black women. These two vascular changes most likely result from estrogen production, often occur together, have no clinical significance, and usual disappear at the end of pregnancy.[8]

Skin tags (molluscum fibrosum gravidarum) are skin-colored, soft fleshy growths, from 1 to 5 mm in length, appearing on the sides of the face and neck, the anterior portions of the chest, axilla, and feet. They usually form in the second half of pregnancy and progress or disappear after delivery. There is, however, some discussion as to whether or not they may not regress, but actually increase. Although unconfirmed, endocrine changes may be the cause.[8]

Increased sweating also occurs near the end of pregnancy and may lead to some types of eczema. Increased weight and thyroid activity have been proposed as factors causing the increased glandular activity, but palmar sweating may be the result of adrenocortical secretion. The effect of pregnancy on sebaceous glands is not consistent. Women often complain of oily skin, but the overall effect of pregnancy on acne is unpredictable. The axillary sweat glands may decrease secretion during pregnancy but possibly produce a rebound effect postpartum.[8]

Pruritus, or itching, affects approximately 20% of pregnant women, either in a localized or generalized fashion. It can begin in the third month and continue to the last, but typically does not continue postpartum.[8]

Hirsutism, to some degree, is seen in most women usually in the early stages of pregnancy, related to increased adrenocorticotrophic hormone and adrenocorticosteroid secretion. Those with darker or more body hair experience greater growth, and hair may increase on the face, arms, legs, and sometimes the back. After delivery, this new, fine hair is replaced by coarse hair. Consequently, by 4 to 12 weeks postpartum, hair loss is noticeable and may continue for several months. In some cases, hair loss occurs in excess. Changes in endocrine balance and stress are some of the many causes for this loss. Regrowth, for the most part, occurs within 6 to 15 months, but the hair may never be as abundant as before pregnancy.

Although not fully understood, nail changes occur as early as the sixth week and may include transverse grooving, softening, increased brittleness, loosening, and overgrowth of the skin beneath the nail (subungual keratosis).

## *Multiple Pregnancies*

Multiple pregnancies occur in 1% of all gestations carried beyond 20 weeks, and account for 10% of all perinatal mortality.[1] The incidence of triplets is 1 in 10,000, and 1 in 1 million for quadruplets. The frequency of twins increases with both maternal age and parity and is more likely to occur after the use of drugs for induction of ovulation, after discontinuing oral contraceptives, and as a result of *in vitro* fertilization. Twins are more common among blacks than whites and among patients with a family history of dizygotic twins (when two separate ova are fertilized by two different sperm).

Multiple gestations are suspected when uterine size is greater than expected for gestational age, but ultrasound and auscultation of the heartbeat can identify twins as early as 6 or 7 weeks. Human placental lactogen levels are higher in twin pregnancies than they are in normal single ones. Monozygotic twins occur as a result of division of one fertilized ovum early in gestation. These identical twins may have four different configurations of chorions (the outermost layer of the amniotic sac and placenta). The most common arrangement is one shared placenta, two amniotic sacs, and one chorion. Next common is two chorions, two amniotic sacs, and two fused placentas; followed by two chorions, two amniotic sacs, and two distinct placentas. The rarest arrangement is one chorion, one amniotic sac, and one placenta.

Twenty-five percent to 40% of all twin pregnancies result in premature labor and delivery due to the volume of intrauterine expansion that exceeds what the myometrium can accommodate. Congenital anomalies, abnormal placentation, and the effect of the uterine contents on cervical integrity may also initiate premature labor and delivery.[1] Perinatal mortality among twins is three to four times that of singleton births because of low birth weight, prematurity complications, intracerebral hemorrhage, respiratory distress syndrome, traumatic delivery, or sepsis. During pregnancy, a mother carrying twins will easily gain 60 pounds, and blood volume increases 50% or more (30-40% with singletons).[1,2] This leads to a disproportionate increase in plasma volume over red cell volume, resulting in hemodilution or "pregnancy anemia."[1] The risk of iron deficiency is two to three times that of a singleton pregnancy because of the increased fetal and maternal demands. Other maternal complications include a greater risk of hemorrhage antepartum, intrapartum, and postpartum because of increased risk of abruptio placenta, placenta previa, and uterine atony, related to complications from surgical deliveries.

## *Exercise*

Exercise in pregnancy is of concern to the physical therapist because of the possibility of exceeding safe metabolic, respiratory, and cardiac thresholds of the mother and fetus. The types of exercises advocated have changed dramatically since the 1930s, when physicians in Great Britain simply encouraged "activity" for expectant mothers, based on an observation that working-class women had easier births.

Recommendations for treatment from research on exercise in pregnancy must be applied cautiously. There are many legal and ethical standards that limit not only the scope of research studies but the relation of results from animal studies to humans. Physiologic parameters that differ between animals and humans, such as heat elimination from sweating versus panting and venous pooling from standing, are but two variables that make it impossible to directly apply results to humans. Therefore, this discussion will focus only on exercise in human pregnancy.

The adjustment to exercise depends upon (1) age, sex, body size; (2) type of exercise, body position, light, moderate, or heavy work; (3) frequency; (4) the environment, temperature, water, altitude, pollution, as well as; (5) the health and nutritional status of the subject. It should also be understood that there are no consistent methods of training nor consistent test protocols. This makes extrapolations from research difficult to apply to activities of daily living. Of importance, however, are maternal physiologic responses to work and exercise, including oxygen consumption, circulation, cardiovascular response, respiration, hormonal changes, body temperature, energy expenditure, and physical work capacity, as well as fetal and placental responses.

### Maternal responses to exercise

Artal has summarized the literature for cardiovascular responses to exercise during pregnancy as follows: (1) there is a slight increase in cardiac output during mild and moderate exercise with a significant drop in maximal cardiac output; (2) there is an increase in stroke volume on any given work load; (3) there may be an increased heart rate at low intensity exercises, a normal heart rate at normal intensity exercise, and a reduced maximal heart rate; (4) there is no

Cardiovascular Changes That Influence Exercise Capacity during Normal Pregnancy

| Function | Nonpregnant | Pregnant | Percentage Change |
|---|---|---|---|
| Blood volume (ml) | 2500 | 3900 | 55 |
| Heart volume (ml) | | | 12 |
| Heart rate (bpm) | | | |
| Rest | 70 | 85 | 20 |
| Exercise | 190 | 170 | 15 |
| Cardiac output (ml/min) | 4500 | 6000 | 30[a] |
| Stroke volume (ml/beat) | 60–70 | 85–90 | 30[b] |
| A-V oxygen difference (ml) | 45 | 40 | 12 |
| Arterial pressure | | | |
| Systolic | 120 | 112 | 5 |
| Diastolic | 75 | 70 | 5 |
| Systemic vascular resistance (dynes/sec/cm⁵) | 1700 | 1250 | 30 |

[a] Greatest during mid-pregnancy.
[b] Greatest by the end of the second trimester.

Figure 4-6: Cardiovascular changes that influence exercise capacity during normal pregnancy (From M. deSwiet en F. Hytten, G. Chamberlain (eds), Clinical Physiology in Obstetrics, Oxford, Blackwell Scientific Publications, 1980).

difference in arteriovenous oxygen difference between work and pregnancy; and (5) there may be an error associated with the prediction of maximal work capacity from a submaximal heart rate. (See Figure 4-6)

The oxygen consumption per unit time ($VO_2$) at rest in pregnancy increases with advancing gestation to a maximum value near term.[13] This increase may be due to a higher metabolic rate, increased tissue mass, or extra work needed to perform vital functions. Increased $VO_2$ during exercise results from increased muscle work involved in changing body position, respiration, and cardiac function.[13] The highest measurements of $VO_2$ have been recorded at term during maximal exercise.[13] Lotgering reported a 10% increase in $VO_2$ during a treadmill test in a pregnant woman, compared to her nonpregnant value. It is believed that there is a training effect evident in pregnancy (unless a sedentary lifestyle is adopted), because every activity requires a higher absolute $VO_2$. In addition to maternal demands, uterine oxygen consumption also increases during pregnancy due to the expanding demands of the fetus and placenta. During exercise, uterine blood flow may reduce markedly, but the uterine $VO_2$ is maintained secondary to hemoconcentration and increased oxygen extraction by the myoendometrium.

Exercising women may experience increasing difficulty as their pregnancy advances because of the inability to transfer oxygen and carbon dioxide from the air to the cells. Along with a significant increase in hemoglobin and cardiac output, there is an excess demand that leads to a decrease in arteriovenous oxygen difference. Nonpregnant women compensate by increasing pulmonary diffusion capacity and increasing alveolar ventilation. The pregnant woman compensates for these physiologic and associated anatomic changes by breathing more deeply. As weight increases during pregnancy, exercise produces a greater oxygen debt, and results in a longer recovery rate.

Artal compared pulmonary responses to exercise at mild, moderate, and $VO_2$max (maximum oxygen consumption) levels (see Figure 4-7 and 4-8). He found that in mild exercise, respiratory frequency was significantly higher than in controls. Overall, pregnant women responded to exercise with increased ventilation at mild and maximal exercise levels. At moderate exercise, they responded with a more efficient ventilation. This may be the result of primary respiratory alkalosis of pregnancy. Pregnant subjects were found to have lower respiratory frequencies and tidal volumes equal to controls.

Hyperventilation, during rest in pregnancy, increases with exercise (see Figure 4-9) and results in a lower carbon dioxide tension, lower bicarbonate concentration and buffering capacity, and a moderate increase in $p$H with a negligible change in oxygen tension.[13,14] In addition to the findings of Artal, research has shown that respiratory frequency during and after bicycling or weightbearing exercises slightly increases, but not significantly. Gas exchange during exercise increases to the same levels in pregnant women and controls as

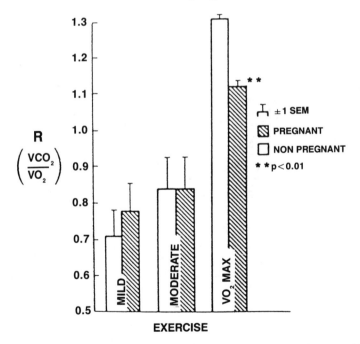

Figure 4-7: Comparison of respiratory exchange ratio (R) during mild, moderate, and $VO_2$ max exercise (from Artal R et al: American Journal of Obstetrics and Gynecology (in press).)

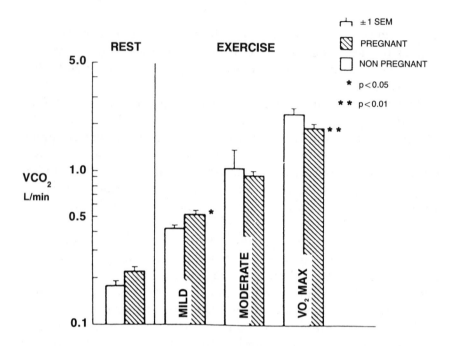

Figure 4-8: $CO_2$ production during mild, moderate and $VO_2$ max exercise (from Artal R et al: American Journal of Obstetrics and Gynecology (in press).)

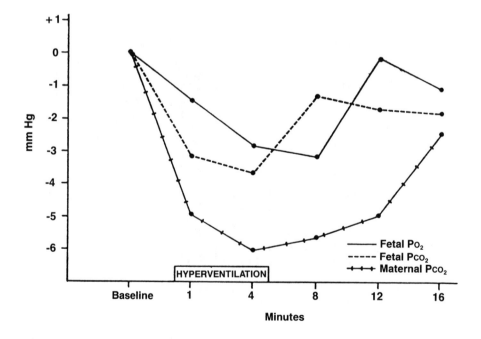

Figure 4-9: The relationship between maternal $PCO_2$, fetal $PCO_2$ and fetal $PO_2$ during maternal hyperventilation (from Miller FC et al: American Journal of Obstetrics and Gynecology 120: 489, 1974.)

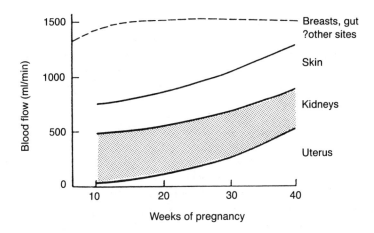

Figure 4-10: Distribution of increased cardiac output during pregnancy (From M. deSwet: en F. Hytten, G. Chamberlain (eds), Clinical Physiology in Obstetrics. Oxford, Blackwell Scientific Publications, 1980).

an effect of increased pulmonary diffusion capacity and increased alveolar ventilation.[15] In a study of pregnant women during moderately strenuous bicycle exercise, lower carbon dioxide tensions were found at rest and during exercise, with hyperventilation displayed during exercise. No change in arterial carbon dioxide content was found during mild exercise in pregnant and nonpregnant women. (See Figure 4-8) Mean arterial blood pressure may increase up to 20% in response to exercise in human pregnancies, mainly because of systolic pressure increases proportionate to the level of exercise at moderate work loads. Increased weight from pregnancy may be a factor in this alteration in pressure. Diastolic pressure decreases about 10% below nonpregnant values in early and midgestation, although systolic pressure decreases only slightly.

During pregnancy, the whole blood volume increases slowly by 50% near term because of a 30% to 60% increase in plasma volume and a 20% to 30% increase in erythrocyte mass.[13,15] Because of this hypervolemia, there may be an increase in mean systemic pressure, which, combined with a decreased peripheral resistance, mediates the increase in stroke volume and resting cardiac output. Plasma volume, however, decreases during exercise (depending on intensity) to a maximal low of 15% at about 60% $VO_2$max. This occurs within the first 10 minutes and does not change with further exercise. In studies of pregnant cardiac patients, it has been demonstrated that heart disease does not affect blood volume or plasma but does reduce cardiac reserve. As a consequence, these patients respond with increased stroke volume and tachycardia.[15]

By using indicator dilution and electromagnetic flow probes with the patient under anesthesia or in a compromising supine position, a dramatic increase in uterine blood flow can be demonstrated. (See Figure 4-10) Because the woman is anesthetized, the actual changes in uterine blood flow may be, in fact, further increased under physiologic conditions.[13,15] Urine tests measuring 5-hydroxyindolacetic acid suggest that there is a decrease in visceral blood flow in pregnant women during exercise compared to controls.[15]

Cardiac output, peripheral resistance, arterial blood pressure, left ventricular work, and arteriovenous oxygen difference adjust to within normal limits during exercise,[13] as long as there is no preexisting cardiac problem. Cardiovascular function is impaired in cases of patients with heart disease and pregnancy-induced hypertension. The increased blood pressure at rest noted in patients with pregnancy-induced hypertension appears to be the result of increased systemic vascular resistance. Vigorous exercise for these patients is contraindicated and needs further study.

Cardiovascular responses to isometric exercises in patients with pregnancy-induced hypertension was studied by Nisell and colleagues.[16] Although the isometric hand-grip test increased blood pressure, heart rate, stroke volume, cardiac output, epinephrine, and norepinephrine concentrations in arterial plasma in both the pregnancy-controlled group and the pregnancy-hypertensive group, these factors did not differ significantly. Nisell and colleagues concluded that pregnancy-induced hypertension does not seem to be associated with exaggerated cardiovascular or sympathoadrenal reactivity to isometric exercise compared with normal pregnancy.[16] The increase in blood pressure appeared to be a response to an increase in cardiac output for both groups.

Cardiovascular conditioning during pregnancy has been of interest as a possible means to shorten or decrease the intensity of labor. Many studies have tried to relate physical fitness to pregnancy outcome,[13,17] and there is some evidence to suggest that physical fitness may shorten labor in multiparas.[17] Results of studies of labor in primiparas are mixed; some show a shorter labor, and others do not.[13] More control is necessary to accurately assess the question of labor duration and level of previous exercise. Lactate levels studied by Erkkola and Rauramo[13] revealed that fit women worked harder during labor and delivery than the non-fit. The study also showed that fit women had higher oxygen-carrying capacities to compensate for metabolic acidosis.

The mother's basal body temperature rises by about 0.5°C immediately following ovulation, increases to a maximal level at midgestation, and, thereafter, decreases to normal.[13] This rise in temperature is due to progesterone, which increases through term. The decline in basal body temperature after midpregnancy reflects the opposing effect of increasing estrogen concentrations. Body core temperature may also be affected by prolonged maternal exercise, which may cause an increase high enough to produce teratogenic effects on the fetus. Animal studies show that core temperature above 39°C may be teratogenic and may result in neurotubale defects. Hyperthermia-induced dehydration may also precipitate premature labor and should be avoided.

There is evidence, as well, to suggest that strenuous exercise during pregnancy may be linked to intrauterine growth retardation.[13,15] Working mothers tend to have babies with birth weights as much as 400 grams lower than babies of nonworking mothers.[13]

Maternal hormonal changes during exercise are transitory, reversible, and have no marked effects. Prolactin has a role in water electrolyte balance, which, in turn, has an effect on energy. It has been found that submaximal exercise during pregnancy will elevate serum prolactin levels significantly for 1 hour. Estradiol and progesterone, the ovarian hormones, will increase during exercise, especially strenuous activity.[15] Low values of estriol reflect fetal distress. After submaximal exercise, there is a significant brief rise in estriol, which may indicate fetal well-being, or an increased flow of estriol-rich, uteroplacental blood.

Various endocrine adaptations occur during maternal exercise, however. Glucose utilization and production increase during exercise. During mild exercise, glycogen rises slightly, but insulin level does not. When exercise is more intense, glycogen levels increase significantly, increasing glycogenolysis and gluconeogenesis in the liver. These increases have a primary role in the physiological adaptation to exercise. Increased glucocorticoids induce lipolysis and possess antiinflammatory properties. Exercise, in fact, may be used to achieve a normoglycemic state in pregnancy.[15] With medical supervision, pregnant diabetics can capitalize on individually-designed exercise programs. However, hypoglycemia is a major problem in diabetics during and after exercise. Studies suggest that prolonged strenuous exercise may induce hypoglycemia faster in pregnancy. In addition, exercise may cause a rise in norepinephrine, which can act as a stimulant to the uterus and possibly induce uterine activity.[15] There are minor changes in cortisol levels during exercise, because mild exercise produces only a minimal adrenal effect; therefore, it appears that the cortisol level has a limited role during maternal exercise.

The basal energy expenditure or metabolic rate of maternal tissues alone, during pregnancy, cannot be measured. During pregnancy, the increases in resting $VO_2$ and metabolic rate are related to changes in lean or total body mass.[15] The nonprotein respiratory quotient in nonpregnant and near-term women, despite fetal growth, is the same or slightly increased (about 0.85).[15] Similarly, during mild bike exercise, the nonprotein respiratory quotient is not significantly higher in pregnant women than in nonpregnant controls. Consequently, the ratio of fat-to-carbohydrate used for energy expenditure remains constant. The metabolic rate appears to vary linearly with $VO_2$.[15]

Artal found, however, that during weightbearing exercise, pregnant women used primarily fat, and proportionately less carbohydrate, as a fuel source. He suggests this mechanism may protect the mother from exercising anaerobically and the fetus from hypoxia. However, with some forms of aerobic exercise, for instance, pedaling in water, carbohydrate stores were the primary energy source.[14] In cases of moderate non-weightbearing exercise on the ergometer, the calculated metabolic costs are slightly, but not significantly, higher during pregnancy.[15]

There is a decrease in physical work capacity in the first trimester, so women with low physical capacity may be functioning at their limit to perform simple activities of daily living. If, however, the pregnant woman's physical work capacity is high, she will probably be able to tolerate greater demands during the first trimester. Weightbearing exercise, however, requires increasing oxygen uptake as the pregnancy advances. Weightbearing exercise increases respiratory frequency more than during nonweightbearing exercise. Minute ventilation and tidal volume also increase at rest, during, and following exercise.[13] Because energy demand with weightbearing exercise increases, and maximum work capacity remains the same or decreases, the absolute intensity of weightbearing exercise should be lowered as the pregnancy advances into the second and third trimesters.

### Fetal response to maternal exercise

Typically, the fetal heart rate is used to assess fetal well-being. Changes in fetal heart rate reflect hypoxic and nonhypoxic stress, sympathetic and parasympathetic activity, or asphyxia. However, a 50% reduction in uterine blood flow would have to occur to cause such changes. The healthy fetus can tolerate brief periods of asphyxia, which may occur during maternal exercise. (See Figure 4-10) The fetus will respond to this asphyxia with increased blood pressure and tachycardia. In this way, blood circulation is facilitated, followed by an increase in $O_2$ and a decrease in $CO_2$ tension. In a summary of published studies on fetal heart rate response to maternal exercise, increases of 10 to 30 beats/minute were recorded. These changes do not vary with increased intensity of maternal exercise or gestational age.[15] In a study by Artal of 354 subjects, 22 had fetal bradycardia during or after exercise (6.2% incidence), 11 of the 22 had abnormal pregnancies (pregnancy-induced hypertension or premature labor), and the other 11 had normal pregnancies.[13]

Maternal exercise is associated with an increase in catecholamines metabolized by the placenta. Only 10% to 15% of these catecholamines reach the fetus, but it has been theorized that they could have a restrictive effect on the umbilical blood flow. The combined effect of possible vasoconstriction from elevated catecholamines and decreased blood to the uterus could lead to fetal asphyxia and result in an initial response of tachycardia and bradycardia with prolonged hypoxia and vagal stimulation. Carpenter and colleagues[18] found that brief submaximal maternal exercise (up to 70% of maximal aerobic power; maternal heart rate less than or equal to 148 beats/minute), on the cycle ergometer, did not affect fetal heart rate. Maximal exertion, however, appears to be followed by fetal bradycardia. Fetal breathing movements are episodic and occur 30% of the time in the last trimester. Hypoxia significantly reduces the frequency of fetal breathing and body movements. Gestation, time of day, catecholamine level, and maternal plasma glucose level affect fetal breathing movements as well. It appears that the frequency of fetal breathing movements may be a more sensitive indicator of fetal well-being than fetal heart rate.[15] Fetal breathing movements appear to increase following maternal exercise but decrease in fetuses suspected to be in distress who are carried by hypertensive mothers. Fetuses who have experienced hypoxia, as well as those enduring labor, exhibit decreased fetal breathing movements. Katz and coworkers[19] measured fetal and maternal responses to immersion exercise (ergometer with water level to the xiphoid process). At 60% $VO_2$max at 15, 25, and 35 weeks of pregnancy, they found, with underwater ultrasound, that the fetus demonstrated body limb motion and fetal breathing movements. Fetal heart rates were normal and unchanged from those at rest. Maternal temperature was unchanged during exercise, or recovery, at all gestational stages. The nature of the immersion exercise eliminates the major problems with decreased uterine blood flow, physical discomfort, and elevated core temperature.[19]

### Placental responses to maternal exercise

The fetus receives a continuous supply of oxygen necessary for growth and development. This supply averages 8 ml/min/kg and is derived from the maternal circulation by diffusion across the placenta. It is possible that maternal exercise may have an effect on this placental oxygen transfer. Many factors contribute to oxygen transfer across the placenta: maternal and fetal arterial $PO_2$, maternal and fetal diffusion capacity, maternal and fetal hemoglobin affinities, maternal and fetal hemoglobin flow rates, vascular regulation of maternal and fetal vessels, and the quantity of $CO_2$ exchange.[13] Unfortunately, because of ethical and technical problems in measuring placental transfer, the only studies are on pregnant ewes. In these animals, 10 minutes of 70% maximal exercise on a treadmill at maximal oxygen consumption caused increased maternal arterial $PO_2$ by 8%, and hemoglobin concentration by 25%. Uterine blood flow decreased by 21%. Fetal and maternal blood pH increased. By the end of the exercise, however, uteroplacental oxygen delivery was unchanged because of the increase in maternal hemoglobin concentration.[15] It cannot, however, be predicted that the same will occur in humans.

# Aging

Most female mammals are able to reproduce until late in life. In the past, women were likely to die at an early age from infectious disease or complications of repeated pregnancies, factors that can now be prevented in large part. Consequently women live longer than past generations. The climacteric signals the transition or phase of a woman's life that begins several years before menopause and ends when ovarian function ceases. Menopause is an episode within the climacteric period, and the postmenopausal stage includes both the late climacteric period and the following years during which atrophic changes occur.

## Climacteric and menopause

After the age of 40, the ovaries start to decrease their responses to pituitary gonadotropin stimulation. Often, in the early part of climacteric, there will be a cycle without an ovum being released (anovulating cycle). With increasing years, ovulation occurs less frequently, eventually ceasing completely, which explains the decrease in fertility in premenopausal women. As long as the ovaries respond to produce moderate amounts of estrogen, there will be episodic bleeding. Levels of gonadotropin increase as ovarian function diminishes.

Menopause can be correctly diagnosed after 1 year of amenorrhea. Although there is variation, the average age for menopause is 51. Within normal limits, some women do stop menstruation as early as 35, while others may continue until 55 or longer.[2] Usually the bleeding decreases over 1 to 3 years, the interval between menstrual periods increases (amenorrhea), and the amount of bleeding decreases. In some women, however, the periods stop abruptly and permanently. Many of the symptoms women experience also occur in men and are not related to hormonal secretion. In both sexes, these symptoms are the result of physical changes and the emotional feelings associated with aging.

One of the first signs of menopause is a vasomotor reaction, commonly called a hot flash. Typically, it will appear suddenly, day or night, with a feeling of heat in the chest, neck, and head, and it will rapidly increase. As menopause approaches, there are several hormonal changes. There is a reversal of estrogen fractions, in which estrone, rather than estradiol, is produced. Estradiol production decreases, most likely due to the decrease in the number of responsive follicles. With more time, ovarian estrogen secretion falls sufficiently, so that the endometrium is not stimulated to produce bleeding.

Other physiologic changes of menopause include decreased thyroid function, hyperparathyroidism, decreased renal function, decreased insulin released due to glucose challenge, and decreased response to catecholamines (affecting vascular tone and metabolic activities). There is a major change in the increased conversion of androstenedione to estrone, along with changes in fat distribution, and excessive hair growth. Neurologic changes include confusion, loss of memory, and decreased balance control, which may lead to falling.[2]

### Reproductive organs

Changes in reproductive organs arise from the decrease in estrogen. The myometrium, the smooth muscle comprising the middle layer of the uterus, thins and gradually becomes the size of that in a prepubertal girl. The endometrium, the mucosal layer lining the uterus, becomes atrophic and thin. The cervix reduces in size, usually over several years, and the secretion of the cervical gland decreases early in the climacteric period. The vagina slowly becomes smaller and its mucosa, thinner. A vaginal smear will reflect cells typical of an estrogen-deficient pattern. Externally, the labia fat is reabsorbed. Consequently, the labia majora are flattened, and the skin may hang. The labia minora may disappear completely. After menopause, the muscular supports of the uterus, bladder, and rectum lose their strength and tone and share a role in the possible evolution of cystocele, rectocele, and uterine prolapse. Stress urinary incontinence may increase, or begin after these anatomic changes occur.

### Cardiovascular

The multiple risk factors associated with coronary heart disease, such as heredity, hypertension, diabetes mellitus, hyperlipidemia, obesity, smoking, decreased activity, and stress make it difficult to fully understand the specific influence of menopause on heart disease. Studies show that the incidence of cardiovascular disease, hypertension, and stroke is lower in premenopausal women than in men of the same age. For men, there is a marked increase in coronary vascular disease after age 40; whereas for women, the risk factors do not increase until after menopause. After this time, the rate of cardiovascular disease in women increases in a linear fashion. Although it has been theorized that ovarian function appears to have a protective effect against cardiovascular disease in young women, there is not an abrupt rise after cessation of ovarian function. Ritterband, in 1962, found that women who had had an oophorectomy were predisposed to coronary heart disease. There have been many studies since to determine the effect of estrogen therapy in the development of atherosclerosis and myocardial infarction in men. Although estrogen has been found to positively alter certain levels of lipoproteins, the potential side effect of thrombosis limits its use.

### Bone change

After 30, bone loss begins and progresses throughout life in both sexes. Women experience an abrupt increase in bone loss after menopause, either naturally from decreased estrogen production or as a result of hysterectomy. Postmenopausal women lose bone on the average of 1% to 2% a year. Consequently, by their 80s, they may have lost half of their total bone mass.

Osteoporosis is a disturbance that indicates increased bone porosity and a widening of the haversian canals.[2] Some interesting statistics arise as a result of this marked loss. Twenty percent of women will have a femoral neck fracture by age 90, 80% because of osteoporotic bone; and it is estimated that as many as 50,000 elderly women die each year from symptoms related to hip fractures. Twenty-five percent of those over 60 develop compression fractures of the vertebrae and long bones, especially in the forearms.

Men have a greater basic bone density and their major bone loss starts about 15 years later than women of the same age.[2] Studies indicate that bone formation by osteocytes and resorption by osteoblasts occur independently.[1] In a postmenopausal woman, there is a delay between the resorption phase and the formation phase, but the total active resorption is not increased. With advancing age, the major problem is a decrease in the rate of total bone formation leading to net skeletal loss.[1,2]

The effects of increased activity have been shown to slow bone loss and demineralization. Bone is the major calcium reservoir of the body, stored in the lacunae, and released on demand. Calcium is an important electrolyte responsible, in part, for mental activity, and an adequate amount of it depends upon intake and absorption from the stomach. This absorption is dependent on the available amount of vitamin D, which is dependent on the kidney enzyme, C1-hydroxycholestrolase, and prolactin, which activates the enzyme. But prolactin levels are decreased at menopause, most likely because of decreased estrogen levels. Consequently, there may be a decreased absorption of vitamin D from the stomach. Contributing to this, as well, may be an intestinal lactase deficiency and an inability to digest milk.[12]

It has been shown that estrogen may stop or slow the process of osteoporosis; however, there are other factors to consider. Osteoporosis occurs more in white than in black women, more in thin than fat, more in smokers than non-smokers, and finally, more in physically inactive females than in active ones.[12]

### Psychologic

With the onset of the climacteric, women are faced with many changes. These marked body changes are often a time of psychologic reflection. This time is marked by loss of function and physical limitation. Childbearing is over. Children are often grown and on their own, and women are facing, in full force, the slowing down and aging process of their bodies. Unlike pregnancy, when the changes are dramatic and last only 9 months; in menopause, the changes are permanent. It is not unusual for women to experience feelings of loss, hopelessness, self-condemnation, depression, anxiety, and tension. A woman may feel less important because, biologically, she is unable to produce. She will often reflect on her own life goals and accomplishments, and possibly experience decreased sexual appetite due to libido changes and discomfort from atrophic vaginitis. A woman, during menopause, may have many fears: death, loneliness, a partner's death, dependency upon her children, helplessness, and physical limitations. These psychologic symptoms are emotional in origin and are not a result of decreasing estrogen. Understanding this period in life, its biologic basis, and the time needed for readjustment, can be reassuring for the menopausal women.

## *Self-Assessment Review*

1. Pregnant women compensate for physiologic and anatomic respiratory changes by _____.
2. During mild and moderate exercise, cardiac output _____.

3. Exercise in pregnant women with impaired cardiovascular function is _____.
4. The vena cava syndrome is _____.
5. Maternal core body temperature over _____ has resulted in _____ and _____ defects.
6. In the first trimester, there is a _____ in physical work capacity.
7. The fetus responds to brief periods of asphyxia with _____ and _____.
8. The cervix is made up of _____ muscle.
9. The corpus luteum is located in the _____ and produces _____ in pregnancy.
10. Chloasma results in increased _____ around the _____ and _____.
11. Oxygen consumption increases _____% in pregnancy.
12. _____ means absence of menstruation.
13. Stress incontinence occurring during the climacteric period is related to the _____.

## *References*

1. Danforth DN: Obstetrics and Gynecology (5th ed). Philadelphia, JB Lippincott, 1986.
2. Wilson JR, Carrington ER, Ledger WJ: Obstetrics and Gynecology (7th ed). St. Louis, CV Mosby, 1983.
3. Niswander KR: Manual of Obstetrics. Diagnosis and Therapy (2nd ed). Boston, Little, Brown & Co, 1987.
4. Freed SZ, Herzig N: Urology and Pregnancy. Baltimore, Williams and Wilkins, 1982.
5. Davidson, JM: The physiology of the renal tract in pregnancy. Clin Obstet and Gynecol 28(2):257-265, 1985.
6. Vilar J, Kestler E, Castello P: Improved lactation digestion during pregnancy: A case of physiological adaptation. Obstet Gynecol 71(5):697-700, 1981.
7. Pritchard J, MacDonald P: Williams Obstetrics (17th ed). New York, Appleton-Century-Crofts, 1980.
8. Wong RC, Ellis: Physiologic skin changes in pregnancy. J Am Acad Dermatol 10(6):929-940, 1984.
9. Kemp BE, Niall HD: Relaxin. Vitamin and Hormones 41:79-115, 1984.
10. Norstrom A, et al: Inhibitory action of relaxin on human cervical smooth muscle. J Clin Endocrinol Metab 59(3):379-382, 1984.
11. Frankenne F, et al: The physiology of growth hormones (GHs) in

pregnant women and partial characterization of the placental GH variant. J Clin Endocrinol Metab 66(6):1171-1180, 1988.

12. Guyton AC: Textbook in Medical Physiology (7th ed). Philadelphia, Harper & Row, 1987.

13. Artal RM, Wiswell RA: Exercise in Pregnancy. Baltimore, Williams & Wilkins, 1986.

14. McMurray RG, et al: The effect of pregnancy on metabolic response during rest, immersion and aerobic exercise in the water. Am J Obstet Gynecol 158(3):481-486, 1988.

15. Lotgering FK, Gilbert RD, Longo LD: Maternal and fetal responses to exercise during pregnancy. Physio Review 65(1):1-36, 1985.

16. Nisell H, et al: Cardiovascular response to isometric handgrip exercise: An invasive study in pregnancy-induced hypertension. Obstet Gynecol 70(3):339-343, 1987.

17. Pomerance J, Gluck L, Lynch V: Physical fitness in pregnancy: Its effect on pregnancy outcome. Am J Obstet Gynecol 119(7):867-876, 1974.

18. Carpenter MV, et al: Fetal heart rate response to maternal exertion. JAMA 259(20):3006-3009, 1988.

19. Katz VL, et al: Fetal and uterine responses to immersion and exercise. Obstet Gynecol 72(2):225-230, 1988.

20. Sinaki M, et al: Relationship between bone mineral density of spine and strength of back extensors in health post menopausal women. Mayo Clin Proc 61(2):116-122, 1986.

# FIVE

# Reproduction

### *Normal Cycle*

Where else to start studying reproductive physiology but at the beginning. And to study reproduction, it is vital to understand the normal menstrual cycle. Man's awareness of the menstrual cycle is as old as man, himself; however, the awareness that this cycle's links to childbearing came later. And the linking of the menstrual cycle to hormonal activity came much later than that. "The classical definition of a hormone is a substance which travels from a special tissue, where it is released into the bloodstream, to distant responsive cells where the hormone exerts its characteristic effects."[1] More recently, the methods of communication by hormones have been further subdivided into paracrine and autocrine to differentiate those hormones that travel through the bloodstream to assorted tissues, and those that communicate locally within cells, respectively. One class of hormones are the steroids, which include the adrenocortical hormones (mineralocorticoids, glucocorticoids, and androgens), as well as gonadal hormones (androgens, estrogens, and progestins).

The follicular granulosa cells and the corpus luteum are responsible for producing estradiol, the major estrogen of the human ovary, in response to stimulation from gonadotropins, follicle-stimulating hormone (FSH), and luteinizing hormone (LH). Gonadotropins communicate paracrinely to the enzyme adenylate cyclase, which in turn, communicates autocrinely to cyclic AMP to stimulate steroidogenesis; and ergo, estradiol production.

Some of the estradiol that is secreted binds in the bloodstream to proteins, but the free form seeks estradiol-specific receptors within cells to transmit the message to the chromatin of the nucleus. Messenger RNA is produced, and the hormone has achieved its goal. It is believed that estradiol can perform this function several times before being metabolized, unlike other sex steroids, such as testosterone, which is released from the cell as an inactive compound.

All three classes of sex steroids are produced by the human ovary: estrogens, progestins, and androgens. Estrogens, specifically 17β-estradiol, produced at a rate of 100 to 300μg/day in the normal, nonpregnant female, exerts a positive feedback effect by stimulating the hypothalamus to release gonadotropin-releasing hormone (GnRH, in the female also known as LHRH). GnRH is secreted from the hypophysis, and in turn, stimulates the gonadotropins.

Prior to ovulation, progesterone, a product of the corpus luteum, is released to join with estradiol to influence the endometrial secretion. The entire role of ovarian androgens is yet unexplained, but great progress has been made in recent years in understanding their complex actions within the female reproductive system. It is generally believed, however, that a small amount of androgen enhances follicular development, whereas an excess inhibits this process by causing follicular atresia and granulosa cell death. The normal female produces about 0.2 to 0.3 mg/day of testosterone; one quarter of that amount is directly contributed by the ovary. The rest comes from the adrenal gland and from an alteration of androstenedione. Follicular development seems to depend on the conversion of androgen to estrogen via FSH stimulation.[1] It is for this reason that the androgens, as well as prolactin and cortisol, are considered by some to be inhibiting or interfering hormones, as opposed to the releasing hormone, GnRH[2].

The balance of the interfering and releasing hormones is the responsibility of the neuroendocrinologic mechanisms of reproduction. GnRH has been detected in the fetus as early as 10 weeks; FSH and LH by 10 to 13 weeks, peaking at about 20 weeks. However, it seems to be the combined effect of genetics and critical body mass that stimulates puberty, gonadotropin secretion gradually increasing about 3 to 4 years before the cycle is well established. Both males and females secrete gonadotropins in a pulsatile fashion; the male secretion staying at a tonic level, and the female secretion cycling with a surge of both FSH and LH about midcycle. The frequency and amplitude of pulsation is critical, and is apparently regulated by a dual catecholaminergic system that balances norepinephrine and dopamine production from the brain. In fact, the anterior pituitary is now believed to secrete GnRH spontaneously, as well as in response to hypothalamic secretions. Dopamine is thought to inhibit both GnRH and prolactin secretion, although GnRH may also directly stimulate prolactin. Norepinephrine is believed to stimulate GnRH. Previously it was believed that the LH and FSH surge at midcycle was related to GnRH secretion in response to estradiol acting on the hypothalamus. Further research has indicated that the regulation of gonadotropins is directed by stimulation of the anterior pituitary by ovarian steroid feedback.[1]

Estradiol increases as FSH stimulates follicle growth and stimulates the rise of the tropic hormones (hypothalamic-releasing hormones and others released from the anterior pituitary). The increase in LH induces ovulation (rupture of the follicle), and the corpus luteum forms. Hence, the menstrual cycle may be divided into the follicular phase, ovulation, and the luteal phase. The follicular phase may be further divided into the primordial, preantral, antral, and preovulatory follicle phases (see Figure 5-1).

It is unclear what governs the number of follicles that grow during a cycle. It has been shown, however, that follicle growth continues during ovulation, pregnancy, anovulatory periods, and at all ages of life.[1] The granulosa-cell covered oocyte selected for ovulation appears to respond to hormonal stimulation, changing in shape and structure to form the preantral follicle. At this stage, the follicle develops a membrane, the zona pellucida, surrounded by the theca

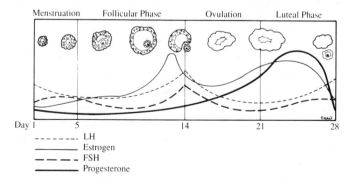

Figure 5-1: Menstrual cycle

layer, and estrogen stimulates gonadotropin production in the granulosa cells. FSH directs the dominance of estrogen over the androgens. And as the estrogen concentration increases, so does the growth of the follicle—now in its antral stage. At this stage, the estrogen/androgen balance is particularly important. In the first 12 days of the cycle, the size of the follicle changes from 4 mm to 20 mm, the follicular fluid volume changes from 0.0 ml to 6.5 ml, and the number of granulosa cells increases from 2 million to 50 million. LH does not appear to any measurable level until day 6 or 7. Prolactin decreases from 60 ng/ml to 5 ng/ml by day 12, and the androgen level theoretically should remain fairly constant. Estrogen and progesterone, of course, increase during the first 2 weeks of the cycle, with levels becoming the same briefly at midcycle.[1] Estrogen production is then explained by the two- cell, two-gonadotropin mechanism: "Though each compartment (theca and granulosa) retains the ability to produce progestins, androgens, and estrogens, the aromatase (conversion of C-19 steroids, androstenedione and testosterone, to C-18 phenolic steroid estrogens, estrone and estradiol) activity of the granulosa far exceeds that observed in the theca. In the antral follicle, LH receptors are present only on the theca cells and FSH receptors only on the granulosa cells."[1]

In addition to this specificity, a variety of growth factors influence cell differentiation, as well as the dominant follicle's own feedback system. This feedback system allows regulation of gonadotropin secretion. The follicular fluid also contains inhibin, synthesized by granulosa cells stimulated by FSH. This peptide is believed to assist in the dominance of one follicle over others. Once inhibin is produced, it acts to stop FSH production at the pituitary, thereby regulating itself. Activin, a releasing substance, does the opposite.

The preovulatory follicle produces estrogen, peaking a day to a day-and-a-half prior to ovulation. The dominant follicle is believed to acquire greater estrogen and FSH concentrations so that the LH surge results in progesterone production in that follicle and an androgen imbalance in less dominant follicles, causing them to yield to atresia. Theca tissue from these lesser follicles produces androgens, causing an increase in androgen levels in peripheral plasma around ovulation. This androgen production theoretically may cause stimulated libido at a time compatible with conception.

*In vitro* fertilization studies have revealed interesting observations about diurnal ovulation patterns. Ovulation appears to occur in the morning between midnight and 11:00 a.m. in spring, in the evening during fall and winter, and between 4:00 and 7:00 p.m., from July to February. Ovulation occurs as the follicular wall decomposes in response to the LH surge. This surge also causes the oocyte to resume meiotic activity, the granulosa cells to luteinize, and prostaglandins to synthesize and promote follicle rupture. A combination of prostaglandins, progesterone, histamine, and proteolytic enzymes is thought to assist follicular wall degradation. Following ovulation, there is a rapid decrease in gonadotropin secretion, although the reason for this is unexplained.

In the luteal phase, the granulosa cells grow larger and become yellow from the pigment, lutein. The corpus luteum forms, becoming heavily vascularized and able to synthesize the three sex steroids. Progesterone levels rise and peak about 8 days after the LH surge, suppressing new follicle growth. This is enhanced by inhibin production. Although it is often believed that the luteal phase is 14 days long, a 1984 study suggests an average of 12 to 17 days. The corpus luteum degenerates toward the end of this phase, unless pregnancy occurs. Pregnancy stimulates human chorionic gonadotropin (HCG) production to maintain luteal steroidogenesis until the placenta can assume this role around 7 to 10 weeks gestation.

## *Prostaglandins*

Anyone who becomes involved in the study of reproduction will undoubtedly hear about prostaglandins. Although prostaglandins were discovered in the 1930s, it wasn't until 1970 that synthetic production was achieved. Arachidonic acid is the basis for the two-double bond family of prostaglandins (PG); however, linoleic acid and pentanoic acid yield $PG_1$ and $PG_3$, respectively. After modification of the naming procedure for prostaglandin compounds from PGE and PGF, representative of their ability to dissolve in ether or phosphate buffer, to an alphabetical system, the prostaglandins of importance to reproduction are $PGE_2$ and $PGF_2$ $PGD_2$ may also prove to be of interest for this field.

Luteal regression occurs if there is no fertilization. It is believed that $PF_2$ is synthesized in the endometrium upon stimulation by follicular estrogen. It is locally transported to the corpus luteum through a connection from the ovary to the uterus. This prostaglandin suppresses LH receptor formation in the corpus luteum, contributing to its degeneration.

## *Periconception*

A special word should be included about the period surrounding conception. Although the effects of teratogenic substances has been recognized for quite a while, especially since the thalidomide tragedy of the 1950s, recent studies suggest that there may be a link between the prepregnancy nutritional status of the mother and the eventual health of the fetus.[3] One study conducted with mothers who took vitamins before conception suggested reduced incidence of myelomeningocele in their infants, as opposed to a group of mothers who received no preconception supplementation.[3] Although this study has not been replicated to date, the idea of encouraging prospective mothers to improve their diets before conception cannot be refuted. Other recent studies suggest that smoking can alter sperm count and integrity. Additional maternal nutrition studies suggest that preconceptional lifestyle may strongly influence fetal health, especially if substance abuse is a factor.

## *Conception*

Hopefully, there's no need to explain how the sperm gains access to the vagina; however, once sperm is introduced into the vagina, the journey becomes even more perilous. The acidic environment of the vagina could spell disaster for the alkaline sperm if not for their ability to mobilize rapidly to the cervical region. The semen forms a gel to protect itself, although the sperm are believed to be immobilized within 2 hours after ejaculation if left in the vagina. The gel is converted by prostatic enzymes to a liquid after about 20 to 30 minutes. Only the sperm enter the uterus, and uterine contractions propel the sperm into the fallopian tube within 5 minutes of insemination. Apparently only 200 of the 200 to 300 million sperm even get close to the egg (less than .001%); the others are either left in the vagina and digested by enzymes, or phagocytosized along the way.

Once the sperm move close to the egg, they undergo a process of capacitation, by which they prepare to penetrate the ovum. The head of the sperm changes to allow specific enzymes to egress for fusion with the egg membrane. Capacitation also causes altered receptor mobility and loss of seminal plasma antigens, as well as increased motility. These factors increase the chances of the sperm to penetrate the ovum and are required for *in vitro* fertilization to occur.

The ova and follicular cells rest on the surface of the ovary until muscular movements cause the cilia of the fimbriae to pick up an egg. To and fro propulsion through the fallopian tube causes the egg to reach the ampulla of the tube after about 30 hours. Any contact by the sperm with the egg occurs in the ampulla. It is believed fertilization occurs through random contact rather than by any mechanism that would attract the sperm to the egg. In the sperm head, the enzyme-containing acrosome undergoes a reaction that results in a fusing of the plasma membrane and the outer acrosomal membrane. As the sperm penetrates the egg, the zona pellucida surrounding the egg from ovulation to implantation appears to prevent additional fertilizations by prohibiting other sperm from entering. This is accomplished by enzymes that harden the extracellular layer and inactivate receptors for sperm.

How then does twinning occur? About once in every 80 births, a dizygotic or monozygotic twinning results either from the discharge of two ova or from the splitting of a single, fertilized ovum. In the case of two ova being released either from two or one ovarian follicle, twins are dizygotic or fraternal. These twins are like any other siblings. It is unclear whether the release of more than one ovum is directed by hereditary factors. The occurrence of monozygotic twinning, however, is believed to be hereditary, as two embryos arise from one fertilized egg. These twins are identical and of the same sex. Multiple births derive from the same circumstances.[4]

Once the male and female pronuclei migrate after the fusion of the sperm and egg membranes, the first cell division occurs. Two to three days after the embryo starts to develop and enters the uterus, implantation in the uterine endometrium begins. The cells of each surface mesh and the embryo becomes firmly situated.[1]

## *Genetics*

A brief review of genetics may be useful for physical therapists dealing with pregnant women or those planning a pregnancy. Although the ramifications of genetic disorders will be discussed more in the chapter on fetal development, it is important here to introduce the idea that those in the obstetric and gynecologic health care team are becoming increasingly liable for genetic counseling prior to conception and during pregnancy.

Human chromosomes number 46; 2 sex chromosomes and 44 autosomes. The female chromosomes include XX sex chromosomes; the male chromosomes, XY. Although the autosomes are paired and numbered by morphologic traits, they are arranged in an arbitrary manner called the karyotype. In the female embryo, one of the two X chromosomes (one paternal and one maternal) randomly becomes inactive, condenses, and is known as the Barr body or sex chromatin. It is the active maternal or paternal X that determines the autosomal trait seen clinically.[5]

Genetic screenings typically focus on three general categories: single-gene disorders (autosomal dominant, autosomal recessive, or X-linked), chromosomal anomalies (cytogenetics), and multifactorial disorders related to both hereditary and environmental factors.[6] Examples of each category are described in Table 5-1.

Prior to conception, then, a number of these disorders can be screened for, and the occurrence of risk calculated, based on familial traits and history. A diagram, called a family pedigree, can map

**Table 5-1. Overview of Genetic Screening Categories**

Single-gene disorder
  Autosomal recessive (homozygous alleles)
    Sickle cell anemia
    Cystic fibrosis
    Phenylketonuria
    Albinism
    Tay-Sachs disease
    Werdnig-Hoffman disease
  Autosomal dominant (heterozygous alleles)
    Huntington's disease
    Myotonic dystrophy
    Osteogenesis imperfecta, types I and IV
  X-linked (mutant gene on X chromosome)
    Dominant
      Vitamin-D resistant rickets
    Recessive
      Becker's muscular dystrophy
      Duchenne's muscular dystrophy
      Hemophilia A and B
Chromosomal anomalies
  Numerical
    Trisomy (21 = Down's syndrome)
    Turner's syndrome (monosomy 45,X)
    Triple X syndrome (47,XXX)
    Klinefelter's syndrome (47,XXY)
  Structural
    Isochromosomes
    Ring chromosomes
    Duplications, Inversions, Deletions, Translocations
    Fragile X
    Inactive X
Multifactorial
  Cardiac defects
  Legg-Calves-Perthes disease
  Scoliosis
  Cleft palate
  Spina bifida
  Dislocated hip

family members and generations affected by multiple or single traits. This information can also help determine homozygosity or heterozygosity of defects. Once a woman is pregnant, the same type of map can be drawn; however, additional tests will help diagnose the possibility that such a disorder exists in this particular fetus.

Prenatal tests are usually conducted via samples of amniotic fluid. Amniocytes are then cultured and "examined cytogenetically, assayed biochemically (for inborn errors of metabolism) or analyzed for DNA changes."[1] Other methods for prenatal diagnosis include alpha-fetoprotein analysis, chorionic villus or fetal tissue biopsy, ultrasound, contrast radiography, and fetoscopy. While a certain amount of risk is associated with each of these procedures, and there may be a considerable wait for results from such tests, women at risk for producing a child with genetic abnormalities may consider the risk worth the answer.

## *Abnormal Cycles*

From the background presented above, it must be clear that conception and regular menstrual cycles are nothing short of a miracle. Things do go wrong sometimes, however, and in a variety of ways. The suffix "rhea" or "rrhea" comes from the Greek "rhoia," "to flow." [7] Abnormalities of flow are termed amenorrhea (absence of flow), dysmenorrhea (painful flow), or oligomenorrhea (infrequent flow occurring no more than every 40 days and no less than every 6 months). However, the list continues with hypomenorrhea (reduced number of days or amount of flow), and cryptomenorrhea (flow obstructed by lower genital obstruction).

Amenorrhea is estimated to occur in less than 5% of women in the normal population, but research suggests that certain groups of women (those imprisoned for great lengths of time, those with nutritional deficiencies, or those who extensively exercise on a regular basis,[8-9] such as long distance runners or ballet dancers), tend to experience menstrual abnormalities at a greater incidence.[1] To further differentiate those cases in which menstruation has not occurred at all versus those in which flow has started but then stops at a later point in the woman's life, the terms primary and secondary amenorrhea have been assigned. There is also physiologic amenorrhea (normal state of no flow prior to puberty). Because treatment for amenorrhea and excessive bleeding (menorrhagia) by physical therapists is limited, the basic causes are summarized in Table 5-2.

Although treatment for these disorders is limited, treatment methods for women with premenstrual syndrome (PMS), dysmenorrhea, and chronic gynecologic pain are currently being explored by physical therapists.[10-11]. Since primary dysmenorrhea is believed to affect between 40% and 95% of menstruating women[112], this population is one that could potentially benefit greatly from therapeutic assistance. Because many women dislike using medication monthly, although medication can be highly effective, an offer of a pain relief mechanism such as transcutaneous electrical nerve stimulation (TENS), instruction in relaxation techniques, or designing exercise programs specific to the patient may provide therapists an opportunity to help these women. This topic will be discussed more in Part II, but basic to providing treatment is an understanding of the pathologic process and symptomatology.

Central to an understanding of PMS is the idea that the symptoms occur cyclically, after ovulation. If symptoms occur irregularly or chronically, PMS may not be an accurate diagnosis. And because recent legal actions against violence have lost to a defense of PMS,

**Table 5-2. Overview of Causes of Menstrual Dysfunction**

| Disorder | Site of Problem | Cause |
| --- | --- | --- |
| Primary amenorrhea | Hypothalamus | Decreased GnRH |
| | | Poor Nutrition |
| | | Exercise |
| | | Stress |
| | Pituitary | Lesions, tumors |
| | Ovary | Tumors |
| | | Polycystic ovary syndrome |
| | | Turner's syndrome |
| | Uterus | Defects |
| | | Urinary tract anomalies |
| Secondary amenorrhea | Hypothalamus | Lack of LH surge |
| | | Stress |
| | | Dieting |
| | | Exercise |
| | | Post-birth control pill |
| | | Decreased GnRH |
| | Pituitary | Tumors |
| | Ovary | Genetic defects |
| | | Autoimmune, thyroid, or adrenal deficiency |
| | | Myasthenia gravis |
| | | Pernicious anemia |
| | | Mumps oophoritis |
| | | Idiopathic early menopause |
| | | Cancer therapies |
| | | Polycystic ovary syndrome |
| | Uterus | Severe endometritis |
| | | Chronic granulomatous disease |
| Excessive bleeding | Hypothalamus | Failure of LH surge unopposed by estrogen |
| | Pituitary | Hyperprolactinemia |
| | Ovary | Menopause |
| | | Polycystic ovary syndrome |
| | | Decreased androgens |
| | | Estrogen-secreting tumor |
| | Uterus | Pregnancy |
| | | Fibroids |
| | | Polyps |
| | | Cancer |
| | | Adenomyosis |
| | | Cystic hyperplasia |
| | | Inflammatory lesions |

practitioners are becoming increasingly concerned with taking a meticulous history before confirming such a diagnosis.[12]

Premenstrual syndrome has many definitions. Among them: "The symptoms usually begin 10 to 14 days prior to the onset of the menstrual period and become progressively worse until the onset of menstruation or, for some women, several days after the onset."[13] "PMS is the cyclical occurrence of various signs and symptoms beginning near or after ovulation and resolving soon after the onset of menses."[12] It is "the cyclic appearance of a large collection of symptoms, occurring to such a degree that lifestyle or work are affected and followed by a period of time entirely free of symptoms."[1] "PMS is defined as a menstrually related mood disorder that includes the cyclic occurrence of symptoms that are of sufficient severity to interfere with some aspects of life and that appear with a consistent and predictable relationship to menses."[6] The lack of a consistent definition adds to the problems of treatment and identification of this syndrome.

The most common symptoms include abdominal bloating, breast tenderness, weight gain, fatigue, depression, and irritability. Headache, constipation, acne, rhinitis, and edema may also occur, as well as more uncommon symptoms like paresthesia, sleep disorders, and wide mood swings.[1214] It has been estimated that over 100 symptoms could possibly be related to PMS. For these reasons, the first step to diagnosis and treatment usually involves the woman keeping a daily menstrual diary.

Since 1931, the theory of hormonal imbalance has been advocated as the cause of PMS; however, researchers have been unable to confirm the exact nature of that imbalance. "The wide discrepancies among studies are due to: lack of a standard definition for PMS (patients enrolled in studies are not homogeneous populations; many are self-diagnosed); failure to measure hormones at frequent, standardized intervals (estrogen and progesterone levels change during the luteal phase; patients and control samples must be matched according to day past ovulation by basal body temperature charts or day of LH surge); and failure to recognize that PMS may have multiple etiologies."[12] Another related theory proposes that the ratio of bound to free circulating hormone may be more important than the absolute concentration. Dalton found lower levels of sex-hormone binding globulin (a specific transport protein to which sex-steroids are bound, and by doing so, become inactive at target tissues) in women with PMS than in controls. This, in turn, would cause an increase in free circulating estrogen, thought to be the only active type. Therefore, the total progesterone/estrogen ratio could be unchanged; while in actuality, the estrogenic activity and symptomatology would increase.[15]

Whatever the causes of PMS, treatment has traditionally involved medication; although recently, innovative physicians and caregivers have experimented with treatments including diet modification, vitamin and mineral supplementation, psychotherapy, and exercise. Diet therapy includes limitation of caffeine and sodium, and an increase of complex carbohydrates and essential fatty acids, despite cravings that might contradict this philosophy. Of the vitamins and minerals, B6 and magnesium are believed to be of some value; but the dosages must be regulated by a physician because of the potential of toxicity. Psychotherapy has been especially valuable for families struggling to understand a family member's mood swings and unpredictable behavior. Finally, but not least important, is exercise.

Physicians and counselors of PMS patients have acknowledged the value of exercise, not only for PMS, but for a variety of health-related ailments. Aside from the physical benefits of exercise, well-known by physical therapists, some physicians are encouraging exercise for other reasons as well. One theory supports exercise as an antidepressant, possibly related to the release of endorphins, believed responsible for promoting a feeling of well-being. endorphin levels rise during the early luteal phase of the menstrual cycle; as the corpus luteum function decreases, the endorphins may decrease and a type of withdrawal, similar to narcotic withdrawal, may account for emotional symptoms.[12] Forms of exercise recommended for PMS symptoms include aerobics, particularly bicycling, swimming, and racewalking. Jogging is not the exercise of choice for premenstrual women because of the potential risk of injury, as well as the possible jarring of pelvic organs and breast irritation. Physical therapists can play a role in designing specific exercise programs to fit in with a woman's current lifestyle, coordinate supportive group exercise programs, or even offer TENS for symptoms of muscular aching and headache.

TENS has already been used in limited testing for patients with dysmenorrhea, painful menstruation thought to be linked to prostaglandin stimulation of uterine contractions. Primary and secondary forms of dysmenorrhea have been defined: primary, associated with normal ovulatory menstrual periods, and secondary, associated with pathology. Secondary dysmenorrhea encompasses endometriosis, pelvic inflammatory disease, and painful menstruation associated with wearing an intrauterine device, among other causes. Besides the local symptoms of dysmenorrhea, women may also experience fatigue, nausea, vomiting, low back pain, diarrhea, headache, or dizziness.

Contractions of the uterus are believed to be responsible for the local symptoms of dysmenorrhea. Using electrical potentials and direct measurement, electrical activity is highest during menstruation and lowest during the follicular phase. High frequency waves occurring every 2 to 4 minutes and lasting 30 to 60 seconds have been recorded, producing intrauterine pressures of 100 mm Hg or more. This type of contraction is comparable to that of some women's labors. In contrast to a normally progressing labor, however, the contractions may be dysrhythmic, sometimes escalating to uterine tetany.

Prostaglandins are synthesized by the endometrium and cause

contraction of uterine smooth muscle. In fact, prostaglandins in greater quantities have been identified in the menstrual flow of dysmenorrheic women.[6] This discovery has led to the successful use of prostaglandin-synthetase inhibitors to relieve menstrual cramping, especially if administered during the first 6 to 12 hours of menstruation when the most severe contractions occur on the average.

Another possible cause of dysmenorrhea is estrogen-progesterone imbalance, but little objective evidence has been collected to support this hypothesis. In addition, placebo administration has relieved certain symptoms in dysmenorrheic patients, suggesting a possible psychogenic component, as well, particularly in women whose mothers had similar menstrual problems. It is more recently the opinion of specialists that psychogenic symptoms may be associated with some dysmenorrheic patients, but that these symptoms are not necessarily the cause of physical complaints.

Still another cause of disabling dysmenorrhea is endometriosis, a pathologic condition of endometrial tissue growth in extrauterine locations such as the ovaries, uterine ligaments, cervix, pelvic peritoneum, rectovaginal septum, appendix, umbilicus, laparotomy and episiotomy scars, and even pleural or pericardial cavities.[6] It has been estimated that more than half the teenagers who report chronic pelvic pain will show evidence of endometriosis during laparoscopic exploration,[6] although the incidence of this condition in the general population is only 1% to 2%. Although the actual cause of endometrial tissue growth in extrauterine sites is unknown, practitioners are becoming more aware of its potential as a cause of infertility, cyclic rectal bleeding, or a number of other clinical signs. Tender nodules may be found in uterine ligaments, especially the uterosacral. Pain during menstruation, especially with referred pain to the rectum, lower sacrum, or coccyx, can be debilitating. Scarring and adhesions are characteristics of this condition, but the extent of involvement does not necessarily coincide with the severity of symptoms. Pain or infertility are the usual indications for treatment, either with medication or surgery.

In the case of a woman with dysmenorrhea, physical therapists can offer TENS, heat, and instruction in exercise. Two studies have recently been published documenting successful treatment of dysmenorrhea with TENS.[10,16-17] The most recent study by Lewers and colleagues attempted to replicate a previous study by Neighbors in which significant differences in relief were found between TENS patients and controls receiving placebo. The Lewers and coworkers study did not replicate this significant difference between groups. However, it was postulated that because their method involved the pre- and post-TENS treatment measurement of electrical conductance activity at auricular acupuncture points (for uterus, endocrine, low back, and ovary), any significant differences in pain relief from TENS could have been overshadowed by that obtained via auricular acupressure. It is also possible that these women's symptoms merely subsided during the time frame of the study (4-hour no medication period, 30 minute treatment/placebo, and pre- and posttreatment auricular measurements, plus 3-hour follow-up, and following next a.m. wake-up). Relief from dysmenorrheic symptoms measured over time may not be valid over an average 12-hour span, if, indeed, symptoms caused by uterine contractions normally subside during this time. However, whether or not this is indeed a placebo/Hawthorne effect, relief via TENS or acupressure can certainly be argued as a less invasive means than prostaglandin-synthetase inhibitors and other medications.

The ultimate cause of less frequent menses and abnormal cycles is menopause. The tricky part of this diagnosis is that menopause may occur any time within a 20-year span for the female population. "About one fourth of women experience spontaneous menopause before age 45 years, about one half experience it between 45 and 50 years, and the remaining one fourth experience it after age 50 years. Many gynecologists, however, are impressed with the frequency with which apparently regular menstruation may persist well into the sixth decade."[6]. The gradual extension of the lifespan of the human female, now averaging about 77 years in Western countries, virtually places the woman in a postmenopausal state for about one third of her life.[6]

With this increasing longevity, new problems for female clients have developed. As a woman ages, the number of follicles with oocytes decreases, and the ovary begins to decrease in size and weight. Follicles tend to degenerate and, in combination with fewer oocytes, the amount of estrogen and inhibin decreases as well. As the inhibin decreases, FSH increases, follicles are stimulated, and short menstrual cycles occur. As the number of follicles decreases and estrogen production level falls, it becomes impossible to induce an LH surge, and ovulation tends to occur irregularly. As steroidogenesis by the follicles decreases, ovarian stroma increases. When combined with adrenal cell production of steroid hormones, a certain amount of steroidogenesis continues, although the level of estrogen and progesterone production is markedly decreased. However, the postmenopausal ovary produces mostly androgens, which are converted peripherally to estrogens. Yet this peripheral conversion cannot compensate for the direct secretion by the ovaries premenopausally of over 90% of the estradiol.

Occurring at the time of menopause is a variety of physical and psychologic symptoms including some strictly associated with menopause and others related to aging. Researchers view the symptoms of menopause in different ways, for instance, as four associated endocrine syndromes: anovulatory cycles, hot flashes, vaginal atrophy, osteoporosis; or as problems related to estrogen withdrawal: or as disturbed menstrual pattern, vasomotor instability, psychologic symptoms, atrophic conditions, varied complaints (headache, insomnia, myalgia, altered libido), and health problems secondary to long-term deprivation (osteoporosis and cardiovascular disease). Hot flashes (flushes), hirsutism, voice changes, vaginal dryness and itching, dry mouth, and loss of skin integrity are among the symptoms related to hormonal changes. Other symptoms of interest to the physical therapist include stress incontinence, with or without frequency or urgency, uterovaginal prolapse, backache, and fractures associated with bony changes. After menopause, the vagina actually becomes smaller, the mucosa atrophies, and cervical secretions decrease. Although urinary incontinence is believed to be caused by poor muscle tone, cystoceles and rectoceles resulting from poor muscular support are thought to be encouraged to develop by waning hormones.[6]

Treatment of specific menopausal symptoms is primarily centered around estrogen replacement therapy, but additional problems sometimes result from this form of assistance. Spontaneous excessive estrogen can cause irregular uterine bleeding, endometrial hyperplasia, and has been linked to endometrial cancer. Estrogen-progestin therapy has been associated with thromboembolism, metabolic disorders, hypertension, and breast tumors, but only at dosages used in oral contraceptives. The amounts of hormone used postmenopausally apparently are low enough that risk for these complications does not increase.[1] As far as urinary incontinence symptoms are concerned, a number of clinics have emerged to assist those in need. The role of physical therapy in this latter treatment, as well as in the treatment of gynecologic cancer pain, will be discussed more fully in a later chapter.

## *Self-Assessment Review*

1. A substance that sends a message to a distant site in the body via the bloodstream is a _____.
2. Intracellular communication is called _____; intercellular communication, _____.
3. Gonadal hormones include _____, _____, and _____.

4. The human ovary produces how many types of sex steroids? _____

5. Estradiol, a major estrogen, is produced by the _____ _____ cells and the _____.

6. Progesterone is produced by the _____.

7. Neuroendocrinological mechanisms regulate the balance of _____ and _____ hormones.

8. The human menstrual cycle may be divided into three phases: _____, _____, and _____.

9. Amenorrhea, chiefly treated with medication, is defined as an _____.

10. Dysmenorrhea, defined as _____, might be helped by physical therapy measures such as _____, _____, and _____.

## *References*

1. Speroff L, Glass RH, Kase NG: Clinical Gynecologic Endocrinology and Infertility (4th ed). Baltimore, Williams & Wilkins, 1989.

2. Federman DD: Ovary. In Scientific American: Endocrinology. Scientific American, 1986.

3. Smithells RW, et al: Apparent prevention of neural tube defects by periconceptional vitamin supplementation. Arch Dis Child 56:911-918, 1981.

4. Warwick R, Williams PL: Gray's Anatomy (35th ed). Philadelphia, WB Saunders, 1973.

5. Ganong WF: Review of Medical Physiology (11th ed). Los Altos, Lange Medical Publications, 1983.

6. Jones HW, Wentz AC, Burnett LS: Novak's Textbook of Gynecology (11th ed). Baltimore, Williams & Wilkins, 1988.

7. Dorland's Illustrated Medical Dictionary (24th ed). Philadelphia, WB Saunders, 1965.

8. Russell JB, et al: The relationship of exercise to anovulatory cycles in female athletes: Hormonal and physical characteristics. Obstet Gynecol 63(4):452-455, 1984.

9. Bachmann GA, Kemmann E: Prevalence of oligomenorrhea and amenorrhea in a college population. Am J Obstet Gynecol 144(1):98-102, 1982.

10. Mannheimer JS, Whalen EC. The efficacy of transcutaneous electrical nerve stimulation in dysmenorrhea. Clin J Pain 1(2):75-83, 1985.

11. Pomerantz E: Premenstrual syndrome: Concerns for the OB-/GYN physical therapist. Bull Sect Obstet Gynecol 11(3):8-9, 1987.

12. Chihal HJ: Premenstrual Syndrome: A Clinic Manual. Durant, Oklahoma, Creative Infomatics, 1985.
13. Lark S: Premenstrual Syndrome Self-Help Book. Los Angeles, Forman Publishing, 1984.
14. Glass RH: Office Gynecology (3rd ed). Baltimore, Williams & Wilkins, 1988.
15. Dalton K: The Premenstrual Syndrome and Progesterone Therapy. Chicago, Year Book Medical Publishers, 1983.
16. Lewers D, et al: Transcutaneous electrical nerve stimulation in the relief of primary dysmenorrhea. Phys Ther 69(1):3-9, 1989.
17. Neighbors LE, et al: Transcutaneous electrical nerve stimulation for pain relief in primary dysmenorrhea. Clin J Pain 3:17-22, 1987.

# Six

# Fetal Development and the Newborn

The physical therapist practicing in the field of obstetrics will undoubtedly have a patient who asks, "Will this treatment harm my baby?" While the number of studies about safety and modality use is severely limited, other basic physical therapy treatments, such as instruction in corrective exercises or in body mechanics, are considered safe. However, to answer some questions clients may have about positioning and general maternal health, a knowledge of fetal anatomy and development is vital. It is also useful for physical therapists to be aware of certain terminology used to describe fetal development to understand obstetrician's chart notes.

## *Growth and Development*

"How could one single cell, until then stored quietly in the body, suddenly give rise to a new human being with every feature that human beings have in common but still not exactly like any other living individual?"[1] Prior to ovulation, the ovum, or primary oocyte, completes its first meiotic division (becomes haploid with 22 auto-somes + 1 sex chromosome); the result is a secondary oocyte and a first polar body (one of the meiotic divisions that receives less cyto-plasm than the other, and is therefore, nonviable as an oocyte). The first polar body eventually disappears, while the secondary oocyte begins a second meiotic division. If fertilized, a second polar body is discarded, and the fertilized ovum (now a diploid of male and fe-male cells) is what remains.[2] During the first week after conception, that single fertilized cell (zygote) travels down the tube as it under-goes multiple mitotic divisions, still within the zygote. The zygote becomes a morula after several mitotic divisions (cleavage), then a trophoblast, and finally a blastocyst, as fluid accumulates, and fluid and cellular matter polarize. About 5 to 9 days after ovulation, the blastocyst burrows into the endometrium (implantation) and draws nourishment from the endometrial blood vessels as the placenta develops around it.

The location of the implantation is of great clinical importance. Most commonly, implantation occurs on the upper, posterior wall of the endometrium of the uterine body. Implantation involves cellular breakdown in the endometrium, closed over by a blood-clotting mechanism. This implantation bleeding may be mistaken clinically or by a woman as the start of a menses. If the blastocyst implants at sites other than the upper one third of the uterus, completion of pregnancy to term may be jeopardized. "In order of frequency they (abnormal implantations) occur as follows: (1) region of the internal os of the cervix, (2) ampulla of the uterine tube, (3) isthmus of the uterine tube, (4) angle of the uterine cavity, (5) infundibulum of the uterine tube, (6) ovary, (7) interstitial portion of the uterine tube, (8) peritoneum of the broad ligament, mesentery of the intestine or rectouterine pouch, and (9) pregnancy in a rudimentary uterine horn."[3] Outside the uterus, implantations are considered ectopic and can rarely reach full term within the abdominal cavity.

From here, the blastocyst differentiates into ectoderm, mesoderm, and endoderm to give rise to the brain, spinal cord, nerves, and skin; skeleton, urogenital system, heart, blood vessels, and muscles; and digestive system, liver, and pancreas, respectively. Rather than reiter-ate the contents of an embryology text, the information that is more useful for the practicing physical therapist regarding the develop-ment of the blastocyst focuses on the anatomy and function of the fetal membranes, the umbilical cord, the placenta, and the fetus, itself.

The fetal membranes include the yolk sac, allantois, amnion, and chorion. The yolk sac and allantois play a role in the development of the placental circulation and umbilical vessels. The amnion is the wall of the amniotic cavity, which holds the amniotic fluid. This fluid is produced by the amnion cells until the fetal kidneys start to function. The fluid is circulated, and the amount increases until the fifth month. Until then, there has been an increase up to about one quart; the volume reduces in the seventh month to allow growth of the fetus. It has been estimated that about one third of this fluid of water, protein, glucose, and inorganic salts is replaced every hour. Within the amniotic fluid, the embryo or fetus floats, is protected from injury, and temperature is regulated. The chorion helps in the establishment of fetal circulation as the decidua (lining of the uterus) in three different layers, fuses into one. The decidua meets the chorion to fill the uterus, except at the cervix where glands secrete mucus to form a mucus plug. This plug forms early to seal off the uterus from outside contaminants until labor begins.

Fusion of the amnion and the chorion creates the umbilical cord. Where this cord meets the ventral wall of the embryo is the umbilicus. Inside the cord is Wharton's jelly, a light blue-green substance, plus the yolk sac, a vitelline duct, allantois, and umbilical vessels. Two umbilical veins bring oxygenated blood from the chorion to the fetus, and two umbilical arteries return the deoxygenated blood from the fetus to the chorion. The umbilical cord is about 3/4 inch in diameter, and about 20 to 24 inches long at term. It is estimated that blood travels through the cord at a rate of 4 miles/hour and completes the trip from placenta, through the baby, and back in 30 seconds. This dynamic force makes the cord stiff and unlikely to knot as the baby moves within the womb.

The placenta is formed by fetal chorion and maternal decidua. The placenta is divided into sections called cotyledons and remains attached to the expanding uterus while thickening and increasing in area. At term, the placenta is flat, discoid, about 8 inches in diameter, about 1 inch thick, and weighs about 1 pound. The fetus is joined to the placenta via the umbilical cord. The placenta is capable of holding about 175 ml of maternal blood, flowing at a rate of 500 ml/minute. Uterine contractions force blood into uterine veins. Placental functions include respiration, nutrition, excretion, protection, and endocrine[3]. The placenta allows oxygen to reach the fetus and carbon dioxide to be carried away. Water, salts, carbohydrates, fats, proteins, and vitamins pass to the fetus, while excreted products pass to the mother to metabolize. The placenta can also protect the fetus from certain bacterial infections, plus it produces progesterone, estrogen, and gonadotropin. The placenta, however, cannot protect the fetus from everything, particularly from certain harmful substances ingested by the mother.

The birth of a normal, fully formed child is nothing short of a miracle when one considers the intricate balance of events that must occur to form all bodily systems accurately. "The normal development of the embryo is an integrated process in which the various organizing influences exert their inductive effects in a coordinated manner, in the correct sequence, at the correct time and place, and in the correct direction."[4] The sequence of systemic developmental events is important, not only to help researchers identify possible teratogenic substances if an anomaly should occur, but to determine clinically the health of the developing fetus. With the advent of diagnostic ultrasound and magnetic resonance imaging, fetal development has become more of an exact science. These events of human development are summarized in Tables 6-1 and 6-2 and in Figure 6-1. In addition to the events summarized in the tables, continued research has yielded interesting information about the fetus. Ultrasound imaging of the fetus has shown that "atropine, cigarette smoking, and frightening the mother produced a fetal tachycardia within 2 to 4 minutes."[5] Also, ductus arteriosus and secundum atrial defects are normally present in utero, and cannot be diagnosed until birth. Experiments have not linked fetal cardiac arrhythmia to congenital heart disease.[5] Craniocaudal development has been confirmed by several investigators. "Fetal movements (at 12 weeks) were characterized as (1) active movements of all body components, (2) sporadic kicking, and (3) strong, pulsed trunk movements that resemble the hiccups of a more mature fetus.... Upper limb movements predominate at 26 weeks. The most powerful movements occurring at this gestational age include foot withdrawal and the lateral trunk incurvation reflex...by 28 weeks, bursts of activity involving the trunk and limbs occur, followed by a resting phase in which, although the fetus may perceive external stimulation, he is unable to react. One month later, spontaneous movements are more powerful and frequent...."[5] Although maternal counting of movements has not proven accurate because of the tendency to count fetal breathing movements, Braxton Hicks contractions, and the mother's own movements, observations by mothers of decreased fetal movement prior to fetal death have been documented in high and low risk mothers.[5]

Unlike fetal body movements, which typically occur as a burst of activity followed by as much as 2 hours of rest, fetal breathing movements normally occur at a rate of 40 to 70/minute.[6] These breathing movements tend to increase after meals and in rate, depth, incidence, and level of organization as pregnancy progresses.[5]

Testing of sensory stimulation *in utero* may prove to be valuable for diagnosis; such tests include using auditory stimuli instead of a

**Table 6-1. Fetal Growth and Developmental Highlights**

| Week of Gestation | Event | Fetal size |
|---|---|---|
| 0–1 | Implantation | 1–36 cells |
| 1–2 | Embryo takes shape | Entoderm, mesoderm, ectoderm differentiate |
| 2–3 | Body forms<br>Heart beats<br>Brain forms two lobes | 1/10 inch |
| 3–4 (1st month) | Head, trunk, arm buds | 1/4 inch |
| 4–5 | Arm buds with hand plates; ears and jaws form; yolk sac useless | |
| 5–6 | Ears form | 1/2 inch |
| 6–7 | Resembles adult with eyes, ears, nose, lips, tongue, teeth buds, fingers, thumbs, knees, ankles, toes; Fetal movements; brain directs other organs; stomach digests; liver makes blood cells; kidney extracts uric acid from blood; first bone cells replace | 1 inch; 1/30 oz |
| (2nd month) | cartilage skeleton<br>Embryo becomes fetus | |
| 9–10 | Total body movements; threefold increase in nerve-muscle connections | 2 inches |
| 12 (3rd month) | Swallows amniotic fluid, fingernails form; eyelids seal; bony ribs and vertebrae form; palate fuses; excretes urine | |
| 12–16 (4th month) | | 6–8 inches; 6 oz |
| 16–20 (5th month) | Grows hair; skeleton hardens; settles into favorite lie | 10 inches; 1 pound |
| 20–24 (6th month) | Permanent teeth buds; eyes open; grip is strong; vernix and lanugo (hair) on body | 13 inches; 1 3/4 pounds |
| 24–28 (7th month) | Deposits adipose tissue under skin | 15 inches; 2–3 pounds |
| 28–38 (8th, 9th months) | Gains weight and length | 20 inches 6–10 pounds |

contraction stress test to determine fetal status. Early research suggested that background noises of the maternal digestive and circulatory systems may calm the infant, but so far these sounds have not achieved the same effect when applied after birth.[5]

## *Fetal-Maternal Physiology*

During pregnancy, the uterine blood flow increases as uterine size increases with fetal growth. However, the increase of blood flow in

### Table 6–2: Fetal Development by System

| System | Time | Event |
|---|---|---|
| Cardiovascular | Day 22 | Primitive tube forms |
| | 4th week | Cardiac activity; cardiac loop |
| | 4-7 weeks | Four chambers form |
| | 7-8 weeks | Heart rate increases from week 4 until now when it decreases due to improved contractility |
| Respiratory | 3-4 weeks | Primordium forms trachea and lung buds |
| | 10 weeks | Left bronchus divides in two, right into three |
| | 11 weeks | Fetal breathing movement |
| | 4th month | 24 bronchial divisions |
| | 13-25 weeks | Canalization |
| | 24 weeks | Alveoli form (this process continues until 8 years) |
| Nervous | | |
| Vision | 5 weeks | Optic cup, lens vesicle |
| | 2-4 months | Retina differentiates |
| | 5 months | Rods and cones form |
| | 10-26 weeks | Eyelids fuse |
| | 30 weeks | Eye responds to light |
| Taste | 7 weeks | Taste buds |
| | 12 weeks | Mature taste buds; swallows |
| | 28 weeks | Taste established |
| Hearing | 18 days | Ear develops |
| | 6 weeks | Cochlea appears |
| | 10 weeks | Cochlea has 2 1/2 turns; Scala vestibuli and tympani |
| | 5 months | Cochlea complete |
| | 6 months | Inner ear functions |
| | 7 months | Eardrum forms |
| | 26-29 weeks | Response to external sounds |
| Touch | 7 weeks | Reflex response to touch |
| | 8 weeks | Receptors to face |
| | 10 weeks | Pressure receptors in fingers; light touch in hands |
| | 11 weeks | Upper and lower extremities respond |
| | 15-17 weeks | Abdomen/buttocks respond |
| | 7 months | Meissner's corpuscles in hand (light touch) |
| | 2nd/3rd trimester | Reflex grasp strengthens |
| Musculoskeletal | 3 weeks | Nerve cells present |
| | 5 weeks | Myotomes give rise to spinal muscles and three muscle layers on thorax/abdomen |
| | 5-8 weeks | Forelimb and hind limb buds grow and angle to form elbows and knees |
| | 6-8 weeks | Spinal reflex arc |
| | 7.5 weeks | First reflex activity (neck contralateral flexion to perioral stimulation) |
| | 8.5 weeks | Thorax/lumbar flexion |
| | 9.5 weeks | Pelvic rotation; mouth opening |
| | 10.5 weeks | Swallowing motions; sucking movements |
| | 11 weeks | Hip movements |
| | 12 weeks | Ankle movements; three motor patterns |

proportion to the growth of the fetus is lacking; therefore, more oxygen is extracted per volume of uterine blood toward the end of pregnancy. The uterine arteries ultimately supply the placenta, which functions similarly to a lung for the fetus. The placental villi act in the exchange of oxygen and nutrition to the fetal blood, and carbon dioxide and fetal wastes to the maternal blood. Fetal circulation differs from that of the newborn and of the adult (see Figure

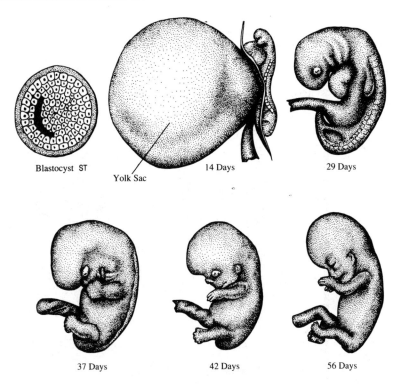

Blastocyst ST    14 Days    29 Days

Yolk Sac

37 Days    42 Days    56 Days

Figure 6-1: Development of the embryo and fetus    © 1989 PARLAY INTERNATIONAL.

6-2). Briefly the difference lies in extra flow from the placenta entering the fetal heart via the ductus venosus to the inferior vena cava. Additional fetal blood shunted to the liver from the umbilical vein flows to the inferior vena cava via hepatic veins, and blood from the gut reaches the ductus venosus from the portal vein. The inferior vena cava opens near the foramen ovale, causing blood to flow through the foramen ovale to the left atrium, while blood entering via the superior vena cava passes into the right-sided chambers. Blood in the left chambers pass into the aorta and then to the head, neck, and upper extremities. This blood appears to be better oxygenated than the blood that passes to the caudal regions via the pulmonary trunk. Little blood flows into the lungs because of the resistance, flowing instead to the patent ductus arteriosus and the descending thoracic and abdominal aortae to the lower extremities. These openings in the ductus arteriosus and in the foramen ovale cause the left and right sides of the fetal heart to pump in parallel rather than in series, as in the adult. Fetal blood then travels to the placenta through the umbilical arteries, and circulation repeats.

At birth, blood flowing through the umbilical cord will continue to diminish over several minutes, although it is believed that most of it reaches the infant within a minute after delivery.[3] Part of the reduction in flow is due to swelling of the Wharton's jelly inside the

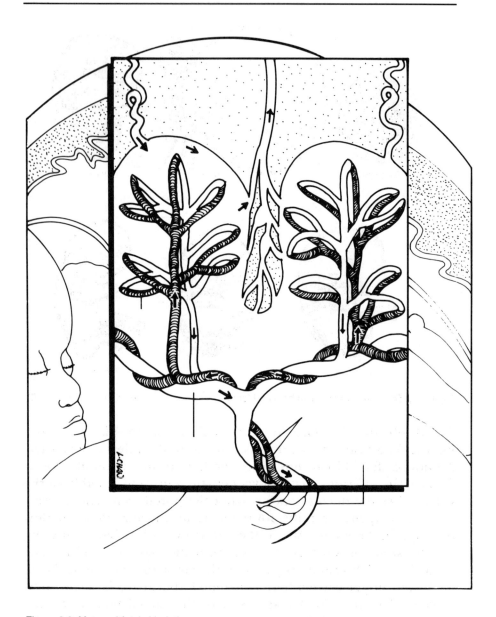

Figure 6-2: Maternal-fetal circulation

cord, which compresses the two arteries and one vein.[7] As the placental circulation stops, peripheral resistance rises until the aortic
pressure exceeds that in the pulmonary artery. The infant becomes
asphyxic, gasps, and these responses added to negative intrapleural
pressure cause the lungs inflate. This first breath apparently draws
in additional placental blood. When the lungs expand, pulmonary
blood flow can increase, pressure in the left atrium rises and shuts
the foramen ovale by pressing on the valve. The ductus arteriosus
also shuts after a few minutes, possibly because of a rise in arterial

oxygen pressure. The complete mechanisms for these closures are unknown, but may be linked to vasoreactive factors.[2] Experimentation with prostaglandins suggests they may play a role in the adjustment of fetal circulation to birth. In any event, peripheral circulation may take longer to establish, and the hands and feet of the newborn may be cold for the first few hours.

After the cord is cut and ligated, the placenta remains inside the uterus for a short time, then peels off the uterine wall and is delivered. This peeling tends to leave a wound on the uterine wall which bleeds for a few weeks after the birth.

## *Teratogens and Environmental Hazards*

In the 1950s, the administration of the drug thalidomide to pregnant females in their third to fifth week of gestation, slammed home the idea that the pregnant female who was exposed to or who ingested certain substances might be risking the health of her baby. Thalidomide is a tranquilizing agent or hypnotic drug and was then used to calm the stressed-out expectant mother. Yet the stress increased considerably when an infant with phocomelia (absence of the proximal part of a limb) was born. The relative rarity of this anomaly enabled epidemiologists to track the teratogen to thalidomide administered early in the pregnancy. This unfortunate incident, however, stands as a hallmark of expanding obstetric and epidemiologic awareness, especially concerning agents that affect the fetus. But rather than learn from past mistakes, the nonsteroidal estrogen, diethylstilbestrol (DES) was used, supposedly to decrease the incidence of miscarriage. This drug was administered from 1940 to 1971 until researchers linked it epidemiologically to congenital anatomic and reproductive anomalies in the offspring of women receiving DES.

A variety of factors can result in abnormal fetal development. Teratology is the study of the those factors, called teratogens, substances that cause congenital abnormalities. And congenital abnormalities can include anything from gross structural defects down to cellular defects. Anomalies may be transmitted genetically, environmentally, or spontaneously. Examples of specific anomalies of each category are listed in Table 6-3. What is important to remember when answering patients' questions about potential birth defects is that not every mother who has a maternal infection will deliver an abnormal infant. In fact, only a very small percentage of children will have birth defects. Neither will every woman who has had a child born with birth defects deliver another the same. In some cases, however, such as genetically based anomalies, some disorders are more likely to occur in any offspring. Mothers with children who

**Table 6-3. Modes of Transmission and Examples of Congenital Anomalies**

| Mode of transmission | Trait | Cause |
|---|---|---|
| Genetic | Sickle-cell anemia<br>Color blindness<br>Huntington's chorea<br>Chromosomal aberrations<br>(Turner's syndrome, Klinefelter's syndrome, Down's syndrome)<br>Tay-Sachs disease | Aberrations of genes or chromosomes; hereditary |
| Environmental | Depends on gestational age at time of exposure | Radiation, maternal infection, maternal nutritional deficiency, chemicals, maternal-fetal blood difference |
| Spontaneous | Depends on gene affected | Possible weakness in genetic strain |

have genetic disorders should be referred to a genetic counselor to determine the risk of producing similar offspring.

It is important, too, for practitioners to keep aware of research in this field. Recent studies have implicated video display terminals on computers, smoking, alcohol, social drug abuse, and chemicals used in the workplace or at home, as potential teratogens. For instance, pregnant women were warned to avoid changing cat litter boxes because of the risk of toxoplasmosis carried in cat feces. In other research, initial suspicions of harm induced by caffeine consumption during pregnancy could not be conclusively proven, at least in regard to certain birth deformities, although there is data for both sides of the issue.[8] Therefore, the well-informed practitioner needs to keep updated to help clients answer questions about nutrition and environmental hazards. The physical therapist may also receive questions about the safety of analgesics, over-the-counter medications, and anesthetics used for labor and delivery, and even about the safety of certain fetal diagnostic procedures (amniocentesis and diagnostic ultrasound). Tables 6-4 and 6-5 list a small sample of proven and suspected teratogenic substances; however, these lists are by no means exhaustive.

**Table 6-4. Confirmed Teratogens**

| Substance | Possible Fetal Effect |
|---|---|
| Alcohol | Microcephaly, growth and developmental retardation |
| Birth control pills | Bony and respiratory tract anomalies |
| Vaccines | Infection in fetus |
| Phenobarbital | Limb or heart defects, mental retardation |
| Cancer drugs | Assorted malformations |
| Cocaine | Assorted malformations |
| Diethylstilbestrol (DES) | Reproductive tract anomalies, cancer |

**Table 6-5. Suspected Teratogens**

| Substance | Possible Fetal Effect |
| --- | --- |
| Smoking and passive smoking | Decreased birth weight |
| Nutritional deficiencies | Inadequate growth |
| Aspirin | Jeopardized hemostasis |
| Prolonged hyperthermia induced by hot tubs and saunas | Neural defects |
| Nasal decongestants | Anomalies |
| Allergy medications | Anomalies |

Clients should be advised to consult their physicians or caregivers if any doubt exists as to the safety of a substance. It is also wise to refer these clients to their caregiver even if a substance used is a confirmed teratogen. For some unexplained reason, teratogenic substances do not always induce birth defects. The substances identified as teratogens are associated with a significant increase in congenital anomalies. But that does not mean that an identified substance will always cause a defect. Legalistically, the practitioner is better off referring questions about general physical and mental health during pregnancy to a specialist in that field.

## Maternal Nutrition, Health of the Newborn, and Role of the Placenta

"The nutrient supply to a fetus is dependent on placental transport."[9] And the ability to transport nutrients increases as pregnancy progresses, especially closer to term as the baby puts on weight. "Morphometric studies in human placentas have shown that the placental thickness decreases, and the surface area continues to increase exponentially until term." The conclusion drawn from these observations is that placental growth meets fetal nutritional requirements. It is believed that most of the protein transfer occurs after 30 weeks gestation; hence, fetal growth can be considered dependent not only on those substances ingested by the mother, but on the size and transport capacity of the placenta.

"The placental transport of nutrients to the umbilical circulation depends on the permeability of the placenta to each nutrient, the maternal-to-fetal concentration gradient for each nutrient, net placental nutrient consumption, and the magnitude and pattern of uterine, placental, and umbilical blood flows."[9] The placenta transports carbohydrates via diffusion, amino acids via active transport, and fats via a number of ways; the mechanism for fetal uptake of lipids is unclear. In fact, the mechanism for transport for most substances of high molecular weight is not totally understood. This applies to maternal antibodies as well as lipids. Vitamins B, C, D and dissolved substances such as sodium, chloride, and potassium transport easily; unfortunately, so do many drugs, some of which are teratogenic.

After the infant is born, metabolic levels increase, and the energy requirement changes from 40 kcal/kg/day to about 115 kcal/kg/day. The infant continues to require this amount for at least the first 6 months. Preterm infants may require 120 to 150 kcal/kg/day to assure continued growth at the intrauterine rate.

Lactose is the infant's main dietary carbohydrate. Lactose breaks down into glucose and galactose with the assistance of lactase present in the small intestine. Although occasionally infants are lactose-intolerant and suffer from diarrhea and malnutrition unless they receive an alternate carbohydrate, all infants require glucose in some form for adequate brain function. About 150 ml/kg/day of breast milk supplies about 4 mg/kg/minute of glucose. This, as is nature's way, coincides with the amount and rate required by the brain tissues.

Whey proteins are the chief proteins in breast milk; in humans, these proteins are composed of lactalbumin, serum albumin, lactoferrin, lysozyme, and immunoglobulin. In general, breast milk has less protein than commercial formulas, and the whey proteins in formulas are usually from cow's milk. Some researchers believe that increased protein may cause metabolic abnormalities, but others argue that increased protein may be beneficial for preterm infants.

"Lipids are a major source of energy, fat-soluble vitamins, hormones, and essential fatty acids for neonates. The essential fatty acids are important for cell membrane integrity as phospholipids and are precursors of prostaglandins and leukotrienes."[9] It is for these reasons that nonfat and diets too low in fat are unhealthy for infants. Linoleic acid is the primary fatty acid in breast milk. With other fatty acids, lipids form, and contribute approximately 50% of the calories in breast milk; however, the lipid content of breast milk varies. It is believed that lipid content is lowest in the morning and at the start of each feeding.

Vitamins and minerals vary in content in breast milk as compared to commercial formulas. In this case, more is not necessarily better. Excess vitamin A, vitamin E or selenium administered to infants can produce metabolic and growth problems by reducing the production of other vital factors. Although breastfeeding is considered the ideal way to care for an infant, realistically not every woman will either be able to or want to breastfeed. Until more is known about biochemical interactions, it is probably wise to advise clients who plan to feed their infant with formula to talk to a qualified pediatric dietician to compare formulas and select one similar to human breast milk.

## *Checking on Baby*

The status of the mother is relatively easy to assess compared to the status of the fetus. Several methods have been devised in recent years to help obstetric attendants learn more than the information gained by fetal heart monitoring and feel more confident that the fetus is healthy during pregnancy and during labor. Tests for early pregnancy include amniocentesis, chorionic villus sampling, and maternal serum alpha-fctoprotein. Other tests for later pregnancy include electronic fetal monitoring; ultrasonography; magnetic resonance imaging; antepartum fetal heart rate testing, which includes the nonstress test and the contraction stress test; fetal movement charting; and, possibly, a biophysical profile, which is a composite score of fetal breathing movements, gross body movements, muscle tone, amniotic fluid volume, and the nonstress test.

Amniocentesis can be used for a variety of analyses. This sampling of amniotic fluid drawn by needle from the area around the baby can be done early to detect genetic disorders, or later in pregnancy to assess fetal lung maturity. Fetal lung maturity is assessed by several other tests, but the most widely used one determines the ratio of lecithin and sphingomyelin (L/S ratio). These substances are phospholipid components of surfactant, which increases alveolar surface tension. A ratio above 2:1 is considered a normal proportion. Amniotic fluid can also be examined for signs of maternal or fetal infection. There is a certain risk of maternal infection and fetal demise from the procedure.

Chromosomal analysis can also be done by chorionic villus sampling of about 30 mg of chorionic tissue drawn by suction catheter through the vagina and directed by ultrasound. Again, a risk is associated with the procedure.

Sampling of maternal serum alpha-fetoprotein is a screening for neural tube defects and has been recently used with encouraging results to detect Down's syndrome.[10] Concentrations of this alpha-globulin synthesized in the fetal yolk sac, liver, and gastrointestinal tract are much higher in fetal serum than in amniotic fluid, and higher in amniotic fluid than in maternal serum, but the ease of sampling maternal serum makes this test more practical.

Another test that used to be performed routinely with maternal blood typing is for Rh incompatibility. An Rh-negative mother may become sensitized if the fetus is Rh positive. Rh immune globulin can be administered several times during pregnancy and immediately after delivery.

Electronic fetal monitoring has become a legalistic necessity during labor and delivery in the minds of many obstetric physicians and nurses. The readout from the electronic monitor assures the physician that fetal heart rate is within normal limits (120-160 bpm) over time and that the uterus is contracting efficiently. Two tracings record fetal heart rate variations and pressure of uterine contractions (mm Hg). The fetal heart is monitored through a sound transducer placed externally or internally and contractions, via a pressure transducer. The internal electrode is attached through ruptured membranes to the fetal scalp. If monitored externally, there are two belts that must be worn (see Figure 6-3). If the woman changes position the reading may be disturbed. Many women find these belts uncomfortable, but a great number of physicians and hospitals require continuous monitoring for medicolegal records. Women who do not want these procedures should be advised to shop around for a physician and hospital that will meet their needs.

Diagnostic ultrasound, to be differentiated from therapeutic ultrasound and surgical ultrasound, is used to determine gestational age and to detect fetal anomalies, intrauterine growth retardation, fetal position, multifetal pregnancy, uterine size, and placental location. There are three basic systems of diagnostic ultrasound, usually in the range of 3.5 to 5 MHz, static B scan, real-time imaging, and the Doppler. The static B scan is a pulse-echo method, real-time is a rapid-pulse scan, and the Doppler is a continuous transmission of ultrasound waves. The echoes received from the sound waves that bounce off the fetal heart are then converted to audible range. With ultrasound, the higher the frequency is, the less the depth of penetration will be. Therefore, the intensity must be increased to maintain the desired depth of penetration with good resolution.[11-12]

Unfortunately, the effects of higher intensity ultrasound on fetal tissue are not well documented. The American College of Obstetricians and Gynecologists has developed guidelines for use of diagnostic ultrasound, but the guidelines are broad and include almost any use except as a routine screening tool.[13] The International Childbirth Education Association published a position paper on this topic to encourage use "only in the presence of medically valid criteria," and discouraged use "in the absence of a high-risk indication."[14] It may be many years before the long-term impact of routine use of diagnostic ultrasound is known. Until then, women should be advised to avoid routine screening with ultrasound. Obstetricians and nurses can listen to fetal heart tones without a Doppler device. This does not imply, however, that if a woman is at high-risk, or there is a question of fetal safety, she should refuse. What it seems to boil down to is trust and respect between physician and client. If a woman feels comfortable and confident of the physician's abilities, she should also be able to ask questions and have them answered in

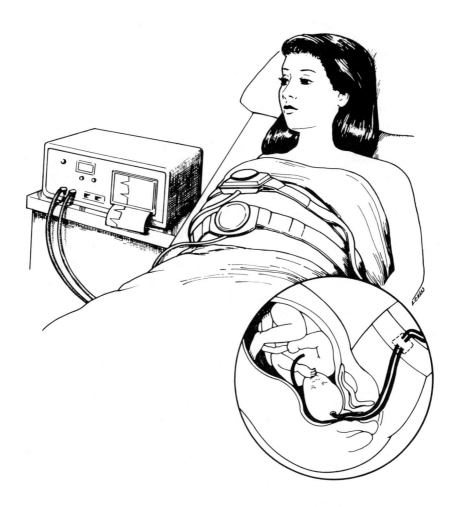

Figure 6-3: Electronic fetal monitor: external and internal (in circle) electrode placements

a logical way. Physicians need to provide facts when asked if a procedure is necessary and whether it is safe for the fetus. And women need to demand these facts before making an informed decision.

Magnetic resonance imaging has recently been used for better resolution of hydrocephalus and other fetal anomalies. It is also believed to be useful for measuring the bony pelvis. Few studies have been done to determine safety and cost-effectiveness.

The stress tests do as their name suggests—place stress on the fetus. Even the nonstress test places stress if the fetus is unhealthy. These tests are done, if indicated, during the last trimester. In the nonstress test, patients are placed in a semi-Fowler position, while maternal blood pressure and pulse and fetal activity and heart rate are assessed in serial readings for 20 to 40 minutes. The test may be reactive or nonreactive; the reactive test results in two to three or more fetal heart rate accelerations in this period. An acceleration is 15 beats/minute above baseline for 15 seconds or longer. The contraction stress test repeats the nonstress test plus stimulates uterine contraction, either by the mother stimulating her nipples or by infusing oxytocin (the substance that should be naturally produced by nipple stimulation and causes uterine contractions). Again fetal heart rate is the criteria for a positive, suspicious, or negative test, but late decelerations are the key. The test is positive if there are repetitive late decelerations coincident with uterine contractions, suspicious if late decelerations are noted but not persistent, and negative if none occur with uterine contractions. A contraction stress test, though, may also be reactive or nonreactive should accelerations occur as well. The predictive value of these tests is debatable in terms of fetal outcome. The worst scenario is a nonreactive positive contraction stress test, suggesting that elective delivery may be needed to save the fetus.[15] The mother must plan to rest in a lateral recumbent position for at least an hour to chart fetal movements. This test depends heavily on the mother's perceptions of fetal movement as she charts gross motions. Four or more fetal movements in an hour are considered normal, although a healthy fetus may move far more often.

The factors associated with the biophysical profile have been explained, except for the amniotic fluid measurement and fetal tone assessment. The examiner looks for pockets of amniotic fluid, greater than 1 cm in size, surrounding the fetus. One or more pockets of this size are normal. The assessment of fetal tone examines active flexion and extension of the limbs or trunk. Each of the five factors of the profile can earn 2 points if normal; if the patient achieves 8 to 10 points, the fetus is considered healthy. A score of 2 or less suggests consideration of elective delivery. Additional tests are constantly being developed. Recent research has introduced prenatal screenings for hepatitis B virus, herpes simplex virus, and congenital toxoplasmosis.

## The Newborn and Newborn Examinations

Immediately at birth, the newborn receives its first medical examination. Several scales have been developed to assess the status of the newborn, but perhaps the best known is the Apgar scale, named after pediatrician Virginia Apgar. This scale assesses the infant's color, respirations, reflex responses, heart rate, and muscle tone. Each category is scored by someone present at the delivery who assigns 0 to 2 points for the five areas at 1 and 5 minutes after birth. Thus, a perfect score is 10, but scores between 7 and 10 at 1 and 5 minutes are considered high. This scale has been in use since the 1950s, and studies have confirmed its reliability and value in predicting neonatal mortality. The most useful aspects of this scale are the categories for heart rate and respirations. Heart rate should be over 100 beats/minute, and respirations should be deep and even, usually with crying as well. It is becoming increasingly obvious, however, that the Apgar scale is indeed merely a screening. Additional problems can arise after 5 minutes, and therefore a more careful examination is necessary.

Most infants delivered in a hospital or clinic will have a thorough examination by a pediatrician or family physician before discharge. This examination includes careful scrutiny of skin, bony development, weight and weight gain, muscle tone, behavior, and neurologic maturation. The Apgar scale is not the assessment of choice to detect subtle differences or systemic dysfunctions that show up later in the infant's life, including the potential effects of anesthesia used during labor or delivery. This observation has been apparent for many years, however, and numerous scales have been developed to assess the infant's health.

Perhaps one of the best known scales is the Brazelton Neonatal Behavioral Assessment Scale, developed by T. Berry Brazelton, M.D. a pediatrician and author of several books on infant care. Like Brazelton's scale, other similar screenings and evaluation tools focus on the neonate's neurologic status, including motor and sensory components, behavior, and reflex activity. Within the physical therapy realm, pioneers like the Bobaths, Rood, Knott, and Fiorentino have offered techniques for assessment and treatment of infants with neuromuscular dysfunction that are based on these neurologic screenings. The reader is referred to pediatric literature for specific testing items.

In addition to tests for neurologic integrity (*e.g.*, Babinski, palmar grasp, pull to sit, placing, Galant, Glabella, tonic neck, Moro), the neonate may be subject to state-imposed tests for phenylketonuria, or a Vitamin K shot to insure clotting, or ophthalmic treatments within 2 hours of birth to prevent venereal disease.

## *Self-Assessment Review*

1. It is of great clinical importance that the placenta implant in the _____ of the uterus.
2. The placenta serves as a means of _____ for nutrients needed by the fetus.
3. Drugs cannot pass through the placenta to the fetus. T F
4. An example of a suspected teratogen is _____.
5. An example of a confirmed teratogen is _____.

6. Pregnant women should be concerned about working with chemicals and computers. T F
7. Commercial formulas are the same composition as human breast milk. T F
8. Newborns need a precise combination of nutrients such as _____, _____, and _____ to thrive and grow.
9. The _____ scale is a screening immediately after birth to assess the health of the newborn.
10. More detailed tests of newborn health include tests of _____.

## *References*

1. Nilsson L: A Child is Born. New York, Dell Publishing, 1965.
2. Ganong WF: Review of Medical Physiology (11th ed). Los Altos, Lange Medical Publications, 1983.
3. Snell RS: Clinical Embryology for Medical Students. Boston, Little, Brown & Co, 1972.
4. Warwick R, Williams PL: Gray's Anatomy (35th ed). Philadelphia, WB Saunders, 1973.
5. Hill LM, Breckle R, Wolfgram KR: An ultrasonic view of the developing fetus. Obstet Gynecol Surv 38(7):375-398, 1983.
6. Rayburn WF, Lavin JP: Obstetrics for the House Officer. Baltimore, Williams & Wilkins, 1988.
7. Flanagan GL: The First Nine Months of Life. New York, Simon & Schuster, 1962.
8. Rosenberg L, et al: Selected birth defects in relation to caffeine-containing beverages. JAMA 247(10):1429-1432,1982.
9. Kennaugh JM, Hay WW: Nutrition of the fetus and newborn. West J Med 147(4):435-448, 1987.
10. DiMaio MS, et al: Screening for fetal Down's syndrome in pregnancy by measuring maternal serum alpha-fetoprotein levels. N Engl J Med 317:342-346, 1987.
11. O'Brien WD: Ultrasonic bioeffects: A view of experimental studies. Birth 11(3):149-157, 1984.
12. Petitti DB: Effects of in utero ultrasound exposure in humans. Birth 11(3):159-163, 1984.
13. American College of Obstetricians and Gynecologists: Diagnostic ultrasound in obstetrics and gynecology. ACOG Technical Bulletin 63:Oct 1981.
14. International Childbirth Education Association: ICEA position paper: Diagnostic ultrasound in obstetrics. ICEA News 22(2):1983.

15. DeVoe LD: Clinical features of the reactive positive contraction stress test. Obstet Gynecol 63(4):523-527, 1984.

# SEVEN

# Labor

What happens to the patient with back pain during pregnancy when she goes into labor? Actually, no literature on this subject could be found, but anecdotal evidence suggests that back pain does not interfere with labor or delivery. In fact, women with back pain during the entire pregnancy may have no back pain during labor, and conversely, women who had no significant back pain during pregnancy may have severe back pain during labor. However, the back pain experienced only during labor, referred to as "back labor," arises from pressure on lumbar and sacral nerves from the fetal head as it works its way into the pelvis and birth canal. The exception to the women described above is the woman with a herniated disc; yet, successful vaginal deliveries have occurred even in this situation. Contrary to popular belief, the physical therapist does have a role in the care of the laboring woman. Pain relief measures that can be provided by the therapist include instruction in positioning, childbirth education, and possibly the use of transcutaneous electrical nerve stimulation (TENS). How then does labor progress, what anatomic features change at this time, and what causes the pain of labor?

## *Pregnancy: Prodrome to Labor*

During the first few months, changes of pregnancy may be imperceptible to some women. In fact, many women do not know they are pregnant during the first month and perhaps partway through the second month until the realization strikes that a menstrual period has not arrived. Other women, however, know from conception; their breasts become tender and swollen, they may have nausea or vomiting, they may need to urinate frequently, appetite may increase, and mood swings may abound. With home pregnancy tests, women can verify their suspicions as early as hormone levels rise high enough to register.

Pregnant women may need to change to maternity clothes at varying times. Some need them early, some not until the end; it depends on the way the weight gain is distributed. By the third or fourth month of pregnancy, the mother probably has felt the fetus moving (quickening), and the uterus has started to enter the abdominal cavity. This shift relieves some of the pressure on the urinary bladder caused by the weight of the uterus, placenta, amniotic membranes and fluid, and the fetus. However, continued growth of the uterus and fetus causes some compression of the mother's internal organs, especially intestines, stomach, and later lungs. In the last trimester, the fetus takes up most of the room inside the uterus, and the uterus takes up most of the room inside the abdominal cavity. The mother may find it difficult to breathe deeply or catch her breath after exertion. That is, until the last few weeks of the pregnancy (see Figure 7-1).

Towards the end of term, the baby may approach the bony pelvis, and the mother may feel as though she can take a deep breath again. This event is lightening and may be accompanied by additional maternal symptoms such as increased pelvic pressure and need to urinate, constipation from pressure on the intestines, and vulvar or rectal varicosities, and edema in the lower extremities related to pressure on blood vessels.

Throughout the pregnancy, and especially starting around the seventh month of gestation, uterine contractions may be felt by the expectant mother. These contractions are thought to be similar to warm-up exercises as the uterus prepares for a long, continuous workout. Sometimes called Braxton Hicks contractions (named after their founders), they may be strong enough in the latter months to cause some cervical effacement or dilation.

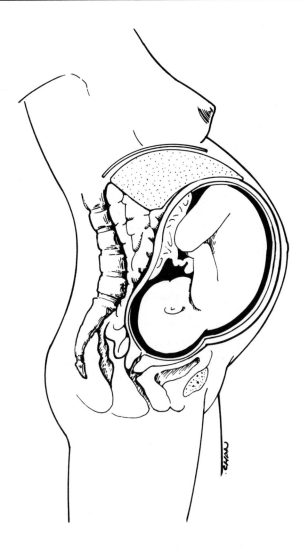

Figure 7-1: Full-term pregnancy

The part of the fetus that lies closest to the cervix is the presenting part; this is most commonly the head, but may be the feet, knees, buttocks, and, occasionally, an arm. Any position, or lie, of the fetus other than head first is considered breech presentation and is a potential complication for delivery and the progress of labor. The obstetric caregiver can tell by physical examination, and by listening to the fetal heartbeat, the position of the fetus. This position may change frequently during pregnancy, but less often as term approaches. Babies have been known to change from breech to cephalic presentation in the beginning of labor, but usually once labor starts position is fixed.

As the fetus draws closer to the bony pelvis it is considered to be floating (freely moving), dipping (presenting part passes into the inlet), or engaged (the presenting part at its widest diameter passes through the pelvic inlet). In the primigravida, or woman in her first pregnancy (as opposed to multigravida), engagement often occurs 2 to 3 weeks before labor. In the multigravida, engagement may not occur until labor starts, or may even occur during labor. In either case, engagement is often associated with cervical effacement. The neck of the uterus thins, shortens, and softens and becomes quite stretchy during labor. In the multipara (a woman who has delivered more than one viable child), the uterus is often thinner and softer; therefore, engagement may not seem to occur as suddenly as it might in the primipara. Also, near the onset of labor, women may lose a few pounds, feel renewed energy and have an intense need to finalize preparations for the newborn. This intense need is known as nesting.

## *Normal Labor*

The onset of labor happens primarily in three ways: rupture of the amniotic sac, bloody show, or contractions that become stronger and rhythmic. False labor episodes occur often, usually mimicking true labor with contractions that get stronger, longer, and closer together. While these contractions may be exciting, and seem like the real thing, it is this false labor that may stop if the woman changes activities (goes for a walk or takes a rest), or, more commonly, after she arrives at the hospital. The contractions of real labor, though, do not disappear with activity. In fact, the woman that experiences real labor contractions may indeed wish she could turn them off.

Bloody show is the passing of the mucus plug that formed early in the pregnancy to seal off the uterus from the external world. As the cervix thins and softens, the plug simply dislodges. When it dislodges, it tends to break free from the uterine wall, and in so doing breaks some of the small blood vessels. As a sign of impending labor though, it is unreliable since it may pass whenever the cervix starts to dilate and soften. Many women never see the bloody show; it may pass unnoticed while using the bathroom.

Rupture of the membranes, however, is a more reliable indicator of impending labor. In fact, if the membranes rupture, the woman will either start labor on her own or it will be started for her via intravenous oxytocin drip anywhere from 8 to 48 hours afterwards. Many labors, however, continue with the membranes intact until the end of the first stage. It is believed that the fluid in the amniotic sac provides a cushion between the fetal head and the cervix, thereby reducing stress on the fetus.

After the membranes rupture, the inside is exposed to the outside, infection is a possibility, and contractions seem to increase in frequency and intensity, because of the firmer pressure exerted on the cervix by the presenting part. The mother may experience either a sudden gush of fluid or a trickle, depending on where the membranes rupture. If the tear is high towards the fundus, there will probably be a trickle with each contraction. If the tear is low, fluid will gush forth, mostly during one or two contractions; however, there is still plenty of fluid left around the baby, and the membranes continue to produce fluid during labor. Women can be advised to investigate the fluid for odor, color, and ability to stop the flow if they are unsure whether the fluid is amniotic or urine.

Although some physicians like to start infusing oxytocin (usually a synthetic pitocin) after 8 hours with no regular contractions, some will wait longer and allow the woman to monitor her temperature at home for signs of infection. Pitocin drip or "pit" can cause contractions in uterine muscle. For some reason, these artificially-induced contractions seem stronger to women who have had previous labor contractions. The woman must also labor with an intravenous line in place, which is uncomfortable for many. The idea behind using pitocin is to stimulate the uterus to start contracting on its own. When contractions start on their own, the pitocin is stopped.

Although some people describe their 24-hour labor, or their 10-hour labor, it is always difficult to compare the two experiences, since the perception of when labor starts can vary greatly. For instance, one woman may consider labor started at the first contraction; another may consider labor started when contractions became regular; another when the membranes ruptured. Studies of length of labor suggest an average first labor of 12 to 14 hours and subsequent labors of 6 to 8 hours. Since these are average figures, however, labor may be longer or shorter; but usually after 24 hours of labor, the health care provider considers intervention by forceps or by Cesarean section. The decision to intervene depends on the fetal and maternal health during labor and on the policies of the physician or obstetric department.

Labor is simply the process by which the uterus expels the fetus. What triggers labor to start is unknown. Theories range from a preset lifetime of the placenta to some type of stretch initiated response as the fetal size increases. This latter theory does little to support premature birth. It is known that oxytocin is secreted around the time of labor onset. This hormone causes uterine contraction. What is even more interesting is that this hormone is purely specific to uterine contraction. Oxytocin is also secreted in response to nipple stimulation, particularly during lactation; and in fact, this response has been tried as a method to stimulate postmature labor, with limited success. It is believed this response is nature's way of returning the uterus to prepregnant size as the mother nurses the infant.

The muscle fibers of the uterus run longitudinally, transversely, and in a figure-eight pattern. Therefore, muscle contraction causes a downward force and an upward pull starting from the fundus and moving caudally to the cervix area. The contractions tend to become stronger, longer, and closer together if labor progresses normally and efficiently. Contractions may start approximately 20 minutes apart and gradually occur less than 1 minute apart, or in an erratic fashion, close to delivery. These contractions may also start out fairly mild and build in intensity; although when a beginning labor contraction is considered mild, it is definitely a relative term. To the woman having a first labor, the early contractions may seem very strong—that is, until she experiences those of later labor.

In any event, the sum force of these contractions is to thin out or efface the cervix, measured as a percentage of complete effacement of 100% (about 0.25 mm thick), and to dilate or open the cervix completely from 0 to 10 cm (diameter of the cervical os) for passage of the fetus. Effacement and dilation are measured manually. The cervix also tends to soften as labor starts or during the weeks prior to onset (see Figure 7-2).

As the contractions occur and the cervix effaces and dilates, the fetus is being assisted down into the birth canal. The descent of the fetal presenting part is measured by station (centimeters above or below the ischial spines; -5 is 5 cm above the ischial spines, +5 is

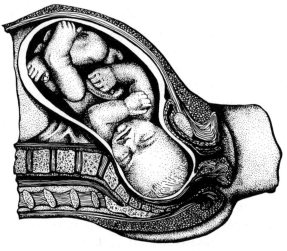

© 1989 PARLAY INTERNATIONAL ▼

Figure 7-2: First-stage labor; cervix starting to dilate

5 cm below or caudal to the ischial spines—see Figure 7-3). When the fetus passes through the cervix, passes through the vagina, and the largest diameter of the fetal head is seen at the vaginal opening in the perineum, the fetus is considered to be "crowning." Prior to crowning, however, the mechanism of labor may be described as follows: in the cephalic presentation, engagement is followed by an attitude of flexion of the fetal neck, then the neck rotates (internal rotation) with the occiput anterior (baby's face to the spine) to fit through the pelvis, followed by neck extension as the head passes under the pubic arch and continues to the outside. After this event, delivery is hopefully imminent, barring any complications in extracting the rest of the body. Once the head is born, the head again rotates (external rotation) to realign with the shoulders, the upper shoulder maneuvers under the pubic bone, then the lower shoulder, and the rest of the body slides out. This is the moment of birth, and, technically, labor has ended.

The easiest way to understand human labor is to divide it into stages and phases. Four stages divide labor into the period of thinning and dilating of the uterine cervix as the baby descends (Stage I), delivery of the infant (Stage II), delivery of the placenta (Stage III), and postpartum (Stage IV). Stage I is actually what is commonly known as labor and is further divided into three phases: early labor or latent phase, active labor or active phase, and late labor or transition. The basic characteristics of the first stage and its phases, as well as relief measures, are described in Table 7-1. These characteristics have been placed in a chart form that has been used as a patient handout for couples attending childbirth education classes. Stages II, III, and IV will be discussed in other chapters.

The early or latent phase of labor is usually the longest because contractions are milder and stay at the peak for a shorter time than later contractions. Again, it is difficult to judge exactly how long this phase will be, but on average, it lasts from a few up to 10 or more hours. During this time, the mother is excited and probably initially

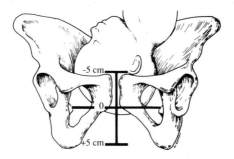

Figure 7-3: Station

**Table 7-1. Phases of First Stage Human Labor**

| Phase | Characteristics | What to do | How to help |
|---|---|---|---|
| Effacement 0–3 to 4cm dilation, 20–5 min apart | Cervix softens, thins, begins to dilate; mild contractions begin; length of phase varies; may see show or fluid leakage; may have backache, nausea | Relaxation; continue light activity at home; deep breathe when can no longer walk, talk; rest; urinate often | Assist in relaxation with touch, imagery; watch for signs of tension; time contractions; observe type of contractions; apply back pressure; prepare for hospital |
| Active 3–7cm dilation, 60 sec long, 3–1 min apart | Cervix opens; baby comes down; contractions increase; 2–9 hours; may feel pressure in low back, groin, perineum | May feel busy or discouraged; concentrate on breathing; change positions; urinate often; conserve energy; use effleurage | Encourage relaxation; relieve tension; help with positioning; breathe with her; watch for hyperventilation; apply counterpressure; give ice chips; praise her; ask about progress |
| Late (Transition) 7–10cm dilation, 60–90 sec long, erratic | Cervix is open; baby enters birth canal (20–60 min); may feel irritable, out of control, hot, dizzy, tingly; may have rectal or perineal pressure, hiccups, nausea, shaky legs, desire to push | Relax body, perineum; remember baby is coming; rest between contractions; change positions; relax; maintain breathing | Help with relaxation and position; time contractions; help her breathe at the start of each contraction; breathe with her; watch for hyperventilation; praise her; apply counterpressure; remind about baby coming |

unsure whether this is true labor or not. The hallmark of this phase is effacement of the cervix and dilation to 3 cm.

Between 4 cm and 7 cm dilation is the active phase of first stage labor. This is typically a busy time for the mother, and not only because the contractions are getting longer, stronger, and closer together. If she is having a hospital birth, it will most likely also be the time that contractions are about 5 minutes apart, regular, and of a stronger intensity than in early labor. It is at this time that physicians usually suggest the woman be admitted to the hospital. Women that attend childbirth education classes learn how to relax, breathe, and deal with the pain associated with labor contractions during admission procedures. Otherwise, this time can be particularly stressful to some women and couples.

Late labor, or transition, is marked by 7 to 10 cm dilation, frequent, lengthy, and intense contractions, and possibly by symptoms of nausea, vomiting, trembling legs, and feelings of discouragement. This is generally the most difficult phase of labor, but also the shortest. At 10 cm dilation, the woman in the hospital is allowed to push, whether or not she experiences any urge to do so. This magic number, estimated by manual measurement, is the signal that the cervix is completely open and ready for passage of the fetus. The transition phase may take about an hour or so, and pushing, an hour or longer, if left alone. Once the fetal presenting part (hopefully the head) passes through the cervix, it enters the birth canal. The vagina is capable of instant expansion to accommodate the fetus as it rotates under the pubic bone and down to the perineum. As the widest part of the fetal head passes through the vaginal opening, crowning has occurred, and delivery is imminent.

Preparation for labor and delivery in the hospital, depending on the policies of the hospital and the policies of the physician, can include enemas, pubic hair shaving, hooking up of an electronic fetal monitor, and many questions. Enemas to cleanse the lower bowel and pubic hair shaving to reduce the risk of infection from bacteria used to be standard procedures. Research has suggested that no greater risk exists without pubic hair shaving and that bowel evacuation is solely to encourage uninhibited pushing by the mother. For these reasons, many physicians no longer insist on these procedures. Other options for labor and delivery exist aside from the traditional hospital birth. Women need to look for hospitals that will let them walk and move around during labor, assume different positions for labor or delivery than standard lithotomy, and receive minimal intervention from nursing staff. Women should also be advised to explore a variety of childbirth education classes that exist to help women reduce anxiety and pain of labor. ASPO/Lamaze, Bradley Method, Read Natural Childbirth, and classes by International Childbirth Education Association teachers utilize different methods to cope with labor. All are based on relaxation and some type of breathing techniques, as well as education about the birthing process. Even if women are introspective and tuned in to the changes in their body during labor, childbirth education classes are probably a good idea to learn varied pain relief methods, to share feelings with other pregnant couples, and to understand what will happen before, during and after labor.

## *Complicated Labor*

Although it may seem that the phases of labor are fairly well delineated and that the normal labor will run a predictable course, labor is like anything else in medicine. There is no such thing as a classic textbook case when it comes to labor. The figures we hear about as being average are just that—average. Researchers do know, however, that in normal labor the contractions tend to get stronger, longer, and closer together; the cervix effaces and dilates at a certain rate; and the fetus moves down against the cervix as labor progresses.

Occasionally, though, contractions do not cause cervical dilation, the fetus does not descend, or other delays in progress occur. These situations present complications in labor and are generally called dystocia.

Premature labor contractions can result in the birth of a premature infant (weight less than 5 pounds 8 ounces) and can be caused by several factors. Among these are premature rupture of membranes, incompetent cervix, trauma, placenta previa, abruptio placentae, or illness. A recent study suggests premature contractions might be linked to maternal standing with little movement.[1]

There is no known cause for premature rupture of the membranes. It occurs in 10% to 12% of women, resulting in a premature infant 20% of the time.[2] In some cases, premature rupture of the membranes is associated with cervical incompetency. But other times, the cervix is unfavorable or unripe (less than 80% effaced and 2 cm dilated).

An incompetent cervix is a weak cervix that may shorten, efface, and dilate during pregnancy. If the patient makes it to labor, progress is often rapid as well. This weakness has been treated a variety of ways: either by cerclage, which involves placing a suture around the cervix; by placing the patient on bed rest; or by using tocolytic therapy if premature contractions occur. Tocolytic therapy employs medications such as ritodrine or terbutaline that inhibit uterine contractions. The drug may be infused and then administered orally in a maintenance dosage. Physical therapists have become more involved with this clientele by providing instruction in bed exercises and transfer methods to reduce intraabdominal pressure and pressure on the cervix.

On the opposite end of the spectrum is the postdate pregnancy, over 42 weeks' gestation. Studies suggest a greater risk of fetal mortality and morbidity from postdate pregnancies than in those delivered at term, probably related to the decay of the placental function.[3] Stress testing and induction of labor have not been associated with reduced mortality, but maternal breast stimulation to induce uterine contractions has shown some success. Another method currently being researched to induce labor is the use of prostaglandins administered vaginally.[4]

Abnormal placement of the placenta is a potentially serious complication causing significant fetal mortality.[5] Placenta previa is an implantation of the placenta low in the uterus that remains low or even covering the cervical os at term. This happens only 2% to 3% of the time.[6] Cesarean section is usually recommended unless the placenta is only marginally covering the os and there is little danger of the placenta preceding the delivery of the infant. If the placenta or the umbilical cord precedes the infant, blood supply and, there-fore, oxygen supply is jeopardized.

Occasionally the umbilical cord will prolapse through the vagina if membranes are ruptured. This presents a hazardous situation as the infant may compress the cord against the sides of the birth canal as it descends.

Abruptio placentae is a premature peeling away of the placenta from the uterine wall. Again, this is a dangerous situation that may require Cesarean section.

Aside from these less common complications of labor are epi-sodes of malpresentation, malposition, uterine dysfunction, pelvic contraction, and passage of meconium. Malpresentation refers to any part, other than the fetal head, that is presenting to the cervix, and therefore will be born first. This presenting part can be a breech (buttocks, knees, or feet first), shoulder, face, or brow of the fetus. Any of these presentations complicate the progress of labor.

Breech presentations prior to labor are fairly common, but re-main that way for delivery only 3% to 4% of the time. When the fetus is breech, the mother may feel kicking against the rectum and fetal movement more in the lower abdomen. Because of the uneven pressure from the presenting part, as opposed to the pressure when the head is down, it has been theorized that the cervix dilates more slowly and labor and descent take longer. However, research does not bear out this theory.[2] The major problem with a breech presenta-tion is that the largest and least moldable part, the head, must be born last. If the pelvic outlet will not accommodate the head, or if the cervix is not dilated completely and the body slips through, the fetus may be jeopardized. For this reason, many physicians elect to deliver breech babies by Cesarean section, especially if the baby appears to be large. Specific types of breech deliveries are discussed in Chapter 8. Basic breech presentations may be complete (knees and hips flexed), frank (hips flexed, knees extended; the most com-mon type), footling (hips and at least one knee extended with the foot coming first) or kneeling (one or two hips extended, knees flexed and coming first).

Fetal heart tones will be heard at different locations depending on the presentation and position. Position refers to the orientation of the presenting part and is designated by stating where a certain point on that part is located in relation to the front, back, or sides of the mother's pelvis. That certain part is called a denominator and is the occiput for the cephalic presentation, sacrum (S) for breech presentations, and scapula (Sc) for shoulder presentations. The most common is the left occiput anterior, abbreviated LOA. For brow presentations, the chart may note Fr for forehead; for face presentations, an M for mentum or chin.

Another way fetal position is described is by lie, that is the orientation of the longitudinal axis of the fetus to that of the mother while standing. Lie may be longitudinal (cephalic or buttocks), transverse, or oblique. Transverse lie that persists is almost always an indication for delivery by Cesarean.[2]

The uterus is subject to a variety of dysfunctions—prolapse, anatomic anomalies, sacculation, torsion, poor quality contractions, or failure of the cervix to dilate. Cervical dystocia may arise from anatomic anomaly, scarring, or carcinoma. Contractions may intensify until the cervix ruptures or detaches. However, if parts of the uterus do not work in synergy, contraction strength diminishes, and labor is slower. The uterus can also develop an inefficient type of tetany that produces few, if any, productive contractions. Incoordinate uterine action occurs most frequently in primigravidas.

A contracted pelvis, at the inlet, midpelvis, or outlet, can also jeopardize labor progress because of bony impedance to the fetus. A past history of pelvic fracture mandates careful examination of the pelvic capacity, hopefully prior to pregnancy. There is also a variety of pelvic deformities linked to spinal deformity and to leg length discrepancy from childhood.

## Maternal Position and State

Contrary to the "flat on the back" position assumed by many laboring women for many years, it is now believed that the instinct to remain upright and moving can help labor progress. In this latter situation, the woman utilizes the forces of gravity to assist fetal descent. Research does exist to support the theory that ambulation shortens the length of labor.[7] Sitting versus laying down in labor also tends to increase the pelvic outlet.[8] Therefore, even if a woman must be strapped to an electronic fetal monitor or intravenous line, she should try to stay upright and change positions fairly often.

Another misconception about labor is the idea that a full bladder impedes the progress of labor. A study on this topic found no effect of a full bladder on uterine activity and labor duration.[9]

## Pain Mechanisms and Relief

Although labor pains were for many years a woman's cross to bear, the acceptance of anesthesia for obstetric practice changed that way of thinking. And with Queen Victoria's approval of and insistence upon using chloroform for her own birthing process, physicians thereby gained approval for use with the common folk.

The pains of labor vary from woman to woman. One woman can have little pain; in fact, it is not uncommon to hear stories about someone who unknowingly delivers a child. These stories may be farfetched, because there are legitimate physical causes of pain in addition to any psychologic overlay. "Labor pain is not of a single intensity but of varying intensities and is usually greatest only for a few seconds at the peak of contractions. Labor pain is not the lancing pain of injury, but rather an aching, cramping pain that can be associated with positive functioning, great pressure, or the accomplishing of an important task."[10] Indeed, what can be more important than the birth of a child?

This pain is not easily forgotten, but in many ways, the pain of labor is welcome; each pain of the uncomplicated labor signals that the infant is closer to being born. It is also a relief to many to have the pregnancy draw to an end, because the baby becomes heavy and wearisome to some women in the last month, in particular. Women may also find they have to get up at night to urinate because of pressure from the fetus on the bladder. Although this may be good practice for those night feedings after the baby is born, the broken sleep tends to wear on many women and bearing the pregnancy becomes tiresome.

Once labor does start, there are real causes of pain (see Table 7-2). As the fetus descends and the uterus contracts, there is increased pressure on organs, tissues, and nerves and increased pull on ligaments, tissues, and muscles. Women may also experience pain in the lower abdomen or in the back related to posterior position of the fetus, inefficiency of uterine contractions, or a cervix resistant to dilation. The uterus that contracts uncoordinately or spasms may cause additional pain as well.

Since the Victorian era, relief of labor pain has shown little progress, although measures have been developed to lessen that pain in varying degrees. Three general categories of pain relief exist: medications/anesthesia, prenatal childbirth education, and more recently, TENS. The latter category is still in its infancy and has not been proven safe for the fetus, nor is it listed as an indication for TENS by the government.

The practicing physical therapist will undoubtedly receive questions about the types of drugs used for labor pain. Basically, these drugs fall into categories of analgesia or anesthesia and are used specifically for either first stage or second stage. Analgesic agents are used to raise pain thresholds or induce sleepiness and are administered either orally or by injection. Anesthetic agents block nerves and are administered by infusion or inhalation. The phase of first stage, during which pain relief is needed, may also determine

**Table 7-2. Causes of Pain in First Stage Labor**

I.  Physiological Causes
    Anoxic uterus due to inadequate relaxation of muscle between contractions of late labor
II. Physical Causes
    A.  From stretching as fetus descends:
        1. Cervix
        2. Fallopian tubes
        3. Ovaries
        4. Peritoneum
        5. Uterine ligaments
        6. Pelvic floor muscles
        7. Perineum
    B.  From pressure (exerted by the fetus and uterine contractions):
        1. Nerve ganglia near cervix
        2. Nerve ganglia near vagina
        3. Urethra
        4. Bladder
        5. Rectum
        6. Nerve Pathways
            *Sympathetic sensory:* Uterine contractions and cervical dilation → sympathetic → uterosacral ligaments → uterine, pelvic, hypogastric, aortic plexuses → dorsal roots T11, T12 → spinal cord.
            *Sympathetic motor:* Uterus → aortic, hypogastric, pelvic, and uterine plexuses to ventral rami of T10–T12.
            *Pudendal:* Anterior S2–4; passes near ischial spine and to urogenital diaphragm; breaks into inferior hemorrhoidal to lower rectum and rectal area, dorsal clitoris to clitoral area, perineal to vulva, skin, fascia, and deep perineal muscles.
            *Posterior femoral cutaneous:* may pass impulses to S2–4
            *Ilioinguinal:* may pass impulses to L1.

the type of medication selected by the physician or anesthesiologist. The dosage required, length of action by the particular drug, or maternal and fetal side effects warrant careful selection (see Table 7-3).

In some cases, analgesia or anesthesia may be titrated or administered more than once during a labor. Or analgesia may be given, later to be followed by an anesthetic for stronger contractions in active labor. It is wise to remember that, while some drugs have less

**Table 7-3: First Stage Medications**

| Type | Action | Example | How Given Time to Work How Long Lasts | Side Effects Mother | Baby |
|------|--------|---------|----------------------------------------|---------------------|------|
| Narcotics | Pain relief | Demerol | IM 5–20 min 1–4 hrs | Nausea Respiration ↓ contractions ↓ | Respiration ↓ |
| Tranquilizer | Relaxant | Vistaril | IM 15–20 min 3–4 hrs | BP ↓ lethargy, sleepiness | Respiration ↓ |
| Barbiturate | Relaxant | Seconal | PO 20–30 min 3–4 hrs | Hangover, lethargy, moodiness, anxiety, effects long-lasting | Respiration ↓ |

pain has been proven entirely safe for the fetus, and all drugs are believed to cross the placenta. Drug companies perform tests under specific conditions of dosage, time during labor, and health of the mother and baby. In cases that do not follow these specific criteria, outcome is undetermined. This does not mean that the physical therapist then warns mothers not to use drugs for labor pain relief.

The role of the physical therapist is to educate expectant parents (without inflicting guilt if the parents decide to use medications) about the risks and benefits of therapeutic drug use and to discuss their concerns with their birth attendant. Parents should be told the effects of medications and anesthetics used by their birth attendant and whether there have been any long-term deficits associated with administration of that drug during labor. There is some evidence to suggest that drugs used during labor may have effects on children, reaching into their school-age years or longer. The decision, then, belongs to the parents to make after they have collected enough information to feel comfortable about using therapeutic drugs during labor without regrets.

Many women who go through labor and birth are disappointed; many are not. Those who are, often say, "Next time it'll be different." This usually means they will obtain a different birth attendant, hospital or setting, or avoid medications. Another factor to consider is that one medication often leads to another and may result in complicating labor. For instance, some drugs slow labor contractions, and because regional anesthesia can also affect motor control, forceps may be required if the mother is unable to push the baby out during delivery. One other point worth mentioning is that the contractions of late labor are generally the most painful, but also, those that last the least amount of time. Often, strong encouragement and support from a spouse or loved one can help the woman bear the last few contractions before the cervix is fully dilated. And, because the contractions of the second stage are usually easier, and involve active pushing, the excitement increases, and the pain decreases.

Despite all the pain, few women who want children avoid subsequent pregnancies because of the labor of the first. The birth of a healthy child, for most women, is worth any amount of pain. Every woman's labor is different, and only she knows the amount of pain she experiences. An informed decision is the goal of education.

Other routes for second stage include pudendal blocks, saddle blocks, inhalation anesthesia, and perineal blocks for episiotomy. These and nature's anesthesia will be discussed in the next chapter.

If a woman decides emphatically that she does not want to take medications unless absolutely necessary, the only other option that is fairly well accepted by physicians, primarily because of consumer demand, is childbirth education. The most popular forms are psychoprophylaxis (ASPO/Lamaze) and variations of relaxation techniques combined with breathing methods.

Psychoprophylaxis is a technique adopted by Dr. Ferdnand Lamaze after he visited Russia, where this breathing and relaxation method was taught to laboring women. Lamaze introduced the idea of the monitrice, or labor attendant, to help women learn these methods. In the 1950s, the method worked its way to the United States, primarily with the assistance of a book *Thank You, Dr. Lamaze,* and promotion by Elisabeth Bing, P.T., who was instrumental in the development of the early childbirth organization and pro-consumer movement. This technique uses physical and psychologic relaxation as a foundation, to which deep, shallow, and paced breathing techniques are added as the pains increase in intensity and frequency. Instructors of other methods utilize relaxation and deep breathing methods more than some Lamaze instructors. Basic philosophies are similar, and classes are eagerly sought by many women. Reasons for the popularity of childbirth education classes center mainly around the need for women to take an active rather than a passive role in the birth of their child. These methods also usually include instruction for the father at the same time, a trend set by Dr. Robert Bradley of the Bradley Method and the American Academy of Husband-Coached Childbirth.

The third alternative for the control of labor pain is TENS. Research on the safety of TENS for use in labor and delivery is scant

### Table 7-4: First Stage Anesthetics: Regional

| Type | Site | Area Numbed | Time to Work How Long Lasts | Side Effects Mother | Baby |
|---|---|---|---|---|---|
| Epidural | Lumbar epidural space | Below navel | 10–20 min 60–90 min | BP ↓ Possible, numbing on 1 side, forceps use | HR ↓ O₂ ↓ |
| Caudal | Sacral below cord | Pelvic area | 10–20 min 60–90 min | Pushing urge ↓ forceps use | HR ↓ |
| Spinal | Spinal fluid | Below injection site | Immediate 60–90 min | BP ↓ Headache, forceps use | O₂ ↓ |

### Table 7-5: First Stage Anesthetics: Local

| Type | Site | Area Numbed | Time to Work How Long Lasts | Side Effects Mother | Baby |
|---|---|---|---|---|---|
| Paracervical | Cervix | Cervix Uterus | 5–20 min 1 hr | Weak or numb LEs | HR ↑↓ |

and inconclusive. [11] Legally, TENS has not been approved for this usage by the Food and Drug Administration. Although some physicians will authorize use of the TENS unit for their patients, a legal challenge of the safety of this has not yet occurred. Because obstetrics is a high-risk profession, malpractice rates for obstetricians are exorbitant. Therefore, the physical therapist practicing obstetrics and using TENS during labor and delivery should be aware of the risks and clarify malpractice insurance coverage with his or her carrier.

Protocol for the application of the TENS electrodes suggests placement on the back over the T10-T12 area during early labor and lower over S2-S4 for delivery to correspond with nerve pathways. Some experimentation has been done suprapubically, but this evidence is mostly anecdotal. The physical therapist interested in conducting a TENS program for obstetric clients would be wise to collect as much documentation as possible to support research in this area. Cases should be well documented and submitted for publication in physical therapy literature.

## Self-Assessment Review

1. Symptoms of pregnancy include _____, _____, and _____.
2. By the third or fourth month of pregnancy the uterus may move _____ into the _____ and relieve the pressure on the _____.
3. Toward the end of term, the fetus may approach the bony pelvis. This event is called _____. Once in the pelvis, _____ has occurred.
4. Warm-up or preparatory contractions of the uterus that begin about the seventh month of pregnancy are called _____.
5. The way the fetus is oriented in the abdomen is described by _____, _____, and _____.
6. Signs of true labor include _____, _____, and _____.
7. Labor may be described by stages and phases. Name and define the stages and phases.
8. Labor may be complicated by problems of _____, _____, or _____.
9. Three ways a woman may obtain relief from labor pain are _____, _____, and _____.
10. The physical therapist using TENS for obstetric clients should obtain physician's authorization, clarify insurance coverage, and _____.

# References

1. Schneider KTM, Huch A, Huch R: Premature contractions: Are they caused by maternal standing? Acta Genet Med Gemellol 34:175-177, 1985.
2. Oxorn H, Foote WR: Human Labor & Birth (3rd ed). New York, Appleton-Century-Crofts, 1975.
3. Elliott JP, Flaherty JF: The use of breast stimulation to prevent postdate pregnancy. Am J Obstet Gynecol 149:628-632, 1984.
4. Jagani N, et al: Role of prostaglandin-induced cervical changes in labor induction. Obstet Gynecol 63:225-229, 1984.
5. McShane PM, Heyl PS, Epstein MF: Maternal and perinatal morbidity resulting from placenta previa. Obstet Gynecol 65:176-182, 1985.
6. Rayburn WF, Lavin JP: Obstetrics for the House Officer. Baltimore, Williams & Wilkins, 1988.
7. Flynn AM, et al: Ambulation in labour. Brit Med J 2:591-593, 1978.
8. Noble E: Controversies in maternal effort during labor and delivery. J Nurs-Midwifery 26(2):13-22, 1981.
9. Kerr-Wilson RHJ, Parham GP, Orr JW: The effect of a full bladder on labor. Obstet Gynecol 62(3):319-323, 1983.
10. Shearer MH: Labor and delivery. In Cooper PJ (ed): Better Homes and Gardens Woman's Health and Medical Guide. Des Moines, Meredith Corp, 1981. PT1
11. Section on Obstetrics and Gynecology, APTA: TENS special issue. Bull Sect Obstet Gynecol, APTA 7(3), 1983.

# EIGHT

# Delivery

Multiple factors determine the duration of labor. These include parity, position and size of the fetus, pelvic shape, cervix malleability, medications or anesthesia, medical interventions, abdominal muscle contractions, contractions of the diaphragm, power of the uterine contractions, and the mother's ability to assist her body in labor and delivery.

## *The Second Stage of Labor*

The stages of labor delineate phases the mother's body goes through during preparation to deliver, delivery of the infant, delivery of the placenta, and return of the uterus to its prepregnant size. The first stage, detailed in the last chapter, includes the time from the onset until the cervix is fully effaced and fully dilated to 10 cm. The second stage encompasses the time of full dilation to delivery of the infant, and usually requires about 20 contractions in the primigravida and 10 or less contractions with multiparas. The median duration of second stage is 50 minutes for primigravidas and 20 minutes for multiparas. Succeeding labors tend to be shorter until the fifth or sixth labor, after which labor tends to lengthen. The shorter labors are credited to a more lax cervix, which offers less resistance. There is, however, an increase in connective tissue in the myometrium after the fifth or sixth delivery that decreases the intensity of uterine contractions.[1]

Pauls, in her study of the relationship between selected variates and the duration of second stage labor (all women were primigravidas with vaginal deliveries and episiotomies), found that about one quarter of the variation in duration related to infant weight (13%) and fetal station (9%).[2] The strength of the abdominal muscles has been thought of as an important variant in the duration of the second stage of labor; however, this study did not substantiate this hypothesis. Maternal positioning, a full bladder, and pelvic floor fatigue are but a few factors that may have an influence on the effectiveness of the abdominal muscles.

The second stage of labor is distinguished by involuntary contractions of the uterus coupled with voluntary pushing by the mother to assist in delivery of the infant (see Figure 8-1). The fetal position changes in the birth canal so that it may accommodate the passageway. Pushing begins after the mother is fully 10 cm dilated, as verified by the physician or midwife. Sometimes the mother will begin bearing down or grunting, signaling that she is experiencing the pushing reflex. She should still be checked for full dilation to avoid possible bruising of the cervix.

The mother is encouraged to work with her uterine contractions, at the same time, relaxing the perineum and allowing the pelvic floor to stretch as comfortably as possible. Once given the go-ahead to push, she should wait until the urge to push is irresistible. She should then take a deep breath and bear down with a steady push, allowing air to escape so that she is not holding her breath against a closed glottis. In this way, she is not susceptible to large fluctuations

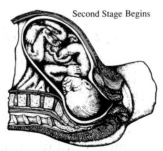

Second Stage Begins

© 1989 PARLAY INTERNATIONAL

Figure 8-1: Second stage of labor. The baby is turning and moving down. The membranes, still intact, are bulging in front of the baby's head.

in blood pressure and is able to maintain respiration while the rib cage, abdominal muscles, and diaphragm interact to supplement the uterine contractions. The mother will often moan and grunt as she releases air through the open glottis. These are natural sounds and should be encouraged to decrease the possibility of prolonged breath holding. When the mother needs to take another breath, she should take that next breath while still maintaining the pressure of the ribs and the abdominal muscles, allowing the diaphragm to ascend slowly. This controlled breathing will decrease the natural backward movement of the infant in the birth canal. Once the baby has crowned, (see Figure 8-2) it may be necessary for the mother to pant, maintaining the baby on the perineum, allowing for the muscles of the pelvic floor to stretch slowly. She will feel an intense burning and stretching, followed by a naturally induced numbness that results when the tissues are fully stretched and blood circulation is depressed. This numbness is referred to as "nature's anesthesia."

An episiotomy may be done when the perineum bulges and the fetal scalp is visible. An episiotomy is an incision of the perineum performed to enlarge the vaginal opening. This is a common, but controversial, obstetric procedure. The two types, midline and mediolateral, are usually performed to prevent extensive lacerations, (see Figure 8-3) fetal head trauma, and postpartum pelvic relaxation from stretching of the endopelvic fascia[3]. Although pain and edema result from an episiotomy, Niswander believes that episiotomies are simpler to repair than lacerations.[3] This, of course, depends on the laceration, but an episiotomy may indeed be larger than a small tear. Perineal massage may help increase the flexibility of the perineum during this crowning phase (when the largest diameter of the presenting part passes through the vaginal opening). Midwives have long advocated perineal massage during pregnancy, labor, and delivery as a way of increasing circulation and increasing flexibility of the perineum. As Niswander states, "Most deliveries can be performed without one (an episiotomy), and the proposed benefits have never been proven."[3]

Second Stage Continues

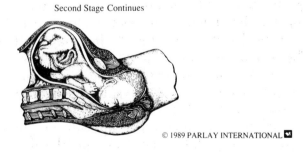

© 1989 PARLAY INTERNATIONAL

Figure 8-2: Second stage continues. The baby's head crowns. Membranes have ruptured.

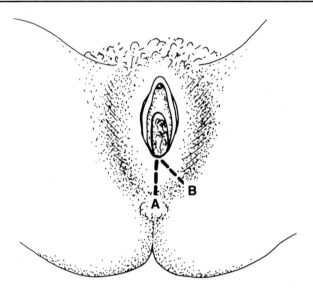

Figure 8-3: Episiotomies: A) midline episiotomy, B) mediolateral episiotomy.

A slow, controlled delivery often results in minimal trauma to the pelvic floor and birth canal. (See Figure 8-4) The mother will be instructed to push the baby out easily, allowing the uterus to readapt to the pressure changes once the baby's head is born. (See Figure 8-5) The shoulders are delivered one at a time, and the mother's bearing down efforts should be controlled for slow, easy delivery. The fetal position changes in the birth canal to accommodate the passageway.

Molding of the infant's head occurs as it passes down the birth canal. The head is usually the widest part of the infant, and this molding, obvious at birth, helps to decrease the overall width of the cranium; molding is possible because the cranial sutures overlap slightly. The cranial bones reapproximate within a few days after birth. The infant's head rotates from a transverse orientation to an anterior alignment (usually occiput anterior, *i.e.*, the presenting fetal occiput faces the anterior of the mother). The vagina expands as the infant's neck extends while passing under the symphysis pubis, which acts as a fulcrum point, and the head emerges. (See Figure 8-4) Between the time that the head is delivered and when the shoulders press on the perineum, the mother may not have an urge to push. The uterus takes a few moments to accommodate to the decreased volume. Yet, the muscle fibers and fundus of the uterus can retract and reduce the size of the uterine cavity within 30 seconds.[4]

Mucus, maternal blood, and amniotic fluid may be seen in the infant's nose or mouth. The midwife or physician will check for loops of the umbilical cord around the neck, slip them off, and aspirate the mucus from the infant's nose and mouth. The infant's head then rotates back toward the original position it had assumed (transverse orientation), and the uppermost anterior shoulder is delivered first. The posterior shoulder, which has been in the hollow of the sacrum, is then delivered. (See Figure 8-5) The rest of the body follows easily. The exact and documented time of birth occurs when all of the infant is outside of the mother's body. This may be before the infant breathes or cries and usually before the cord is cut.

The cord will pulsate for about 2 minutes after delivery, during which time a significant amount of blood will be transferred, depending on the position in which the baby is held. If held at or below the vagina, the placental transfusion may be as much as 100 ml; if held above the mother's uterus, the amount of blood will be much less. The cord should generally be clamped between 20 to 40 seconds postdelivery. However, the cord should be cut promptly if the mother received general anesthesia, or if there is maternal-fetal blood group incompatibility, severe fetal asphyxia, or obvious cardiovascular anomalies requiring resuscitation.

## *The Third Stage of Labor*

The third stage of labor is the delivery of the placenta. Although this occurs in a short period of time, there are many hazards for the mother. Postpartum hemorrhage is the leading cause of maternal death, and manipulations required to decrease blood loss increase the possibility of infection, which can result in illness or death. The placenta will usually separate from the uterine wall spontaneously, 5 to 10 minutes after delivery of the infant, when the sudden reduction in the size of the uterine cavity results in a reduction of the placental site. The placenta, which is noncontractile, cannot change its surface area and, at this time, becomes separated from the uterine wall. If the placenta has not separated after 10 minutes, the attendant will manually remove it with adequate anesthesia administered to the mother. The placenta is examined for possible abnormalities that might suggest congenital anomalies of the newborn. After separation, gentle, firm fundal massage and gentle traction on the cord will assist in delivery of the placenta. Pressure on the abdomen prevents uterine inversion.

After delivery of the placenta, local anesthesia is administered to the perineum for the episiotomy repair. External fundal massage is continued in recovery to help decrease blood loss by encouraging contraction of the uterus. Early suckling of the infant on the mother's breast also increases uterine contractions and is encouraged as soon as possible. Oxytocin may be given to augment uterine contractions, decrease uterine size, and, thereby, decrease blood loss. Oxytocin is often given to women who are susceptible to postpartum hemorrhage (*e.g.*, previous twins, over 35, grand multiparity, hydramnios, prolonged labor, general anesthesia, and postpartum hemorrhage after a previous delivery). Recovery care should continue for at least 1 hour; with 15-minute observations of pulse, blood pressure, consistency and height of the fundus, and amount of uterine bleeding (slight, moderate, heavy).

## *Alternative Birth*

The expectant couple has many options to consider when designing the birth of their baby. They can choose location, who will be present, and often the type of pain management they wish to use if labor is uncomplicated. They may even consider alternative delivery methods or positions.

Options for location include birthing rooms, birthing centers, home births, hospital labor and delivery rooms, or hospital birthing rooms. Hospital birthing rooms are comfortably-designed for labor and delivery. Some feature rocking chairs, decorated bathrooms, and special beds to give the appearance of home. The bed may be sectioned, so that the lower half can be removed and stirrups added, if needed, for delivery. Most complications, however, would necessitate a move to the delivery room. Birthing centers are usually located within 10 minutes of a nearby hospital. Here a family-centered approach to delivery may take place, where mothers may labor with assistance from family and midwives. If a labor or birth is complicated, the mother can be transferred quickly to the local hospital. Birthing centers and even some hospitals now offer programs to prepare siblings to view the birth. These classes generally present discussions of mother's limitations, terms, such as uterus and placenta, labor and delivery, and adjusting to the new family. The sibling is usually forewarned about the possibility of seeing blood and hearing the different sounds of childbirth. Many sessions also include discussion of potential feelings of being left out, sibling rivalry, and jealousy.[5] How much the sibling or siblings are involved in the labor and delivery process depends on the parents. The presence of siblings at birth is a controversial topic, because some believe that children will be frightened at birth and unable to understand its complexities. It appears, however, that with proper explanation and communication of the vast motions and events in a birth, children are able to understand, give support, and bond with their new sibling.

An increase in home births has been noted since the 1970s. This trend has been examined to document consumer dissatisfaction with hospital childbirth and excessive use of technology.[6] The safety of the mother and child is the major concern in any out-of-hospital delivery. In a Michigan study,[6] it was found that better educated women are more likely to make informed choices about their deliveries and take necessary preparations, and that women who choose to deliver at home tend to have higher birth weight babies, a factor that leads to a significant decrease in neonatal mortality. Nevertheless, guidelines are necessary for safe home births. Burst suggests that five criteria must be met to insure safety in alternative out-of-hospital birth settings: (1) attendance by a home-care professional; (2) adherence to strict, stringent screening and transfer criteria; (3) appropriate care at birth; (4) immediate transport be available; and (5) immediate availability of a consulting physician in a hospital.[7]

In the United States, physicians seem to favor mothers positioned on their backs for delivery. In this dorsal lithotomy position, with the mother's legs in stirrups, physicians have easy access to the perineum; unfortunately, prolonged pressure by the stirrups may cause nerve palsies or thrombosis in leg veins. In England, the left lateral side-lying position is preferred; this position physiologically avoids compression of the inferior vena cava by the gravid uterus. Oriental women have long preferred giving birth in the squatting position. This position has the advantage of using gravity to assist the descent of the infant through the birth canal, plus eliminates compression on the inferior vena cava, and allows expansion of the pelvic opening.

Birthing chairs, adjustable recliners with an opening in the seat, were brought back into popularity in the late 1970s as an effective compromise between mothers and obstetricians. The chair may be raised and lowered so that the obstetrician or midwife has maximal ease in delivering the child; and because the mother is upright and assisted by gravity, there is no compression on the inferior vena cava, and perineal support is maintained. There appears to be no change in the length of second-stage labor or time spent in bearing-down efforts while using a birthing chair.[8,9] There have been, however, some cases of vulvar edema resulting from the prolonged use of birthing chairs.[10]

## Pain Management for Delivery

The goal of pain management is to help the mother to easily and effectively work with her body to safely and comfortably deliver her infant. Methods include psychoprophylaxis, analgesics, and narcotics. The mother works with the contractions, bearing down without holding her breath. Forced muscular efforts while breath holding, known as the Valsalva maneuver, may cause large fluctuations in circulation and respiration, and are discouraged. Pushing with a partially closed glottis will lead to the production of a guttural sound. When the presenting part stretches the pelvic floor (as long as there is no anesthesia given), the brain receptors are stimulated to release oxytocin and, thereby, further stimulate contractions.

During delivery, the mother and her partner who have attended childbirth classes will find they use what they have learned. These classes prepare them both for the physical and psychological aspects of childbirth. Not all women have the benefit of partners or classes, however, in which case the midwife, physician, or other attending staff may act as a support person. In delivery, the support person can provide the mother with feedback about the intensity of her pushing efforts, progress on how she is doing, and general encouragement. Because fetal monitors can sometimes detect the beginning of a contraction before the mother can, this technology, if necessary, can be used by the support person, as well, to help the mother prepare for the next contraction. Whether an electronic monitor is used or not, the mother must be encouraged overall to listen, trust, and work with her own body. Her job is to assist the uterine forces by contracting her abdominal muscles, while at the same time relaxing and opening the pelvic floor to allow passage of the infant. Pain during delivery will be increased by fear of the unknown, previous unpleasant experiences, anxiety, insecurity, and anger. The mother may reduce her pain and discomfort, through education, and, as a result, gain confidence, better understand the birth process and need for outside support, learn relaxation, breathing exercises, and distraction techniques, plus develop realistic expectations.

In addition to standard childbirth pain relief methods, some women can use hypnosis for pain relief. They initiate the hypnotic trance once in labor, and continue it throughout delivery. Hypnosis probably works as a pain reliever through suggestion, conditioned reflex, education, and motivation.

If there is evidence of fetal distress, expulsive efforts need to be assisted at the time of delivery, and the need for pain relief is immediate. A mixture of 50% nitrous oxide and 50% oxygen may inhaled during contractions. If there is a need for Cesarean section, however, choices include general anesthesia, subarachnoid block, and epidural analgesia.

General anesthesia is chosen when there is a contraindication for conduction anesthesia, or there is a need for rapid delivery. It is believed that uterine relaxation is maximal with general anesthesia, but it has the disadvantage that the mother needs to be intubated to prevent aspiration of vomitus. Antacid may be given to counteract the effects of aspirations, should they occur, and an injection of thiopental 4 mg/kg may be used with an injection of a muscle relaxant (*e.g.*, succinylcholine 1 to 1.5 mg/kg) to facilitate intubation. Muscle relaxants have a low transmissibility across the placenta due to their low lipid solubility, high water solubility, and high ionization. Anesthesia is maintained with inhalation of enflurane, halothane, isoflurane, or similar agents.

Subarachnoid blockage is used for Cesarean section when there is no critical fetal distress or urgency. Spinal anesthesia has the advantage that the mother is awake, and her reflexes are intact; therefore, aspiration pneumonia is less of a problem. There is a lower risk of cardiovascular or central nervous system toxicity, as well. This regional anesthetic is given in one dose, injected into the subarachnoid space to achieve a dermatomal block up to T5. This produces anesthesia for all the pelvic organs and nerves supplying the pelvis and abdomen. The injection may consist of 5% lidocaine, 1% tetracaine, or 0.75% bupivacaine, and a 7.5% dextrose mixture. The main disadvantage is that spinal anesthesia may cause maternal hypotension. To counteract this problem, the uterus is displaced to the left so that good venous return to the heart may be maintained. Epinephrine can be administered in 10 mg increments to maintain blood pressure between 90% and 100% of its original level. Blood pressure is continuously monitored, and oxygen can be given by mouth, if necessary.

Epidural analgesia for Cesarean section can be dangerous because of the increased possibility of cardiovascular and central nervous system toxicity. It is superior to spinal anesthesia, because encroachment on respiratory function is less. With continual, carefully titrated dosage, the block can be maintained for postoperative analgesia as well. Generally, epidural success rate for Cesarean section is lower than with the spinal and is more complicated, but it is valuable in conditions where sudden and marked fluctuations in blood pressure impose a great risk.[3]

## *Complicated Deliveries*

Complicated deliveries often follow dysfunctional labor, precipitous labor, or dystocia secondary to pelvic and fetal factors. Danforth describes the four "Ps" that are concerned with influencing the success and failure of delivery: (1) the powers, which represent the expulsive forces of the contracting uterus; (2) the pelvic architecture and its boundaries; (3) the passenger (the fetus) as it passes through the pelvis and birth canal; and (4) the psyche of the mother, which has an important impact on the force and duration of labor and delivery.[1]

Precipitous labor and delivery occur in 10% of all deliveries.[4] This indicates completion of the first and second stages of labor in less than 1 hour. It occurs more in multiparas than in primigravidas. The infant is sometimes injured during this rapid, uncontrolled labor because of the force on the presenting part. The baby should be delivered in as safe a place as possible, and no anesthesia should be given to delay delivery. The diagnosis is often made by serial pelvic exams that reveal a rapid cervical dilation accompanied by severe, violent contractions. There is no known etiology for precipitous labor. Patients who have had one precipitous labor are prone to subsequent ones, however. The infant needs to be evaluated, postdelivery, for possible fetal intracranial bleeding and depression.

A breech presentation is one in which any part other than the fetal head is the presenting part. The fetal sacrum becomes the designated reference point. There is a 4% incidence of breech presentation. Breech births are defined by the posture of the lower extremities of the infant: frank breech, complete breech, footling breech. A frank breech (see Figure 8-6) refers to hips that are flexed and legs extended, so that the feet are at the level of the chin. In a complete breech (see Figure 8-6), the infant's legs are fully crossed at the level of the buttocks, so that it is sitting in a tailor fashion. A footling (single or double) or incomplete breech (see Figure 8-6) means that one or both of the feet and legs are extended through the birth canal.

Breech presentations that can be delivered vaginally should meet the following criteria:

Second Stage Ends

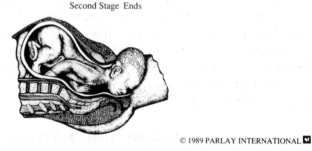

© 1989 PARLAY INTERNATIONAL

Figure 8-4: Second stage ends as the baby's head emerges from the vaginal opening and lifts upward.

Birth

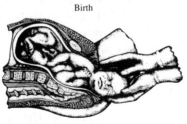

© 1989 PARLAY INTERNATIONAL

Figure 8-5: The baby's head turns as it is being born, and the shoulders rotate.

1. fetal weight is between 2500 to 3500 gm, [11]
2. the pelvis must be able to accommodate the fetus without hyperextending the fetal neck during vaginal breech delivery (the risk of spinal cord transection is 25%),
3. labor progression must be normal (labor longer than 18 hours will often proceed to a Cesarean section),
4. fetal heart rate patterns must be normal and fetal monitoring continuous, and
5. prepregnancy weight must be less than 180 pounds (with increased maternal size, there is an increase in perinatal morbidity due to inability to estimate fetal weights),
6. a complete or footling breech presentation associated with a high risk of prolapsed cord requires the cervix to be completely dilated to avoid entrapping the fetal head.

The mortality of vaginal breech deliveries is 5.5 times that of infants presenting head first. The major causes of perinatal deaths in breech births are cord prolapse, other cord complications, tentorial tears, and cerebral hemorrhage of the after-coming head. The molding of the infant's head, which usually takes several hours, must occur in moments. As a result, sudden stresses that may be highly damaging are placed on the infant's cranium. This is especially true in a preterm infant whose head is larger than the presenting part, and the cervix and lower uterine segment are dilated only enough for the passage of the presenting part.Other injuries include damage to the spinal cord, liver, adrenal glands, or spleen (from abdominal manipulations), and delayed responses to injury that can include cerebral palsy, learning disorders, and cerebral dysfunction.

If a vaginal delivery is selected, the infant is allowed to deliver to its umbilicus, usually with a wide episiotomy. The umbilical cord is pulled down to prevent any tension. The infant's thighs are flexed and abducted to deliver the feet and legs, then traction is applied to the infant's body with a downward rotation of the chest, away from the shoulder to be delivered. The fetus's arm is flexed across its chest and splinted; then, with traction and 180-degree rotation, the posterior shoulder is advanced to the anterior position, and that shoulder and arm are delivered. The head is often delivered by forceps with gentle flexion and suprapubic pressure, which will assist in maintaining the infant's head in flexion during the descent.

Shoulder dystocia is a serious obstetric problem that occurs when the infant's shoulders are too large for the pelvic inlet. Diagnosis is made after the head is delivered and downward pressure exerted on the head meets with obstruction from the pubic bone. The incidence of shoulder dystocia is 1.5 in 1000 deliveries; and in babies over

4000 gm, 17 in 1000 deliveries.[2] An ultrasound evaluation of the bisacromial-to-head/diameter ratio has been suggested as a screening for shoulder dystocia. Infants with an estimated weight of more than 4500 gm should be delivered by Cesarean section. Management includes a large episiotomy and fundal pressure and attempts to dislodge the anterior shoulder while exerting modest pressure on the fetal head. Stretching of the fetal neck can result in brachial plexus injuries. Flexion of the mother's leg (MacRobert's maneuver) has the effect of straightening her sacrum relative to the lumbar spine, which may free the impacted shoulder. Other maneuvers involve delivery of the infant's posterior shoulder first or purposely fracturing the infant's clavicle, a difficult procedure to perform.

## *Forceps*

Two types of obstetric forceps are used today; classic forceps with cephalic curves or pelvic curves, and specially-designed forceps for specific problems, such as breech birth or unusual head presentations. In the past, forceps were applied to the pelvis without regard to the position of the fetal head. This application is rarely used today (unless under most extraordinary circumstances), because it places forces on the head that the fetus cannot tolerate. Generally, in modern obstetrics, if the forceps cannot be applied properly to the fetal head, a Cesarean section is indicated. Conversely, in a cephalic application, the forceps are placed along the occipitomental diameter of the head (occiput to chin). Forceps may also be used for the after-coming head as in a breech presentation.

Low forceps or outlet forceps are used to supply the final force needed to deliver the infant's head through the vaginal opening. If the infant's head does not emerge after it has descended to the pelvic floor, forceps can be indicated, especially if there is prolonged pressure on the fetal head. The following four criteria must be met before forceps are to be used: (1) the scalp must be, or has been, visible at the introitus without separating the labia, (2) the skull must have reached the pelvic floor, (3) the sagittal suture must be in the sagittal plane of the pelvis, and (4) the membranes must be ruptured. Anesthesia and an episiotomy are part of this procedure.[1] Because of the controversy over when low forceps can be used safely, a standardized description of use has not been developed.

The American College of Obstetricians and Gynecologists defines other forceps operations. Mid-forceps is the application of forceps to the fetal head after it is engaged.[1] Danforth suggests that definition be expanded to include that mid-forceps delivery be limited to use when the fetal head lies at a station between 0 and +3.[3] Mid-forceps delivery has changed greatly in the last 19 years. Reviews of mid-forceps delivery have revealed a high incidence of neonatal death and increased frequency of long-term intellectual deficits among the survivors. A high-forceps operation was previously used to apply forceps before the fetal head was engaged in the pelvis. This type of procedure deferred to Cesarean section and is now obsolete.

Vacuum extraction has been found, in some cases, to be less traumatic than forceps to the infant and the birth canal. The extractor consists of a cup, a rubber hose, and a pump. The cup is inserted into the vagina without an episiotomy and secured to the occiput of the infant. The air is pumped out so the cap forms a partial vacuum to the fetal occiput. Traction is then applied to the hose sufficient to pull the head through the birth canal. The vacuum extractor has been found to be easier to use in multiparas and in patients with a transverse arrest than in primigravidas or in those with an occiput posterior presentation.[3] Although this device shows a great deal of promise, it has shown an alarming association with shoulder dystocia and hematoma.

## Cesarean

Cesarean section, or laparotrachelotomy, refers to delivery of fetuses 500 gm or more by abdominal surgery requiring an incision through the uterine wall. Cesarean sections are one of the earliest operations known and have been traced to Rome during the reign of Numa Pompilius 715-672 B.C. He decreed that any woman who died late in pregnancy was to have the child removed from her womb. This law continued under Caesar, when it acquired the name *lex caesarea.* Another explanation for its name, is from the Latin words, *caedare* (to cut), and *caesareus* (abdominal birth).

Attempts were made in the 17th and 18th centuries to save the mothers; all but a few died from hemorrhage or infection. In the mid-1800s, Edoardo Porro discovered that by doing the Cesarean hysterectomy, he was able to circumvent the problem of uterine hemorrhage and save the mother as well as the child.

Prior to 1960, Cesareans were performed only when a mother was dying, to deliver a viable infant, or to save the mother's life when labor was obstructed. Between 1960 and 1965, the reported Cesarean rate was 5% of all deliveries made. Today, hospitals and clinics report a range of deliveries by Cesarean section from 12% to 25%.[1,3] Expectedly, perinatal mortality has decreased with the rise in Cesarean sections; however, there is a three to four times greater risk of maternal mortality with a Cesarean than with a vaginal birth (8-10 deaths per 10,000 with Cesarean delivery versus 2.7 deaths per 10,000 deliveries with vaginal deliveries).[3]

The four general indications for Cesarean section are: 1. when delivery of the infant is necessary but cannot be induced 2. when labor is unsafe for the infant or mother 3. when fetal and maternal dystocia contraindicate a vaginal delivery 4. when an emergency situation demands immediate delivery, and a vaginal delivery is not possible. Specifically, indications for a Cesarean include failure to progress, pelvic disproportion, malpresentation, fetal distress, pregnancy-induced hypertension, mothers with placenta previa or abruptio placenta, prolapse of the umbilical cord, diabetes mellitus, herpes progenitalis, severe Rh incompatibility, failed forceps delivery, failed induction of labor, and sometimes repeat Cesarean section.[3]

There are two major techniques for performing a Cesarean section. In cases of prematurity, before the lower uterine segments have formed sufficiently, in placenta previa, and when the infant is lying in a transverse position, the incision is made longitudinally in the anterior wall of the uterus. Often, these incisions extend into the fundal area, constituting a classical type of Cesarean section (see Figure 8-7A).

In this classical incision, the Cesarean operation proceeds rapidly with the layers of the abdomen opened and the abdominal wall retracted, bladder reflected, vessels clamped, and pads put in place to decrease the amount of amniotic fluid entering the peritoneum. The underlying veins in the broad and cardinal ligaments are avoided, because the incision is made laterally without entering the broad ligament. Fingers are insinuated between the uterine wall and the fetal head. The most preferred incision in the United States is the low-segment approach (see Figure 8-7B), because it is associated

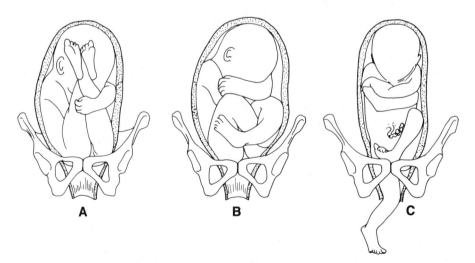

Figure 8-6: Types of breech presentations: A) Frank breech, B) Complete or full breech, C) Single footing breech.

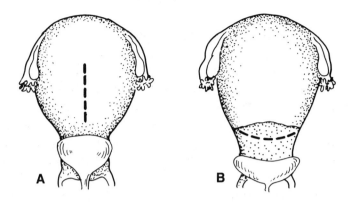

Figure 8-7: Cesarean sections: A) Classic incision, B) Transverse incision made in the lower portion of the uterus with the bladder displaced downward.

with a lower immediate and later morbidity. The incision is made in the peritoneum overlying the lower uterine segment. The bladder is dissected away from the lower segment, and the deeper incision is made to the uterus transversely in the noncontractile portion. With pressure on the fundus, the fetal head pushes up through the incision, and the nose and mouth are then suctioned. The shoulders are delivered one at a time after this. After the fetus is extracted, it is placed head down to facilitate drainage from the mouth and nose and decrease the chance of aspiration. The cord is clamped and cut. The placenta is removed and layers of the uterus and abdominal wall are approximated and sutured in layers. Oxytocin is given to augment the uterine contractions. Care is given to the mother's legs to decrease the risk of developing thrombophlebitis and thromboembolism. Spontaneous movements of the legs and early ambulation are strongly suggested.

## Vaginal Births After Cesarean

Despite the famous dictum of 1916 made by Edward Cragin, M.D., to the Eastern Medical Society of New York, "Once a Cesarean section, always a Cesarean section," more and more women who have had Cesarean births now demand a chance to deliver vaginally. In response to this demand, the New York State Health Department has started a statewide program to reduce the rate of Cesarean sections. In 1988, Cesareans accounted for 20% of all New York births. State medical experts, however, believe that many of those were unnecessary, and they have set up an independent team to review each Cesarean procedure.[12]

The major concern for vaginal birth after Cesarean (VBAC), is the increased possibility of uterine rupture (i.e., the uterine surgical scar will be unable to withstand the forceful labor contractions). Rupture of the uterus is very serious but occurs only once in every 1500 to

2000 deliveries, most often as the result of a rupture of a scar from previous Cesarean sections or from direct trauma.

Rarely, in labor, the anterior lip of the uterus may be pinched as the head descends between the pubic bone, often following cephalopelvic disproportion. The uterus may become edematous and rupture at the lower segment and may tear the entire cervix (annular amputation). The entrapped lip may be freed by the physician or midwife by disengaging the head and pushing the anterior lip upwards with the fingers. Injuries to the lower segment of the uterus can result from cephalopelvic disproportion or malposition. Because the presenting part cannot descend through the pelvis, muscle fibers in the upper segment continually contract and retract. The lower segment is then thin and stretched to the point of separation.

Traumas causing rupture include excessive oxytocin in patients with obstructed labor and those from surgical delivery, such as version, breech extraction, and manual removal of the placenta.[4] Symptoms include sudden abdominal pain followed by blood loss. Treatment consists of surgery, Cesarean section, blood transfusion, and, possibly, a hysterectomy if there is extensive rupture.

The incidence of uterine rupture following VBAC actually ranges from 0.0% to 2.8%. Seventy percent to 80% of women who do not have a recurrent indication for the primary Cesarean have a successful vaginal delivery. However, this rate is definitely decreased in those who had a prior Cesarean section because of cephalopelvic disproportion and may be reduced further in women with a history of failed induction.

In women with a classic Cesarean section incision, there is a substantially increased chance of uterine rupture over those with a low transverse scar. If rupture occurs, it is more likely to be a complete rupture and result in perinatal death. There has been no objective evidence to support the thought that multiple Cesarean sections predispose women to increased uterine rupture in subsequent pregnancies. An extensive review of the literature from 1950 to 1980 showed some surprising results about vaginal deliveries in patients with prior Cesareans. It was found that with a properly conducted vaginal delivery after Cesarean, there was a 0.7% incidence of uterine rupture, a 0.93% incidence of perinatal mortality, and no maternal deaths associated with uterine rupture. In 1974, however, 99% of those patients who had a previous Cesarean section were delivered by repeat Cesareans in American hospitals. Although controversy continues about the safety of vaginally delivering breech presentations and twins after previous Cesarean sections, a review by Lavin shows that many breeches and twins have been delivered successfully in women with prior Cesareans.[13]

In VBAC, use of oxytocin is believed to increase the risk of uterine rupture and decrease the chance of a successful delivery. There are apparently no ill effects, but physicians' opinions are divided as to whether to artificially rupture amniotic membranes or not. If ruptured, internal fetal monitors may be used early. The use of anesthesia for VBAC is also debated. Some believe that with anesthesia, the mother's inability to perceive pain, especially in uterine rupture, would be masked. Lavin, however, emphasized the unreliability of abdominal pain as a symptom of uterine rupture, and this pain may actually be secondary to peritoneal adhesions, round ligament tension, hypersensitive bladder, or scarring of the abdominal wall.[13]

The duration for labor in VBAC was found to conform to the norms for delivery of patients without a history of Cesarean section, and there is no evidence to support the routine use of forceps. Postpartum exam is encouraged to assess scar integrity, but the medical need for this test is uncertain. Most agree that the following criteria must be met to be a candidate for VBAC:

1. no indication for Cesarean section in the current pregnancy
2. previous low transverse incision, documented in hospital records
3. mother is admitted to hospital when labor begins
4. mother is blood-typed and cross-matched
5. mother is carefully monitored, and the obstetrician is present during labor
6. the facility and personnel must be ready to perform an immediate Cesarean, if needed
7. the mother must be counseled about risks and benefits, and informed consent must be obtained.[1314]

Because over 90% of all Cesareans in the United States today are performed with a low transverse incision,[15] chances are increasing that women will not have a repeat Cesarean section simply because they needed one in the past. The benefits of such a trend will be increased participation by the parents in delivery, less recovery time, more comfort, and reduced financial costs.

## Multifetal Birth

Most mothers with twin gestations will go into labor by 37 to 38 weeks and those with triplets and quadruplets at 35 and 34 weeks, respectively. Consequently, more than 50% of all twins will be delivered at 37 weeks and will weigh less than 2500 gm. Presentation is very important in the delivery of twins, because statistics show that the first twin will present head down in 80% of all cases, but the second in only 50%. Other combinations (first twin to second twin) occur with varying frequencies: cephalic-cephalic, 39%; cephalic-breech, 37%; breech-breech, 10%; cephalic-transverse, 8%; breech-transverse, 5%; and transverse-transverse, 1%.

Another potential combination (also a complication) is fetal interlocking, which occurs in 1 of every 817 twin deliveries. This usually occurs at or below the pelvic inlet, and usually the first twin is breech. The neck of the first baby is elongated and locked above the head of the second. Other entanglements, termed collisions, occur above the pelvic brim. When both heads try to descend at the same time, neither is able to enter the pelvis. Usually, Cesarean section is indicated for a collision situation or where twins are conjoined.

When a vaginal delivery is desired with twins, the physician or midwife must be skilled in podalic version. Podalic version describes the external or internal manual manipulation of the fetal position while *in utero*. Forty percent of second twins require a manipulative delivery. It is suggested that a Cesarean section be done when one twin is of low birth weight or when either infant is in a malposition. Low birth weight, prematurity, and intrauterine growth retardation put the malpositioned fetus at a higher risk for head entrapment and complications of a traumatic delivery.

With twins, the cervix only needs to dilate once, but the uterus must contract for both deliveries. The first twin is delivered as any infant previously described. There is some discussion, however, regarding how long to wait before delivery of the second infant. Classic obstetric instruction suggests a wait of 5 to 20 minutes after the first twin,[1] unless there is bleeding or fetal distress. Noble states that a midwifery text from the last century describes a 4-hour wait before intervention. She further points out that until recently, 30 minutes were generally allowed to elapse between births, so that the uterus could adjust and prepare for the next delivery.[16]

However, the membranes of the second twin usually rupture (depending on the sac configuration) within 5 minutes after delivery of the first twin, and longer waits for the delivery may result in placental insufficiency, premature separation, cervical retraction, and cord accidents.[6] The second twin will most likely change position after delivery of the first and be delivered either head first, breech, or by Cesarean. If the second is in an undesirable position and cannot be helped by internal or external inversion or is distressed, Cesarean section is performed in about 40% of the cases. Occasionally, low forceps may be needed to facilitate delivery.

After either spontaneous or manual delivery of the placenta, it is inspected to determine zygosity and any vascular communications between the twins. Oxytocin is given to augment uterine contractions. Because the uterus is arranged in layers, contraction of the layers cuts off any bleeding vessels and prevents hemorrhage from the placental site. The uterus is manually explored for rupture which may have occurred during the manipulative maneuver. A fundal massage is also given to stimulate uterine contractions. Early suckling of the twins at the mother's breast will stimulate uterine contraction.

## Repair of Lacerations and Episiotomy

The birth canal, cervix, vagina, and perineum should be inspected for lacerations after delivery. Some damage to the soft tissue structures (of the birth canal and surrounding organs) usually occurs after every delivery, especially in primigravidas, because the firm tissues are more resistant to the delivery of the infant. Perineal lacerations are categorized into four types, depending on their depth:

1. a first-degree laceration extends through the skin and superficial structures above the muscles
2. second-degree lacerations are tears that extend through the muscles of the perineum
3. a third-degree laceration tears into the sphincter
4. a fourth-degree laceration includes a tear in the anterior wall of the rectum, as well. These injuries occur if the vaginal opening is stretched too quickly or overdistended during delivery, usually by the infant's head. If the perineum is torn, the lower vagina is also injured, and tears that involve the medial surfaces of the labia minora bleed profusely because of the many veins in this area. Any tears in the perineum are repaired immediately, the layers of tissue approximated by absorbable sutures. Special care is given to the repair of third- and fourth-degree lacerations. Local anesthesia is administered to the perineal wall before intestinal sutures are placed. Frequent ice packs on the perineum after stitching will reduce swelling and increase the mother's comfort. It is suggested that the stools be kept soft for several days so that the sutures are not overstressed during elimination.

Vaginal lacerations may result at the level of the ischial spines or in the vault of the vagina. Vaginal tears are usually circular and result from using forceps in a rotational manner. These lacerations may bleed profusely and are repaired with catgut sutures. Careful investigation is warranted to insure that all tears are inspected and repaired. Injuries to the anterior vaginal wall may be accompanied by injuries to the bladder neck and urethral wall, if they are compressed against the posterior surface of the pubic bones or pushed ahead of the infant's presenting part.

If the pelvis is small, the delivery precipitous, or the infant unusually large, more damage than usual will occur. As the uterus contracts, the soft tissue structures are pushed ahead and will eventually stretch and become injured. Injury to the bladder may also occur if it is distended or if the presenting part is high. The mother should be catheterized if she cannot void.

If posterior lacerations are not repaired to give support to the rectal walls, the levator bundles will retract laterally and destroy the perineal body, thereby eliminating the normal support of the lower vagina. When standing, the weight of the abdomen will then increase the descent of the rectal wall; it will increase with each rectal movement and result in a rectocele (rectum protrudes into the vagina and forms a large pouch). After menopause, with the withdrawal of estrogen hormones, a preexisting rectocele will increase rapidly.

An episiotomy decreases the resistance of the muscles and fascia posteriorly, and endopelvic fascia may be injured even if the skin and vaginal wall appeared uninjured. As the head descends through the vaginal canal, the levator bundles are separated, and the levator fascia is stretched. Often, the fascial layers will tear, allowing the levator to separate and laterally retract. This is especially true if the labor is forceful and the structures are torn apart rather than stretched slowly. If the mother has a narrow pubic arch, the infant's head cannot fit closely beneath the symphysis, and it will be forced backward toward the posterior pelvis putting added strain on the soft tissues. Wilson advocates episiotomy to avoid posterior wall injury, the use of regional or local anesthesia before episiotomy, and that episiotomy be done before the tissues have been injured. He argues that episiotomy performed on an overstretched, blanched perineum offers no protection to the deep fascia and muscles, also stretched to the maximum.

## *Injuries Involving Uterine Support*

The cardinal ligaments rarely become torn during labor and delivery, but they may be stretched a great deal if labor is delayed by cephalopelvic disproportion, or if delivery is forced before full cervical dilation. If the supporting ligaments are stretched or injured during labor and the vaginal wall compromised, the uterus can invert and distend towards the introitus. In a first-degree prolapse, the cervix lies between the ischial spines and the vaginal opening. In a second-degree prolapse, the cervix protrudes through the vaginal opening. The cervix in the third-degree position is completely pro-lapsed, and the vaginal canal is inverted. The advanced stages of uterine prolapse seem to occur in postmenopausal women with atrophied tissues, causing diminished uterine support. Treatment consists of surgical repair through the vagina to reposition a cysto-cele, rectocele, and the uterus. After delivery, a cystocele may de-velop where the bladder protrudes downward into the vaginal canal as a result of the supporting structures in the vesicovaginal septum losing their integrity. The weak anterior vaginal wall will descend due to the force of gravity and weight of the abdominal contents when standing. Added stresses from straining, lifting, and coughing, along with the added weight of the bladder, will stress the septum until the bladder bulges into the vagina. Cystoceles that produce a bulge in the vagina and cause difficulty voiding are often repaired surgically through the vaginal levator sling.

Some women develop a mild incontinence after the delivery of a child, often the result of injury during childbirth to the urethrovesi-cal junction and urethra. Anatomically, the posterior urethrovesical angle changes, and the relationship of the urethra to the pubis changes (see Chapter 12). The amount of incontinence depends on how much damage was done and the amount of recovery that has taken place postinjury. Multiparous women may experience stress incontinence during menstruation, and in cases of extreme dysfunc-tion, the incontinence may continue throughout the entire month.

### Retrodisplacement of the uterus
Retrodisplacement, wherein the uterus rests posteriorly, may result from congenital anomaly, from adhesions from pelvic inflammatory disease or endometriosis, or may develop after childbirth when sup-porting structures are injured. If the retrodisplaced uterus is en-larged, there may be low back pain, pelvic pressure, dyspareunia, and interference with rectal evacuation. Treatment may include a pessary to hold the uterus in place, which remains in place for 2 to 3 months.

### Injury to the pelvic joints
The symphysis pubis tends to separate to some extent during deliv-ery. If, however, there is a great deal of force used, or if the baby is unusually large, the symphysis pubis may be injured. If so, the mother will experience severe pain in the symphysis pubis and pos-sibly the sacroiliac joint on weightbearing. The pubic bones will appear abnormally separated and the symphyseal area may be ex-tremely tender. Increased mobility is noted and the bone ends may shift several centimeters when the woman shifts weight from one

foot to the other. Urine may be bloody from injury to the bladder neck and urethra. Treatment includes instruction in comfort positions and mobility instruction, plus immobilization of the pelvic girdle by a tight binder. The mother is also advised to avoid widely abducted legs, walking on uneven terrain, large strides, and exaggerated pelvic movements. Heat and activities to decrease pain and increase healing are recommended.

Occasionally, the coccyx can become dislocated or even fractured during delivery. The mother will most likely complain of localized pain in the coccyx area and, possibly, radiation down both legs. With digital manipulation through the rectum, the dislocated coccyx can be felt overlying the sacrum and may be reduced. Ice or heat, and perhaps a donut pillow or TENS, plus instruction in comfort positions may help relieve pain.

## Genital Fistulas

Genital fistulas, requiring surgical repair, are abnormal openings between two internal organs. Fistulas of the vesicovaginal, vesicocervical, or vesicouterine (opening between the bladder and the genital tract), rectovaginal fissure (opening between the rectum and the vagina), or ureterovaginal (opening between the ureter and vagina), can be caused by injuries during labor and delivery, surgical trauma, or radiation. Vesicovaginal, rectovaginal, or ureterovaginal fistulas can result from intrapartum injury or from later avascular necrosis in response to the crushing of pelvic organs between the presenting fetal part and the bony pelvis. Diagnoses are confirmed by clinical exam and by cystoscopy and pyelography.

## Self-Assessment Review

1. Cephalopelvic disproportion refers to _____.
2. A third-degree laceration of the perineum is a tear _____.
3. A cystocele is _____.
4. _____, _____, and _____ may influence the duration of the second stage of labor.
5. Stress incontinence often results from injury during birth to the _____ and _____.
6. Breech birth refers to a presenting part _____.
7. Shoulder dystocia occurs when _____.
8. VBAC means _____, and the major risk is believed to be _____, although studies do not prove this to be true.
9. Four generalized indications for Cesarean are:

_____, _____, _____, and
_____.

10. Usually, mothers with twins will go into labor by
_____ or _____ weeks.

## *References*

1. Danforth DV, Scott JR (eds): Obstetrics and Gynecology (5th ed). Philadelphia, JB Lippincott, 1986.
2. Pauls J: The relationship between selected variates and the duration of second stage labor. J Obstet Gynecol PT 10(4):6-9, 1986.
3. Niswander KR (ed): Manual of Obstetrics Diagnosis and Therapy (3rd ed). Boston, Little, Brown & Co, 1987.
4. Wilson JR, Carrington ER, Ledger WJ: Obstetrics and Gynecology. St. Louis, CV Mosby, 1983.
5. Malecki MP: Mom and Dad and I are Having a Baby. Seattle, Pennypress, 1982.
6. Simmons R, Bernstein S: Out-of-hospital births in Michigan 1972-79. Public Health Regs 98:161-170, 1983.
7. Burst H: Issues and concerns of healthy pregnant women. Public Health Regs (Suppl) 102:57-61, 1987.
8. Stewart P, Hillan E, Calder A: A randomised trial to evaluate the use of a birth chair for delivery. Lancet 1:1296-1298, 1983.
9. Liddell HS, Fisher PR: The birthing chair in the second stage of labour. Aust NZ J Obstet Gynecol 25(1):65-68, 1985.
10. Goodlin RC, Frederick IB: Postpartum vulvar edema associated with the birthing chair. Am J Obstet Gynecol 146(3):334, 1983.
11. Queenan JT, Hobbins JC (eds): Protocols for High-Risk Pregnancies (2nd ed). Oradell, New Jersey, Medical Economics Books, 1987.
12. Effort launched by New York to reduce Cesarean sections. PT Bull Feb 22, 1989:7.
13. Lairn JP, et al: Vaginal delivery in patients with a prior Cesarean section. Obstet Gynecol 59(135):135-148, 1982.
14. Keolkirk K: Vaginal Birth after Cesarean. Seattle, Pennypress, 1981.
15. Eglinton GS, et al: Outcome of a trial of labor after prior Cesarean delivery. J Reprod Med 29(1):3-8, 1984.
16. Noble E: Having Twins. Boston, Houghton-Mifflin, 1980.

# NINE

# Postpartum

The puerperium is generally thought of as beginning following the delivery of the placenta and ending about 6 to 8 weeks after that, although some references suggest the postpartum period ends with the resumption of the menstrual cycle. In nursing mothers, the puerperium is not as clearly defined because lactation delays ovulation for weeks or months. Many dramatic changes occur during this time as the uterus shrinks, the birth canal and perineum repair, and the endocrine system rebalances.

## *The Uterus*

At delivery, the uterus weighs about 1000 gm and measures 14 cm long, 12 cm wide, and 10 cm thick, about the size it is at 16 weeks of pregnancy. Within a week, it weighs 500 gm and decreases in size so that it again lies within the true pelvis. This decrease is attributed to the decrease in both the amount of cytoplasm and size of the individual cells.[1] Uterine contractions increase in intensity after delivery, probably because of the decreased uterine volume within the surrounding, contracting myometrium. After the first 1 to 2 hours, these contractions are diminished and become uncoordinated. However, when oxytocin is released in response to the baby's suckling, the uterine contractions (after pains) can once again become smooth, intense, and coordinated and continue through the beginning of the puerperium. They can become quite severe in the multipara.

Exfoliation occurs at the placental site of attachment. The shedding of the endometrial tissue prevents scar formation. The outermost layer of decidua becomes necrotic after the first few days. Consequently, the sloughed tissue of serum and leukocytes makes up the vaginal discharge. Within the third week postpartum, the cells of the endometrial glands (in the remaining decidua) grow across the bare surface and complete regeneration of the area.

Lochia is the name given to the vaginal discharge after delivery. It undergoes many changes during the next 4 to 6 weeks. In the first 6 to 8 days, it is called lochia rubra because of its bright red color and consists of decidua, blood, and trophoblastic material. For the next several days it becomes more serous and darker and is termed lochia serosa; it is made up of sloughed tissue, leukocytes, old blood, and serum. During the following 2 weeks, the lochia becomes whitish-yellow, and is composed of decidua, leukocytes, epithelial cells, serum, bacteria, and mucus. This latter form of lochia is called lochia alba because of its whitish color.

The cervix constricts and returns to its prepregnancy shape in about 2 weeks postdelivery. The cervix undergoes dramatic remodeling from a maximally effaced and dilated condition at delivery to its normally closed position. The vagina resumes its nonpregnant size by 6 to 8 weeks. The introitus is red and swollen, especially locally around an episiotomy or lacerations. Ice packs initially help decrease pain and swelling of the perineum. After 1 or 2 days, sitz baths and careful cleaning, perhaps with a water-filled squeeze bottle, are recommended to help avoid infection and irritation to the healing sutures of an episiotomy and to promote healing. It is believed that pelvic floor exercises started immediately after delivery will help to restore the perineum by increasing circulation and tightening stretched perineal muscles.

## Urinary Tract

There is often trauma to the urethra and bladder after the birth of the baby through the vaginal canal. The bladder wall may be swollen and hyperemic, and there may be slight bleeding in the muscle. The bladder may also be insensitive to the intravesical pressures that stimulate urination. This insensitivity will be even more marked if anesthesia has been used in labor. The mother must empty the bladder frequently to avoid over distention and to help the bladder return to normal function. Some women need a catheter.

Due to diaphoresis during the first week postdelivery, urinary output will greatly exceed intake. The glomerular filtration rate remains elevated to handle the increased urine flow, often reaching 3 L per 24 hours.[1] Physiologic proteinuria may appear during the first week and less often, glycosuria, but these usually resolve within a few days. The ureters and renal pelves return to their normal prepregnant size within 6 weeks.

## *Gastrointestinal Tract*

There is a minor slowing of intestinal motility, in an unmedicated birth, which may be intensified if the mother received anesthesia. Early ambulation, a diet rich in fiber, and a mild laxative will assist in normal motility. If there has been a third- or fourth-degree laceration into the rectal sphincter, laxatives are often prescribed to eliminate straining the rectal wall during bowel movements. In addition, mothers often experience hemorrhoids following delivery due to the increased pressure on the rectal veins from pushing. Sitz baths, laxatives, commercial preparations, and pelvic floor and abdominal exercises tend to stimulate healing and decrease swelling of mild hemorrhoids.

## *Circulation*

An initial heat loss in the postpartum mother results from delivery of the infant and placenta and loss of amniotic fluid, possibly resulting in shaking and chills. Cardiac output after the first minute postpartum may increase approximately 40% to 50% above prelabor values, but should return to nonpregnant values by 2 to 3 weeks postpartum. These changes are due to fluctuations in stroke volume. There is little change in blood pressure, however. With the decreased size of the uterus and descent of the diaphragm, normal cardiac access is restored, and an electrocardiogram at this time will show normalized features.[1] Blood volume changes will depend on the amount of blood lost during delivery and the amount of extravascular water excreted. In the first 72 hours, there is a greater decrease in plasma volume than in cellular components. Consequently, there is a slight increase in the hematocrit level as compared to immediate postpartum levels. Volume changes and reduced pressures often result in the resolution of lower extremity or vulvar varicosities after delivery.

## *Musculoskeletal*

Postpartum abdominal muscle tone is very slack, and the muscles may not provide adequate support for the trunk, specifically for the low back. Ligaments are still under hormonal influences as well. Therefore, the back is at greater risk for injury due to this lack of support and lack of protective ligaments. The ligaments usually return to their shortened length during the postpartum weeks, but until that time, abdominal exercises should be performed in a stable position to avoid over stretching ligaments or exacerbating a rectus diastasis.[2]

To accommodate the expanding uterus, the linea alba becomes stretched and softened because of the hormonal influences of pregnancy. This places the abdominal muscles at a disadvantage, and often the rectus abdominis muscles will separate from the uniting linea alba. If not during pregnancy, a rectus diastasis can instead develop during the second stage of labor, particularly if there is excessive breath holding during pushing. Consequently, by the third day postpartum, the abdominal wall should be checked for rectus diastasis. The woman lies on her back with her knees bent. She raises her head and shoulders until her neck is about 8 inches from the floor, the chin should be tucked and the arms stretched out front. The therapist should check the presence of a bulge in the central abdominal area, which is evident when the muscles have parted. If so, the numbers of fingers that can be inserted horizontally into the gap at the level of the umbilicus, 2 inches above and 2 inches below, defines the amount of separation between the taut rectus muscles. Any separation of more than two fingers wide constitutes a restriction on any type of curl-up or leg lowering exercises (see Chapter 13). Trunk rotational exercises should be avoided until there is no rectus separation. Unless there is significant rectus diastasis, however, abdominal exercises with the pelvic floor contracted should be started within the first 24 hours to restore abdominal tone. A jackknifed position (sitting straight up from a supine position) and double leg lifts should be avoided, because of the possibility of increasing a separation between the rectus abdominis muscles or injuring the low back.

## *Exercise*

Exercise in the postpartum period is a key to rapid and maximum muscle function and restoration of the mother's health. Postpartum, the body must adjust to sudden weight loss, change in center of gravity, and accompanying postural adjustments. Fundamentally, the pelvic floor and abdominal muscles deserve a great deal of attention, but the rest of the trunk is undergoing changes as well, related to postural readjustment. The low, mid, and upper back, buttock, and deep hip muscles should be exercised to facilitate their return to normal. If attention is not paid to a complete exercise program, the mother may run the risk of pelvic floor dysfunction, decreased gastrointestinal motility, back and neck discomfort, fatigue, and possibly a poor self-image. Pelvic floor and abdominal exercises can begin as soon as the infant is delivered.

However, mothers should receive clearance from a physician before beginning an exercise program, because there are some conditions that may limit or contraindicate certain activities. These include myocardial disease, congestive heart failure, rheumatic heart disease (class II or above), recent pulmonary embolus, acute infectious disease, uterine hemorrhage, severe hypotensive disease, diabetes mellitus, radicular arm or leg signs, sacroiliac pain, excessive vaginal bleeding, and marked rectus diastasis.[3,4] Abdominal exercises should be prescribed after the abdominal wall has been fully evaluated for rectus diastasis. In a noncomplicated delivery, specific exercises should be given for proper restoration (strength, endurance) of pelvic floor; abdominal muscles; posture; upper, mid, and low back muscles; buttock muscles; and deep hip muscles (see Chapter 13).

A general exercise program should include aerobic conditioning, during which the mother monitors her pulse (see Chapter 13). Participation in a postnatal exercise class, swimming, walking, bike riding, or any combination of these will help her continue a general conditioning program. Additionally, she should practice conscious relaxation daily for 20 minutes to increase her overall endurance and feeling of well-being.

## Emotional Adjustments

On the third day postpartum, 70% to 80% of women will go through a transient depression, sometimes known as the "postpartum blues." Contributing to this emotional depression are the emerging physical body changes, endocrine upheaval, and readjustment of intracellular fluid level, coupled with adjustments to parenting responsibilities and the infant's demands. Usually this depression is gone within a few days, but rarely, serious psychiatric disorders do occur. If the mother's lingering depression interferes with her effectiveness and her ability to cope with day-to-day responsibilities, a psychiatrist's help must be obtained. Psychological problems of this nature may have a long-reaching history. True psychoses after delivery can occur when a constellation of psychotic factors has been set up prior to pregnancy; the stress of pregnancy and delivery become the precipitating and nonspecific factors.[1]

## *Lactation*

During pregnancy, high levels of estrogen block the secretion of milk and cause an adherence of prolactin to breast tissue to prevent its milk-producing effect on the epithelium.[1] After delivery, the high levels of estrogen and progesterone, human placental lactogen (HPL), and insulin are decreased, and milk engorgement begins in 2 to 3 days. Sucking enhances milk production by signaling the brain to release prolactin and oxytocin. The prolactin stimulates the let-down reflex in the breast. It is believed that the tactile nerve endings in the areola send a stimulus to the hypothalamus, resulting in an increase in production and transport of oxytocin to the posterior pituitary, where it is released into the circulation.[1] Oxytocin signals the alveoli and ducts in the breast to contract and squeeze milk through the nipple. The level of prolactin is gradually decreased during the first weeks of pregnancy. By the fourth or fifth month, the prolactin level has returned to its nonpregnant value. The factors that maintain milk production after this point remain unclear.[1]

There are three types of human milk, the first being colostrum, a clear or yellowish fluid, containing more antibodies, serum chloride, potassium, protein, minerals, and fat soluble vitamins than mature milk. This milk will often leak out of the breast prenatally, but mothers should not encourage expression. It is believed that colostrum readies the infant's intestinal tract for later milk and helps to clean out the infant's digestive tract, by stimulating the elimination of the meconium that fills the gastrointestinal tract of the infant at birth. On the second or third day, the breasts become gorged with milk. Frequent feedings will decrease the distended breasts. Transitional milk comes next and lasts up to 2 weeks postpartum. It changes over a 2-week period to a higher fat and lactose content, thereby increasing its total caloric value. Mature milk, the last to come, 2 weeks postdelivery, decreases in fat content in the latter part of the first year, and works in concert with the additional nutrition the baby receives from other sources.

The composition of milk changes in response to the different stages of lactation, time of day, time within a feeding, and a mother's level of nutrition. Usually, the milk fat comes in the later part of a feeding. In addition, there is an additional rise in fat between the morning and mid-afternoon feedings.

A mother's nutrition, rest, and fluid intake are crucial to a good supply of milk. The nursing mother will need 500 calories more a day than what she was eating before she was pregnant, along with 20 gm more of protein for milk production. If the mother is not nursing, an injection of estrogen and testosterone is given to inhibit milk production. Supportive bras, cold applied to the breasts, aspirin, and a lowered fluid intake, will decrease the engorgement of the breasts.[5]

The breasts in a nursing mother will retain 2 or 3 pounds until weaning. Breasts may leak before and after delivery, and some women use nursing pads inside their bras. Mothers can often toughen their nipples during pregnancy, preparing them for nursing by frequently pinching, rolling, and gently rubbing them with a towel. Because the newborn will nurse on demand, the nipples are subjected to a great deal of manipulation and moisture, which encourages cracking and soreness. To prevent mastitis or cracked and sore nipples the mother should allow nipples to dry between feedings, feed the baby frequently so that the breast does not become full, use good nursing positions, break suction correctly, avoid use of soap or oils on the nipples, get plenty of sleep, and maintain good nutrition.

If only one breast is sore, the baby should nurse on the unsore side first. When both sides are sore, the milk should be expressed until a letdown reflex occurs. This will make the milk more available for the infant and, thereby, decrease the intensity of the baby's initial suckling. Heat and breast massage can decrease sore breasts, as well. If the nipple does become sore or cracked, a breast shield or a 1 to 2 day rest from suckling on that side may help relieve symptoms. The affected breast will probably need to be pumped or milk expressed to maintain the milk production.

Comfortable clothing, such as tops that facilitate nursing, are helpful. Sometimes mothers have difficulty allowing their milk to let down in public. Although a hungry, crying baby can change the mind of even the most modest woman, a mother can usually find a private place to nurse or can drape a cloth over the top of the baby's head and across her own shoulder to facilitate the letdown reflex by decreasing her own embarrassment.

## *Going Home*

The health of the mother and infant and the location where delivery occurs often determine when they go home. Traditionally, women recuperated at the hospital for at least 1 week. Now, after an uncomplicated birth, women and their babies leave the hospital in 2 or 3 days. At a birthing center, they often leave within a few hours to rest at home.

Once home, fatigue is common, and additional sleep and rest are needed for several days. Early ambulation, whether at home or in the hospital, decreases the chance of thrombophlebitis and improves bowel and bladder functions.[6] New mothers should start pelvic floor and gentle abdominal exercises immediately and continue them at home to increase the tone and supportive functions of these muscles.

## Sexuality

Sexual intercourse can be resumed when the bright red bleeding ceases, or at least after 4 to 6 weeks. Contraception is necessary to avoid another pregnancy. Although the hormones produced by breastfeeding women delay ovulation, it is impossible to tell exactly when ovulation will occur. Breastfeeding is not a substitute for birth control. Low-dose contraceptives have been used in women who are not nursing and who have been screened for contraindications. Diaphragms can be fitted at the postpartum checkup at 6 weeks. In the meantime, condoms can be used, but they are not 100% safe for preventing pregnancy. It is a good idea for women to discuss this with their doctors or nurses prior to delivery.

## Postpartum Checkup

The postpartum checkup is scheduled for 6 weeks after delivery. The physician will check involution of the uterus and vagina and integrity of the cervix, perineum, and pelvic support. The abdominal tone and breasts are assessed as well. Lab work may include examination of cervical cells, assessment of hematocrit level, and a urinalysis. Blood pressure and weight are measured, and the woman's medical and emotional health will be screened.

## Following Cesarean Delivery

Because of the high Cesarean section rate in the United States, physical therapists should be trained to assist in the recovery of these women. A mother delivering by Cesarean section will have many of the same physical discomforts associated with any major abdominal surgery or with vaginal delivery. Although there will be no episiotomy, the same changes occur in the uterus, pelvic floor, and urinary and gastrointestinal tracts. Most women will be taken to the recovery room after a Cesarean section, until they have recovered from anesthesia, and will have their vital signs monitored until they are stabilized. While in the recovery room, the parents can bond with their new child, while the mother recovers under supervision. Usually, the intravenous line and catheter remain in overnight, and may be in for as long as 48 hours.

Attention must be given to adequate lung expansion, prevention of wound infection, and a significantly decreased intestinal motility coupled with the residual effects of anesthesia. Clamps or stitches, used to approximate the abdominal wall, are removed around the sixth day, after which, barring any problems, the mother may go home. The mother who undergoes a Cesarean section will have a longer recovery physically. Common postoperative problems, such as gas, severe pain, and fever, may require medication. For moderate pain, however, the mother might use medications or TENS for pain relief so she can get out of bed and begin walking. TENS applied on the lateral aspects of a low transverse incision has been found to significantly decrease the amount of narcotics needed post-Cesarean.[7] Normal contraindications for TENS use must be followed. Preoperative fitting of electrodes and instruction would be ideal to acclimate the mother to the idea of the apparatus and to gather a baseline for the pain level needed.

Characteristically, post-Cesarean mothers lean forward when walking to protect the incision. This slouching posture will be further emphasized when she carries, changes, or breastfeeds the baby. The mother must begin to ambulate in the first 12 to 18 hours to increase intestinal motility, decrease muscle stiffness, and prevent thrombophlebitis. These mothers should also be started on a physical therapy program the first day in the hospital, and have their exercises monitored and graded throughout their stay.

The mother can be taught to splint the incision by placing one hand on top of the other over the incision with her wrists placed just anterior to the iliac crest. The therapist can also make a splint pillow for her from two towels folded in a square, wrapped, and taped to hold position. By holding the incision firmly with this pillow the mother will feel more secure and be better able to walk with good posture. The mother should be told that walking and gentle exercises will not pull apart the incision and that activity stimulates healing by increasing circulation.

Pelvic floor exercises and gentle abdominal exercises can be started on the first day. It is helpful if the mother has been prepared for a Cesarean delivery during her labor and delivery classes. She may be relieved that a Cesarean section was done, especially after a long labor or fetal distress, but she may also feel that she has failed at her own plan or image of giving birth. Here, her self-esteem and confidence may be altered, affecting her parenting and recovery.

Cesarean support classes are often given in the hospital. Support from her partner, doctor, family, and friends will assist her in her readjustment. She needs to know that she could not have had an effect on the outcome of her labor, nor that she is to blame. It is also important for her to know that one Cesarean birth does not always mean another. She will need to adjust her daily activities and conserve her energy. The post-Cesarean mother should have all the time she needs to fully recover before performing household tasks. These mothers are usually not restricted from climbing stairs, but should limit their use. Women should be shown how to brace the pelvic floor and abdominal muscles, using the legs and buttocks to propel the body up stairs.

## *Self-Assessment Review*

1. What are the primary uterine changes postdelivery?

2. The _____ is made of serum leukocytes, sloughing endometrial tissue, and blood.

3. Increased urinary production postdelivery is due to _____.

4. Cardiac output returns to prepregnant level by _____ postpartum.

5. Instructions for stair climbing for post-Cesarean mothers should be _____.

6. Immediate post-Cesarean exercises include _____ and _____.

7. _____ and _____ hormones are necessary for milk production.

8. Tingling around the nipple and ejection of the milk from the breast is called the _____.

9. Name four key areas of muscle restoration following delivery.

10. Name four conditions that may limit or contraindicate exercise following delivery.

## *References*

1. Danforth DN, Scott JR (eds): Obstetrics and Gynecology (5th ed). Philadelphia, JB Lippincott, 1986.

2. Noble E: Essential Exercises for the Childbearing Year (2nd ed). Boston, Houghton-Mifflin, 1982.

3. Artal R, Wiswell R (eds): Exercise in Pregnancy. Baltimore, Williams & Wilkins, 1986.

4. Section on OB/GYN APTA: Perinatal Exercise Guidelines. Alexandria, Bull Sect Obstet Gynecol, APTA, 1986.

5. Walker M, Driscoll JW: Breastfeeding Your Baby (2nd ed). Wayne, New Jersey, Avery Publishing, 1981.

6. Niswander K: Manual of Obstetrics. Boston, Little, Brown & Co, 1987.

7. Brown G, Viviano J, Machek O: Management of postoperative pain in obstetrical and gynecological procedures. Bull Sect Obstet Gynecol, APTA: 7(3):8-11, 1983.

# TEN

# Maternal Disorders and Diseases

A high-risk pregnancy has been identified as that in which maternal or fetal factors may adversely affect the outcome, and a system to identify these high-risk factors has helped avoid adverse outcomes many times. Some factors, such as diabetes, grand multiparity, need for Rh immunization and preexisting heart conditions can be identified before conception or in the first trimester, and management of these risk factors decreases the mortality and morbidity rates of mother and child. However, in other situations, risk factors may develop as the pregnancy advances, such as problems related to multiple fetuses, preeclampsia and hypertension.[1]

Prior to the late 1960s, the management of high-risk pregnancy was by trial and error. Pregnancies were often terminated by induction or Cesarean section at a gestational age that provided the fetus and mother the best chance to survive. To calculate this, an estimate was made, at each week of gestation, to determine the risk of intrauterine demise compared to the subsequent risk of neonatal death if termination was delayed. Danforth explains, for instance, that all pregnancies that were complicated by diabetes were interrupted at 37 weeks, the point in gestation at which cumulative risk of intrauterine and neonatal death was the lowest. He points out, however, that a great number of otherwise normally developing fetuses were delivered prior to their full maturation, proving beneficial in a reduction of fetal mortality in high-risk patients, but often causing prematurity-induced neonatal morbidity or mortality. [2] When Rh incompatibility was recognized in the 1960s as a risk factor for pregnancy, high-risk pregnancy clinics were developed. In addition to Rh-negative patients being screened for antibodies and being treated by specialists in Rh immunization, methods were devised to perform amniotic fluid analysis and intrauterine transfusions to remedy not only Rh incompatibility, but to analyze maternal and fetal status.

## *Death and Mortality Rates*

Unfortunately, maternal and fetal death are part of any discussion of high-risk pregnancy and complicated pregnancy. To understand the difference between death and mortality rates, the physical therapist must first examine the many terms that define and categorize the time of fetal or infant demise. A *live-born infant* is one who shows signs of life: breathing, cord pulsation, voluntary muscle movement, or heartbeat upon complete expulsion from the vagina, regardless of the duration of the pregnancy. *Fetal death,* or stillbirth, refers to the death (no life signs) of a fetus, 500 gm or more, prior to the complete expulsion from the vagina, again, irrespective of the duration of the pregnancy. *Hebdomadal death* is death of a fetus, 500 gm or more, within the first 7 days of life. *Neonatal death* means death of an infant within the first 28 days of life. This infant must weigh 500 gm or more or have completed 20 weeks' gestation to be considered viable. *Perinatal death* includes both fetal and neonatal death (*i.e.,* death of the fetus before or during delivery and death of a liveborn infant within the first 28 days of life).

Mortality rates are actually ratios comparing the number of deaths to a particular number of births. It is also important to note that, in some cases, number of births can mean live and stillborn. *Fetal mortality* describes the number of fetal deaths per 1000 births. *Neonatal mortality* includes the number of deaths per 1000 births of liveborn infants in their first 28 days. *Perinatal mortality* is an inclusive term referring to the number of fetal and neonatal deaths per 1000 births. *Infant mortality* describes the rate between the 28th day and the end of the first year of life.

*Maternal death* is death from any cause during pregnancy or up to

42 days after its termination. A direct maternal death is one that results from an obstetrical complication, and an indirect death is one that results from a previous illness or disease. The *maternal mortality rate* (usually reported as maternal deaths/10,000 live births) has decreased over the years. (Note that in Figure 10-3, maternal mortality is reported as deaths/100,000 live births.)

Reporting of vital data in the United States has been the legal responsibility of the individual states. It is the responsibility of the person who attends the birth or death to report that event to legal authorities. At the time of reporting, additional data is required, including age, length of gestation, and cause of death. There is a variability between the states in terms of measuring a gestational period. Some measure by gestational weight and some by gestational age; however, legally, gestations that exceed 20 weeks duration, or fetuses of 500 gm in weight, are reported as fetal deaths. There are no statistics for total fetal deaths, because most states do not require that deaths from pregnancy of less than 20 weeks be reported. Spontaneous abortions, however, account for 10% to 15% of all pregnancies.

Fetal mortality in the United States has declined to a low of 8.9 in 1981 (see Figure 10-1). Antepartum fetal evaluation and intrapartum fetal monitoring are believed to have contributed to the reduction in fetal deaths. Major causes of fetal death are complications of the membranes, cord, or placenta; anoxia; complications of pregnancy; congenital anomalies; gestational growth problems; illness of the mother; and complications of labor and delivery.

Neonatal mortality has also dropped since 1930 (see Figure 10-2). In 1983, the United States was at an all-time low of 10/1000 live

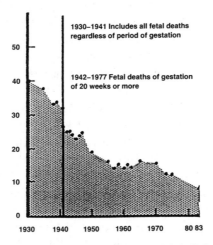

Figure 10-1: Stillbirth rates. (fetal deaths per 1,000 live births), United States 1930 to 1983, (Vital Statistics of the United States, 1930–1983, vol 2, Washington, DC, US Department of Health and Human Services)

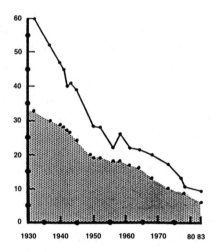

Figure 10-2: Neonatal deaths and infant mortality rates (deaths per 1000 live births), United States, 1930 to 1983 (Vital Statistics of the US, 1980–1983, Vol 2, Washington, D.C., US Department of Health and Human Services)

births. Perinatal centers have contributed to the decrease in neonatal mortality by managing high-risk pregnancies. Most neonatal deaths are associated with high-risk pregnancies—those complicated by diabetes mellitus, hypertensive disorder, multiple fetuses, antepartum bleeding, and hydramnios. The major problems during delivery are abnormal presentations, placenta previa, abruptio placentae, and prolapsed cord. The major cause of neonatal death is impaired oxygenation, which may cause respiratory distress syndrome, hyaline membrane disease, conditions of the placenta, pneumonia, congenital anomalies, and birth injury.

Seven percent of all live-born infants have functional or structural defects. Half of these are diagnosed in the postnatal period. The rest will be diagnosed weeks or years later. Socioeconomic factors do play a part in perinatal mortality, which is higher in poor than in middle and upper class women. Poor women tend to be more malnourished, be more anemic, have less opportunity for good medical care, and have a shorter time between pregnancies.

In 1981, there were 80.5 maternal deaths for each 100,000 live births in the United States (see Figure 10-3). Hemorrhage, eclampsia, and preeclampsia are still the most common causes of death among pregnant women. Others include complications of labor and delivery, hypertension, ectopic pregnancy, antepartum hemorrhage, and abortion. Other complications of pregnancy are unknown factors, other medical illness, and hyperemesis. With more sophisticated care offered to pregnant women since the recognition of obstetrics and gynecology as a specialty, there has been a decrease in maternal deaths. The use of antibiotics and blood transfusions; improvement in anesthesia and quality of prenatal care; along with the opportu-

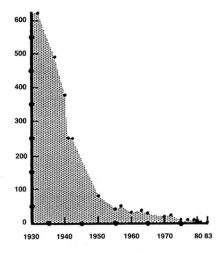

Figure 10-3: Maternal mortality rates. (Deaths per 100,000 live births), United States, 1930 to 1983. (Vital Statistics of the United States, 1930 to 1983, Vol 2, Washington, DC, US Department of Health and Human Services)

nity for safe, legal, abortions have resulted in a significant decrease in maternal deaths.

The physical therapist specializing in obstetrics may either work directly on a ward for mothers with high-risk pregnancies (usually patients are on bed rest or receiving tocolytic therapy), or may work with mothers who may later develop signs of high-risk pregnancy. Therefore, it is important for the physical therapist to be familiar with some of the most common maternal disorders. This chapter does not present every disorder that may occur, but does list and briefly describe in the text and tables[2,3,4] selected problems organized by bodily system and the effects of these problems on pregnancy.

## Cardiac Diseases and Disorders

About 1% of all pregnant women have organic heart disease, about half of it rheumatic in origin. Advances in treatment have decreased the incidence of valvular lesions and the total number of pregnancies affected by heart disease. However, the incidence of congenital malformations has risen and such malformations, plus cardiomyopathies and other cardiac diseases, are responsible for the other half of cardiac-related problems in pregnancy.[5] The New York Heart Association classification system for patients with cardiac disease also applies to pregnant women: Class I, asymptomatic; Class II, symptomatic with heavy exercise; Class III, symptomatic with light exercise; Class IV, symptomatic at rest. Patients of Class III and IV are believed to be at high risk for complications during pregnancy.

For patients with cardiac disease, the goal of prenatal care is the detection and prevention of major complications of arrhythmias, embolisms, and congestive failure. Prenatal visits are required more frequently and patients may need extra rest to reduce cardiac work. Diuretics and sodium restriction may be indicated if the patient has a tendency toward congestive heart failure, and patients may be given iron supplements to prevent any kind of anemia. Patients are hospitalized at the first sign of preeclampsia, increased blood pressure, or proteinuria. During labor and delivery, pain relief measures diminish the amount of cardiac work by 20%. Valsalva maneuvers are contraindicated, and the presenting part should descend to the pelvic floor by the force of uterine contractions alone. Forceps are often used to facilitate delivery. It is generally agreed that epidural anesthesia is contraindicated because of risk of hypotension and reduced venous return to the heart. Epidurals are also contraindicated in patients with hypertrophic cardiomyopthy. Cesarean section should only be done for obstetric emergency in patients with cardiac diseases.

Mitral stenosis is present in 90% of the pregnant patients with rheumatic heart disease. Overall morbidity from mitral stenosis is 1% during pregnancy. In severe cases, mortality rates have been as high as 15%. Pregnancy exacerbates mitral stenosis by causing physiologic tachycardia (the increased volume leads to increased pulmonary capillary blood volume) and by causing a need for increased cardiac output, with increased left atrial and pulmonary capillaries. There is also an increased incidence of atrial arrhythmia during pregnancy. A pregnant woman with mitral stenosis of long duration and pulmonary hypertension should avoid pregnancy.

Mitral insufficiency accounts for 6% of pregnant patients with rheumatic heart disease. Women tolerate the pregnancy well as long as there is not a severe mitral regurgitation or atrial fibrillation. Prophylactic antibiotics are indicated during labor and delivery.

Aortic stenosis accounts for 1% of pregnant patients with rheumatic heart disease. Women with mild aortic stenosis will tolerate pregnancy well, but severe aortic stenosis is a threat to maternal life. Mortality is as high as 17%. Venous return of the heart must be maintained by avoiding the supine position and by avoiding excessive blood loss at the time of delivery.

Another 2-3% of pregnant patients with rheumatic heart disease have aortic insufficiency. In pregnancy, the shorter diastole reduces the amount of blood regurgitating from the aorta into the left ventricle, and does not increase blood volume as previously believed.

Patent ductus arteriosus is now a rare maternal complication, but it used to be a common congenital lesion. Most patients with this lesion tolerate pregnancy well. Shunt reversal is the major pregnancy-associated risk. If shunts totally correct the problem, patients with patent ductus arteriosus have no increased risk during pregnancy.

Tetralogy of Fallot is the most common form of cyanotic congenital heart disease. It is composed of pulmonary stenosis, ventricular septal defect, and dextroposition of the aorta with right ventricular hypertrophy. This tetralogy accounts for 5% of cardiac malformations present at birth. Patients with such a malformation can undergo corrective surgery and have successful pregnancies. In uncorrected cases, cyanosis during pregnancy can lead to intrauterine growth retardation and more complicated outcomes.

Atrial septal defect is the most common congenital lesion seen in pregnant women. Shunting of blood from the left to right atrium leads to an increased load on the right ventricle and increased pulmonary blood flow. Most of these women will demonstrate right ventricular hypertrophy; heart failure is uncommon in persons under 30. Patients with atrial septal defect tolerate pregnancy, but the major risk is shunt reversal during pregnancy, secondary to obstetrical hemorrhage or incorrect use of epidural or spinal anesthesia.

Pregnant patients who have undergone corrective surgery for ventricular septal defects are usually symptom-free, but larger defects may cause shunting of blood from the left to right ventricles with an increase in pulmonary blood flow. There is a significant risk of bacterial endocarditis, and again, the major risk is shunt reversal. Most of these women, however, do well in pregnancy.

Mitral valve prolapse is a common congenital heart defect that occurs in 6% to 10% of women of childbearing age. The mitral valve tends to prolapse during ventricular systole and leads to mitral regurgitation. A click-murmur syndrome is heard on auscultation. Although most women improve during pregnancy because of the increased blood volume and decreased peripheral vascular resistance, the American Heart Association still advises the use of antibiotics prophylactically. Symptoms include palpitations, anxiety, fatigue, chest pain, and lightheadedness; but pregnancy is generally well-tolerated.

Cardiomyopathies and other diseases affecting the heart can be acute or chronic, some first diagnosed in pregnancy due to the extra load on the heart.

During pregnancy, cardiac surgery is rarely indicated and is avoided other than in an emergency life-saving measure. Although maternal mortality is not increased significantly, there is a 30-50% increase in fetal mortality during open-heart surgery.

Over 150 cases have been reported since 1952 in the literature of women who have undergone cardiac valve replacement surgery prior to their pregnancies. During pregnancy maternal mortality has

**Table 10-1. Effects of Cardiomyopathies and Other Diseases on Pregnancy**

| Disease | Symptoms | Effects on Mother | Effects on Fetus |
|---|---|---|---|
| *Hypertrophic cardiomyopathy* (hypertrophy of the left ventricle; also known as obstructive cardiomyopathy or idiopathic hypertrophic subaortic stenosis; autosomal disorder; mitral regurgitation) | Sudden death at any age from sudden arrhythmias or tachycardia; no specific symptoms before death; pregnancy well-tolerated | Unpredictable occurrence; most patients treated with beta blockers | Fetal growth monitored by ultrasound, because beta blockers may cause intrauterine growth retardation |
| *Marfan's syndrome* (autosomal dominant disease with abnormal connective tissue due to dysfunctional protein metabolism) | Involvement of any organ; death usually from cardiac complications; mitral valve prolapse common; increased risk of aortic dissection and rupture during pregnancy; joint deformities; weakness of aortic root | Maternal mortality 50%; risk increased if aortic root >4 cm; pregnancy contraindicated; managed by beta blockers; avoidance of bearing-down effort and forceps delivery | Fetal growth monitored by ultrasound, because beta blockers may cause intrauterine growth retardation |
| *Peripartum cardiomyopathy* (rare: 1/1500–1/4000 pregnancies; etiology unknown; most common in black multiparas; preeclampsia in 7% of patients) | Enlarged heart, development of congestive heart failure during last mo of pregnancy (7%), in 1st 3 mo postpartum (82%), in 4th or 5th mo (11%); ECG tracing of ventricular CHF* | Maternal mortality 10%-15% if heart returns to normal; 85%, if not; future pregnancy contraindicated | None |
| *Primary pulmonary hypertension* (rare disease associated with > 50% mortality) | Progressive constriction and fibrosis of the pulmonary arterioles and muscularization; pulmonary artery pressure high; progressive RVH*; dyspnea, syncope, chest pain; death due to arrhythmia | Death any time, but most often in last mo of pregnancy and early puerperium from increased blood volume and cardiac output, with RV failure arrhythmias; future pregnancy contraindicated | None |

*CHF, congestive heart failure; RVH, right ventricular hypertrophy

been low, but management of problems, which are many, has been difficult. Maternal and fetal risk factors depend on what valve has been replaced and the type of replacement used. For instance, pregnancy is not contraindicated for patients with aortic valve replacements. The hemodynamics after aortic valve replacements are different from those occurring after placement of mitral valve prostheses. The fetal mortality rate, however, is increased in mothers with mitral valve prosthesis. Anticoagulants, which may be necessary through-

out the pregnancy for the mother's safety, may seriously jeopardize
fetal health.

Myocardial infarction (MI) rarely occurs during pregnancy (reported cases total 68 in the period from 1922-1987). Continuation of
pregnancy depends on the size of the infarct. Small and large in-
farcts require individual evaluation. Mortality rates range from 30%
to 40%. The mortality rate from MI increases the later in pregnancy
it occurs. Patients with a history of MI or angina should be have a
full cardiac evaluation before beginning pregnancy. (See Table 10-1)

## *Pregnancy-Induced Hypertension*

Pregnancy-induced hypertension is symptomatic of various disorders with a common factor of increased mean arterial pressure
(MAP). For example, pregnancy-induced hypertension could mean a
blood pressure of 140/90 mm Hg during the second half of pregnancy in a usually normotensive woman—a 30 mm Hg rise in systolic blood pressure or a 15 mm Hg increase in diastolic pressure
over baseline values. To establish the diagnosis, the examiner needs
to find increased blood pressure changes on at least two occasions, 6
or more hours apart.

If proteinuria is present, the pregnancy-induced hypertension is
reclassified as preeclampsia. There are five classifications of hypertensive disease in pregnancy: (1) gestational hypertension (2)
chronic hypertension (3) chronic hypertension with superimposed
preeclampsia (4) preeclampsia (5) eclampsia.

Gestational hypertension is defined as a rise in the MAP above
106 mm Hg, occurring after 20 weeks of pregnancy, without proteinuria. This hypertension disappears after delivery. Gestational
hypertension may be hard to distinguish from chronic hypertension,
if the patient is not seen for obstetrical care prior to the 20th week.

Both chronic hypertensive and normotensive women will have a
decrease in blood pressure during the middle and early third trimesters of pregnancy. Therefore, if patients with unrecognized chronic
hypertension are seen for the first time at the 24th week of pregnancy, they may appear normal; but early in the third trimester, the
blood pressure may rise to an unrecognized hypertensive level, making it impossible to distinguish between pregnancy-induced hypertension and chronic hypertension. There are, however, clinical findings that can help determine if the disorder is chronic in nature: (1)
retinal hemorrhages and exudates; (2) plasma urea nitrogen concen-
trates above 20 mg/dl; (3) plasma creatinine concentration above 1
mg/dl; and (4) the presence of renal disease, collagen vascular disease, diabetes mellitus, or other disorders that predispose a woman
to chronic hypertension. Chronic hypertension is suspected if blood

pressure is above 140/90 mm Hg, if hypertension is detected earlier than 20 weeks, if hypertension dates to prior to the pregnancy, and if hypertension is not accompanied by proteinuria.

Chronic hypertension with superimposed preeclampsia is characterized by hypertension starting before the 20th week of pregnancy with the addition of proteinuria and edema in the latter half of pregnancy. This disorder occurs in 13% of treated chronic hypertensive patients.[3]

Preeclampsia denotes hypertension, proteinuria, and edema, usually occurring in primigravidas after the 20th week of pregnancy. Degrees are mild, moderate, and severe. In the mild form, MAP is less than 106 mm Hg (140/90 mm Hg), diastolic pressure increases more than 15 mm Hg on 2 occasions 6 hours apart with patient at bed rest, and there is proteinuria or edema. In moderate preeclampsia, MAP is 106 mm Hg (140/90 mm Hg) to 126 mm Hg (160/110 mm Hg, or a rise of blood pressure greater than 30 mm Hg systolic or greater than 15 mm Hg diastolic). Increased proteinuria and edema of the lower extremities may also be noted. In severe preeclampsia, MAP is greater than 126 mm Hg (160/110 mm Hg) on two occasions 6 hours apart with the patient at bed rest, proteinuria is greater than 5 gm/24 hours, and the patient complains of headaches and blurred vision. There may also be right upper quadrant pain, oliguria, pulmonary edema, and edema of the face, hands, and lower extremities.[3]

Eclampsia is characterized by generalized seizure activity with hypertension and proteinuria in the pregnant patient. This seizure occurs within the first 24 hours postpartum. No one is able to accurately predict which patients with pregnancy-induced hypertension will develop eclampsia. Its etiology is unknown, although three major theories of causes exist: (1) increased vasoconstrictor tone, (2) abnormal prostaglandin action, and (3) immunological factors. It is likely that the disease process begins with vasospasm and then leads to a reduced blood flow to the uterus and other organs. Reduced intravascular volume and, ultimately, hypertension develop.

## *Vascular Disease*

There are three causes of venous thrombosis and pulmonary embolism: (1) changes in blood clotting factors, (2) vessel wall damage, and (3) venous stasis. Some blood clotting factors are increased, others decreased, during pregnancy. Vessel wall damage may occur during delivery, especially during Cesarean section. Prolonged use of stirrups for a vaginal delivery may also lead to vessel wall damage in the patient's legs. Pooling of blood in the lower extremities is common in pregnancy: this increased venous distensibility occurs in the first trimester; and by 28 weeks of gestation, the venous pressure in the legs is 2 times nonpregnant values. Additionally, the enlarging uterus interferes with venous return from the legs, thereby reducing the velocity of venous flow by half. Consequently, the incidence of thromboembolic disease during early pregnancy is only slightly increased, but as pregnancy progresses, and at term, the incidence is about 50% above nonpregnant values. In the early puerperium, the incidence is five to six times higher than it is in a nonpregnant woman.

Varicose veins, often a familial trait, increase 11% to 25% in pregnancy.[1] The cause may relate to the hormonal changes of pregnancy and to the mechanical obstructions to blood flow by the increasing size of the uterus. Varicosities usually become evident at 10 to 12 weeks of pregnancy; and symptoms include a feeling of heaviness or discomfort in the legs, usually after walking, possibly accompanied by incapacitating pain. Stasis and ulceration may accompany the pain. Varicosities occur more frequently with subsequent pregnancies and may predispose the mother to thrombophlebitis. There is no effect on the fetus. Management includes pressure-graded elastic stockings, bed rest with feet elevated, dorsiflexion and plantarflexion exercises performed frequently throughout the day, and avoidance of binding stockings or socks. Hemorrhoids are rectal varicosities that can cause pain, itching, and bleeding during bowel movements. Resolved preexisting hemorrhoids may become symptomatic during labor, and especially after delivery.

One fifth of pregnant women may develop vulvar varicosities due to a 30-fold increase in the circulation by third trimester and increased pressure through the iliac vein branches as the weight of the uterus increases. These varicosities are not hazardous to mother or fetus, although maternal discomfort is common and rupture may produce a hematoma. Varices will regress after delivery, and discomfort can sometimes be reduced pressure by pressing pads to the labia.

The saphenous veins are frequently affected by superficial venous thrombosis, which is more common than deep vein thrombosis. Superficial venous thrombosis occurs in patients with varicosities. Redness may be present, and pain is evident along the course of the vein. Conservative management, as mentioned above, is helpful. This disorder is rarely associated with embolism, and there is no effect on the fetus.

Pregnant women show an increased susceptibility to deep vein thrombosis. It is difficult to diagnose, and the onset is usually abrupt, occurring more often in the puerperium. On examination, one leg may be at least 2 cm larger in circumference than the other. There may be a temperature difference between legs, as well. A Doppler ultrasound and limited venography will confirm the diagnosis. Treatment consists of bed rest with the bed elevated on 8-inch blocks to decrease the edema and application of heat. Pelvic thrombophlebitis occurs in 0.18% to 0.29% of pregnant women and 0.1 to 1.0% of postpartum women.

Pulmonary embolism occurs in 16% of patients with deep venous thrombosis without coagulation, and in 19% with coagulation. A threat of abortion may occur as the result of iliac vein obstruction, but usually, the fetus is unaffected. Pulmonary embolism is a dangerous complication of venous thrombosis, Cesarean section, forceps delivery, and advanced maternal age. The risk of pulmonary embolism during pregnancy and the puerperium is 5.5 times greater than for nonpregnant women. Without anticoagulation medicine, mortality is extremely high. Pulmonary embolism is the main nonobstetric cause of postpartum death, and maternal hypoxia experienced during pulmonary embolism causes fetal death or impairment.

Few arterial diseases are unique to pregnancy. Raynaud's Phenomenon usually undergoes remission during pregnancy, and medications that can cause arteriospasm are to be avoided. Dissecting aneurysm of the aorta may occur in the last trimester of pregnancy or in the puerperium, as a result of an increase in blood volume and associated with coarctation of the aorta induced by hypertensive stress. There may be a familial history of this disease that causes chest pain, and prognosis for mother and fetus is grave; maternal death is frequent. Management is usually surgical. Splenic artery aneurysm is more frequently associated with grand multiparity and can result in rupture, leading to intraperitoneal hemorrhage. Prognosis for mother and fetus is grave. Management involves blood transfusion and laporotomy to remove the spleen and aneurysm.

## *Endocrine Disease*

Perhaps the most devastating diseases of pregnancy can be linked to endocrine dysfunction. The regulation of endocrine function determines fetoplacental influences vital for blood flow, nutrition, and organ differentiation. It may even be true that the fetus, through endocrine mechanisms, signals the start of labor. Diabetes and gestational diabetes are among the most common endocrine diseases influencing pregnancy, but disorders of the thyroid, parathyroid, adrenal, and pituitary glands, described in Table 10-2, can also cause complications.

Niswander describes diabetes mellitus as a "chronic metabolic disorder characterized by relative or absolute lack of circulating

## Table 10-2. Effects of Endocrine Diseases on Pregnancy

| Disease | Symptoms | Effects on Mother | Effects on Fetus |
|---|---|---|---|
| *Cushing's syndrome* (rare in pregnancy; women usually anovulatory; excess glucocorticoids due to adrenal adenomas or carcinomas | Weight loss, edema, nausea, vomiting, weakness, hypertension, easy bruisability, acne, increased hirsutism, carbohydrate intolerance | Spontaneous abortion; premature labor | High perinatal morbidity and mortality |
| *Addison's disease* (adrenal insufficiency; patients rarely conceive) | Fatigue, anorexia, nausea, vomiting, hypotension, increased pigmentation, fasting hypoglycemia | Dehydration and electrolyte imbalance; delivery indicated; with glucocorticoid replacement; good prognosis | Small-for-gestational-age infants; depressed adrenal function at birth |
| *Pheochromocytoma* (rare in pregnancy; adrenal medulla tumor; catecholamine excess) | Hypertension, headaches, palpitations, sweating, weakness, weight loss, glycosuria, nervousness, tremor | Possible remission between pregnancies, but manifestations more severe with each pregnancy; high maternal mortality, usually during or after delivery; Cesarean and concurrent tumor removal indicated | High fetal mortality |
| *Graves' Disease* (hyperthyroidism; 0.2% incidence in pregnancy) | Weakness; heat intolerance; tachycardia; resting pulse 100 beats/minute | Possibly life-threatening; fever; dehydration; nausea, vomiting, mental confusion; increased risk of preterm labor | 1%-2% thyrotoxicosis rate if untreated |
| *Autoimmune thyroiditis* (Hashimoto's thryoiditis; antithyroid; mxydema; rare in pregnancy) | Fatigue, cold intolerance, excessive weight gain, hoarseness, dry skin, coarse hair, constipation, myalgia | Rise of spontaneous abortion; with hormone replacement, excellent prognosis for mother and fetus | Two-fold stillbirth rate |
| *Thyroid Nodules* (incidence same as in nonpregnancy) | Hard nodule, painful gland, enlarged lymph nodes, hoarseness | Possible englargement of thyroid; rule out malignancy, surgery may be indicated | No effect on gestation |
| *Hyperparathyroidism* (rare in pregnancy) | Polydipsia, constipation, nausea, vomiting, hypercalcemia, fatigue, muscle weakness (may be asymptomatic) | Subperiostial bone resorption; maternal mortality rare; premature labor 20% | Mortality rates 25%–30% (half stillbirths); 15–50% devleop neonatal tetany |
| *Hypoparathyroidism* (secondary to thryoid or parathryoid surgery; rare in pregnancy) | Hypocalcemia, numbness, tingling, weakness, tetany, carpopedal spasm, mental aberration | Increased need for calcium in pregnancy and in labor; breastfeeding not recommended | If untreated, risk for neonatal hyperparathyroidism |

**Table 10-2. Continued**

| Disease | Symptoms | Effects on Mother | Effects on Fetus |
|---|---|---|---|
| *Sheehan's syndrome* (postpartum pituitary necrosis due to blood loss during delivery) | Rapid breast involution; decreased pigmentation; loss of axillary and pubic hair | Possible failure to lactate; possible amenorrhea | No effect if treated |
| *Diabetes insipidus* (inadequate production of antidiuretic hormone by posterior pituitary gland; incidence 1/16,000–1/80,000) | Polydipsia, polyuria | Possibility of disease worsening in pregnancy; symptoms alleviated by lactation | No effect if treated |
| *Acromegaly* (rare in pregnancy) | Possible tumor expansion, visual field loss, severe headaches, nausea, vomiting | No effect on pregnancy | No effect on fetus |
| *Microadenomas* (prolactin-secreting tumors) | Possible headaches, visual field disturbances | No effect on pregnancy; treated with bromocriptine, if enlarges | No effect on fetus |

insulin resulting in hyperglycemia and glucosuria, increased protein and fat catabolism, and the tendency in some patients to ketoacidosis."[4] Some complications of diabetes mellitus include neuropathy, retinopathy, vascular disease, and polyneuropathy. The etiology of diabetes is unknown. It has been theorized that genetic and acquired mechanisms play a role in this multifaceted disease.

Many advances in the last 12 years have been made to help the pregnant woman with diabetes mellitus. Maternal mortality has been almost eliminated, and maternal morbidity has been reduced significantly. For patients who are insulin-dependent, the perinatal mortality rate has approached the rate for normal gravidas. Traditional management of the pregnant diabetic patient has included an elective, premature delivery date between 36 and 38 weeks gestation,[6] but because of advances in antepartum fetal monitoring, more diabetics can be brought to term with successful outcomes.

The rate of glucose intolerance in pregnant women ranges from 3% to 12%, with 0.1% to 0.5% dependent on insulin.[1] Glucose values are not controlled by diet. Fasting plasma values greater than 100 mg/dl or mean plasma glucose values above 120 mg/dl require insulin treatment.[7] The mother may experience some change in sugar control, such as hyperglycemia, hypoglycemia, and changes in quantity of insulin needed. She may also experience some pregnancy-induced hypertension, increased urinary tract infections, and polyhydramnios (an excess of amniotic fluid). These changes are manageable and do not change the maternal diabetic prognosis. The rate of uterine growth and possible signs of preeclampsia are all monitored throughout pregnancy.

The problems that can complicate a pregnancy when the mother is insulin-dependent are of more concern to the fetus's well-being than the mother's. The infant may develop microsomia, congenital anomalies, respiratory distress syndrome, neonatal hypoglycemia, hypercalcemia, hypomagnesemia, and hyperbilirubinemia; sometimes death occurs. The degree and presence of these problems are related to the maternal glucose levels. To provide the best environment for the fetus, the maternal glucose level should be monitored daily and should be maintained below 120 mg/dl. The status of the fetus should be monitored during pregnancy, its age determined, and all possible efforts to bring it to maturity be made. Delivery of the infant should be early and safe; the infant should then be assessed by a skilled neonatologist. Fetal well-being may be monitored by contraction stress test, nonstress test, and daily maternal assessment of fetal activity.

Gestational diabetes is defined as diabetes that first appears during pregnancy. This occurs in about 3% of all pregnancies. All pregnant women should be screened for diabetes with a 50-gm oral glucose load. If blood drawn 1 hour later exceeds 135 mg/dl, then a 3-hour glucose tolerance test is indicated. If it is determined that the pregnant woman does indeed have gestational diabetes, a diabetic diet, and possibly insulin, will be needed. Class A diabetes is the classification given to pregnant women who have an abnormal glucose tolerance test but do not require insulin treatment. This accounts for 90% of all diabetics in pregnancy.[1] These patients' fetuses are at no higher risk for demise than those of nondiabetic obstetrical patients. Their fetuses are not electively delivered early, but their glucose levels are monitored every 2 weeks. If a Class A diabetic pregnant woman has required insulin in a previous pregnancy, has had either a previous stillbirth or previous hypertension, or develops preeclampsia in the current pregnancy, she is managed as an insulin-dependent diabetic. Her classification, however, does not change.[6]

## Renal Disease

Pregnancy causes marked changes in renal function. Disorders affecting renal function in pregnancy may be classified as infections, obstructions, acute renal failure, and chronic renal disease. The most common renal complication during pregnancy is urinary tract infection[1] characterized by ureteral dilation and relative obstruction. A resulting static column of ureteral urine and elevated glucose and amino acids in the urine facilitate bacterial growth. Because asymptomatic bacteriuria occurs in 2% to 10% of all pregnant women, and, if untreated, can lead to pyelonephritis in 25 to 30%, pregnant women should be screened periodically. Cystitis occurs in 1% of pregnant women. Symptoms include urinary frequency, pus, and painful urination.

Pyelonephritis (inflammation of the kidney) occurs in 1% to 2.5% of pregnancies. Symptoms are fever, bacteriuria, pus in the urine, costovertebral angle tenderness, vomiting, nausea, chills, urgency, frequency, and painful urination. The right kidney is more commonly affected. Acute pyelonephritis is often associated with premature labor, and the recurrence rate is high.

Urinary calculi (kidney stones) appear in 0.05% to 0.35% of pregnancies. Pregnancy does not increase the risk of stone formation. Although there is minimal risk of stone formation, urinary infections occur in 20% to 45% of pregnant patients with calculi. Symptoms include blood in urine, loin pain, flank pain, and severe or unresponsive pyelonephritis. Ureteral obstruction is rare in pregnancy. There have been reported about 10 cases in pregnancy of acute renal failure caused by obstruction from a gravid uterus, associated with a single kidney or uterine overdistention.

Incidence of acute renal failure has decreased dramatically in the last several decades. Preexisting renal failure is the cause of most acute renal failure in pregnancy and is related to dehydration, septic shock, or transfusion reaction. Factors in pregnancy that are associated with acute renal failure, most often occurring in the third trimester, include preeclampsia, placenta previa, and abruptio placentae. Severe hepatic dysfunction and jaundice may accompany acute renal failure. Most patients with acute renal suffer from renal insufficiency, and mortality is high.

Idiopathic postpartum renal failure may occur 3 to 10 days postdelivery in otherwise healthy patients. There is a high incidence of morbidity and mortality, dialysis is required, and surviving patients will have renal impairment.

In chronic renal disease, the incidence of fetal loss is 4.1% to 7% in normotensive mothers and 45% in hypertensive mothers. About one quarter of pregnant women with chronic renal disease are hypertensive and moderate decreases in renal function may occur. Pregnancy, in general, however, does not increase progression of renal disease. Pregnancy outcome in women with chronic renal disease varies.

Women with renal complications from collagen disease (*e.g.,* systemic lupus erythematosus) can have successful pregnancies, but in chronic glomerular nephritis, the outcome depends on the degree of renal failure and the amount of hypertension. Patients with diabetic nephropathy demonstrate no greater incidence of maternal mortality nor increased renal disease. Polycystic kidney disease and renal tuberculosis also appear to have no adverse effects on progression of disease or pregnancy, and women with one kidney can tolerate pregnancy. On the other hand, women with pelvic kidney (kidney misplaced into the pelvis) run a greater risk of urogenital tract malformation and dystocia at delivery.

Women with severe kidney disease who regularly receive renal dialysis rarely conceive; and patients who do get pregnant are at high risk. A recent study of 56 pregnancies in which the mother had a renal transplant reported 44 live newborns: 31 deliveries were uncomplicated, and of the fetuses, 4 had congenital abnormalities, 4 had respiratory distress, 2 had adrenal insufficiency, 2 septicemia, and 1 seizures. Patients with severe kidney disease are susceptible to infection and fetal anomalies because of immunosuppressive drugs used post-transplant. Criteria for pregnancy, developed by Davidson and Lindheimer, should be met before pregnancy is recommended to renal transplant mothers: (1) general good health 2 years after transplant (2) status compatible with good obstetric outcome (3) no significant proteinuria (4) no evidence of graft rejection (5) no evidence of hypertension (6) no evidence of pelvicalyceal distention on a recent intravenous pyelogram (7) serum creatinine of 2 mg/dl or less (8) therapeutic drug regimen consisting of 15 mg/dl or less of prednisone and 2 mg/kg/d, or less, of azathioprine (immunosuppressant drug).[4]

## Respiratory Disorders

Upper respiratory infections occur at the same rate in pregnant women as in nonpregnant women. The mother needs to increase fluids and rest, but she should avoid cough suppressants and antihistamines. Half of all pneumonias in pregnancy are preceded by an upper respiratory infection. During the major influenza epidemics of 1918-1919 and 1957-1958, mortality of pregnant women increased. The cause of death was influenzal pneumonia, rather than subsequent bacterial infection. Other than during those epidemics, there have been no studies to link influenza with an increase in maternal or fetal mortality or associated congenital anomalies. Treatment for the mother is the same as for upper respiratory infection. Interestingly, there are no data to suggest that vaccines from a killed virus for influenza yield any teratogenic effects on the fetus. Indications for a flu vaccine are the same as in a nonpregnant woman; but, nonetheless, the use of the vaccine in pregnancy is controversial.

General treatment for pneumonia includes use of expectorants, percussion and vibration, postural drainage, rest, fever-reducing drugs, avoidance of narcotics and cough suppressants, and correction of hypoxia. Hypoxia is not tolerated by the fetus, and correction of fluid electrolyte imbalances is vital. Bacterial pneumonia is usually treated with penicillin and the above supportive measures. Microplasma pneumonia is often treated with erythromycin, because tetracycline has been linked to fetal teeth staining, inhibition of fetal bone growth, and congenital anomalies, and, therefore, is contraindicated. Viral pneumonia requires the aforementioned supportive measures, but there is no specific drug treatment available for varicella pneumonia. When chicken pox pneumonia is complicated by a bacterial superinfection, it is associated with mortality as high as 41%. Neonatal mortality rate is as high as 34%. Fortunately it is not a common infection during pregnancy, because most mothers are immune from childhood exposure. Aspiration pneumonia in the mother calls for suction by endotracheal tube, and blood gases need to be closely monitored. Drugs are given to reduce bronchospasm.

A catastrophic event that mimics acute respiratory distress is amniotic fluid embolus. This type of embolus most often occurs in the multigravida mother late in the first stage of labor when the membranes have ruptured and the amniotic fluid is forced into the maternal circulation. Often the first sign is a sense of suffocation, dyspnea, general distress, agitation, and unexplained cough. The patient will develop chills and fever, cyanosis, and tachycardia; and pulmonary edema develops quickly. It is estimated that there is an 80% chance of fatality.

Pneumomediastinum tends to be a disorder that occurs during labor, but it may also occur during pregnancy. It involves increased alveolar pressure as a result of forceful expulsions with a closed glottis, accompanied by alveolar rupture and splitting of the air along the perivascular spaces into the mediastinum. The patient senses sudden onset of chest pain with a crackling, crunching sound (Hamman's sign) associated with heartbeat that may increase during systole. There is an increased presence of air in the subcutaneous tissues of the upper chest and neck 25% to 35% of the time. Without infection or increased mediastinal or intrapleural pressure, it is usually benign and resolves spontaneously.

Asthma is a chronic obstructive lung disease characterized by hyperreactive airways, increased airway secretion, and bronchospasm. Between attacks, the resultant obstruction may be partially or completely reversible with improvement in symptoms. There are two types: extrinsic asthma, an allergic phenomenon; and intrinsic, a nonspecific type. Symptoms are brought about by respiratory infections, emotional stress, exercise, and cold air. There are patients who have mixed types of asthma with both extrinsic and intrinsic characteristics. Asthma is believed to be a disorder of the autonomic nervous system's control of the respiratory system and occurs in 1.3% to 1.4% of all gestations. Typically, the disease is variable and unpredictable. There seems to be a slight tendency for the disease to improve in the first trimester and get slightly worse in the last trimester.

Women with severe asthma have about an 80% exacerbation rate during the current and subsequent pregnancies. Symptoms include shortness of breath, wheezing, and coughing. On auscultation of the chest, there is an increased expiratory phase and generalized wheezing. Most studies indicate an increased neonatal mortality among infants born to asthmatics; death results from increased frequency of low birth weight, premature labor, and episodes of severe attacks, inducing marked maternal hypoxemia with fetal hypoxia. Treatment during pregnancy is the same as in a nonpregnant state. Bronchodilators or corticosteroids are given for brief episodes. Typical blood gases reveal respiratory alkalosis due to hyperventilation with reduced $PCO_2$ and elevated arterial $p$H. This maternal alkalosis brings about a marked reduction in uterine blood flow and hypoxia. In one study, 5.7% of infants with asthmatic mothers developed asthma within the first year of life. Another 18.4% developed severe respiratory disease during the same period. In severe asthmatics, 28% of the pregnancies were associated with perinatal death, 35% produced low birth weight babies, and 12.5% of the infants were neurologically abnormal at one year of age.[7]

Chronic obstructive lung disease, chronic bronchitis, and emphysema are not usually seen in pregnant women. Treatment is the same as in a nonpregnant woman except to avoid tetracycline. Conduction anesthesia, rather than inhalation anesthesia, is indicated for labor and delivery. The rate of tuberculosis in pregnancy is 1% to 3%. Symptoms include malaise, cough, persistent low-grade fever, weight loss, night sweats, hemoptysis and chest pains, apical rales, cavernous breath sounds, and pleural effusion. Prognosis for the mother is the same as for a nonpregnant woman. If she has active disease, she should be treated. There is no teratogenic effect with INH (isoniazid), even when given during the first trimester. If the mother is treated, the fetus probably will not develop complications, because congenital tuberculosis is rare; however, if the mother is untreated, there is a 50% chance the child will develop tuberculosis in the first year of life, as well as a significant risk of death. If the mother has inactive disease, treated in the past, no treatment is required. If untreated, a mother should receive INH after delivery. If a mother's symptoms are covert in the previous 24 months, the risk of developing an active disease is 3% to 5%; she should begin INH for 1 year, starting after the first trimester. Breast-feeding is considered safe for women taking antituberculosis drugs.

Cystic fibrosis is a congenital, hereditary disease marked by dysfunction of any of the exocrine glands, resulting in an increase in sodium and potassium concentration of sweat and an overproduction of mucus. Women with cystic fibrosis, who conceive and carry pregnancy to term, are generally older than nonpregnant cystic fibrosis patients. Perinatal mortality is 11%, and premature labor occurs in 27%, both 4 times greater than normal. Symptoms include increased sodium and potassium production, sweating, cough of a chronic nature, and production of increased mucus. Cyanosis, dyspnea, and a vital capacity of less than 50% of predicted values are poor prognostic signs. Cor pulmonale and pulmonary hypertension in cystic fibrosis patients are absolute contraindications for pregnancy. These patients are more susceptible to bacteriologic pulmonary infection and almost always require chest physical therapy throughout their lives.

## Infectious, Gastrointestinal, and Dermatologic Diseases and Disorders

Another strong determinant of fetal well-being and infant health is the maternal response to infectious disease, gastrointestinal disturbance, and dermatologic disorders. Many infectious diseases can be easily contracted by the mother, particularly if she has other children. Sexually-transmitted diseases also can have devastating consequences for the pregnant woman and her baby. Highlights of selected infectious diseases are listed in Table 10-3 and selected gastrointestinal and dermatologic disorders in Tables 10-4 and 10-5.

## Reproductive Tract Disorders

Alterations in the reproductive tract can occur during pregnancy as a result of uterine pressure on the vessels, tumors, congenital anomalies, and pelvic infections.

Retrodisplacement of the uterus (backward displacement of the uterus) occurs fairly often in the early months of pregnancy. If retrodisplacement occurs at the ninth or tenth week, however, the uterus may become lodged by the hollow of the sacrum, resulting in compression of the urethra and bladder neck. Knee-to-chest position may help dislodge the uterus, or, if that fails, anesthetic procedure may be performed.

Similarly rare is torsion of the uterus, associated with considerable pain and pathology such as myomas, ovarian cysts, adhesions, or

## Table 10-3. Effects of Infectious Diseases on Pregnancy

| Disease | Symptoms | Effects on Mother | Effects on Fetus |
|---|---|---|---|
| *AIDS* (acquired immunodeficiency syndrome; transmitted by blood and body fluids sexually and transplacentally) | Hypergammaglobulinemia, weight loss, lymphadenopathy, hepatosplenomegaly, diarrhea | Spontaneous abortion rate 25%–50%; hypoxia; premature labor; prognosis poor | No fetal malformation noted; transplacental transmission; prognosis poor |
| *Coxsackie virus* (type A similar to common cold; type B, severe chest wall pain) | Minor respiratory symptoms | Usually self-limiting; no effect on mortality | Type A, no effect on fetus, type B, myocarditis, encephalitis, mortality, tetralogy of fallot |
| *Cytomegalovirus* (in U.S., 50% adults seropositive; herpes virus; infects 50%–60% of women in childbearing ages) | Low-grade fever, malaise, lymphadenopathy, enlarged liver and spleen; may be asymptomatic | Self-limiting infection; no increase in morbidity or mortality in pregnancy | Fetus infected through the placenta or at birth when passing through infected birth canal; possible mental retardation, hearing loss, microcephaly, intracranial calcification, enlarged liver and spleen; stillbirth |
| *Epstein-Barr virus* (serologic diagnosis) | Malaise, fatigue, muscle soreness and tightness, fever, infections, swollen glands | Unknown | Unknown |
| *Hepatitis* (type A, infectious; B, viral; C, serum; 15–180 day incubation) | Malaise, fever, anorexia, nausea, vomiting; chronic liver disease; jaundice; itching; rash, myalgia, lymphadenopathy | Spontaneous abortion and prematurity | Congenital abnormalities; paralysis, convulsions; jaundice; 34% mortality |
| *Herpes simplex virus 1 and 2* | Type 1, cold sores; Type 2, genital blisters | Premature labor; Cesarean section recommended | Transplacental transmission rare; possible fetal contact with infected genital tract in delivery; possible skin lesions, general infection, brain damage, encephalitis |
| *Malaria* (transmitted by anopheles mosquito) | High, spiking fever, headache, myalgia | Abortion possible in severe attacks, prematurity, stillbirth | Growth retardation; fever, enlarged liver and spleen, seizures, jaundice, pulmonary edema 48–72 hours after delivery |

**Table 10-3. Continued**

| Disease | Symptoms | Effects on Mother | Effects on Fetus |
| --- | --- | --- | --- |
| *Mumps* (vaccine contraindicated in pregnant women; contagious disease; 2–3 week incubation) | Generalized infection; swollen parotid glands; possible aseptic meningitis, meningoencephalitis, adenositis, pancreatitis | Spontaneous abortion first trimester | No increase in congenital malformations; possible endocardial fibroelastosis |
| *Poliomyelitis* (rare disease in pregnancy; vaccine should be avoided during pregnancy) | Lower motor neuron paralytic motor disease; fever; nausea; vomiting; nasal inflammation; sore throat; hyperesthesia; muscle pain | Spontaneous abortion | Paralysis, neonatal poliomyelitis; mortality rate 25% |
| *Rubella* (German measles; vaccine decreased number of cases; 15%–20% of childbearing women do not have antibody; 3-mo wait required before pregnancy after vaccine; highly contagious; incubation period 14–21 days) | Erythematous raised rash; lymphadenopathy; arthralgia; arthritis; fever; cough | Spontaneous abortion and stillbirth 2–4 × more frequent | Congenital rubella syndrome; 70% chance of direct infection of fetus in first trimester; risk of fetal malformation or death ranges 10%–34%; cataracts, blindness, cardiac anomalies, deafness, mental retardation, cerebral palsy, encephalitis, cleft palate, hemolytic anemia, birthmarks, hepatosplenomegaly, thrombocytopenia purpura |
| *Rubeola* (measles; slight increase recently; attenuated vaccine given 1957–1967, requiring revaccination; highly contagious disease incubation 10–12 days) | Small, irregular red spots on face and extremities; fever; encephalitis in 1/100 cases | Spontaneous abortion rate high; premature delivery | Death within 2 years; congenital malformations |
| *Streptococcal infection* (group A, puerperal fever; B, genital tract) | Symptoms of bacterial infection; treatment with penicillin required | Endometritis, chorioamnionitis, septic abortion, pelvic peritonitis, premature rupture of membranes | 25% neonatal sepsis, meningitis; pneumonia |

**Table 10-3. Continued**

| Disease | Symptoms | Effects on Mother | Effects on Fetus |
|---|---|---|---|
| *Toxoplasmosis* (common worldwide infection, usually from cat feces and poorly cooked infected meat) | Asymptomatic lymphadenopathy; sore throat, myalgias, macular rash; enlarged spleen and liver; pneumonia; meningitis | Morbidity and mortality unaffected; 10%–15% increase in spontaneous abortion in first and second trimesters | First trimester, lowest incidence of congenital infection; highest in third trimester; possible stillbirth or premature birth; possible mental retardation, hydrocephaly, microcephaly, corioretinitis, convulsions, blindness, deafness |
| *Varicella* (chicken pox or later shingles, herpes zoster) | Prodromal symptoms of fever, malaise, rash, possible pneumonia; 1/3 of adults develop pneumonia | Mortality 41% | Mortality 34%; anomalies; neurologic deficit, mental retardation; seizures, paralysis, limb atrophy; cutaneous scars; rudimentary digits; convulsions; cortical atrophy |

uterine anomalies. The uterus rotates on a radial axis of 45% or greater. Cesarean section is often advised, but fetal mortality is high, and maternal mortality occurs in 50% of all cases.

Uterine sacculation, prolapse, and inversion are extremely rare disorders, but can produce pain and premature labor. If the uterus sacculates, it can result in severe anteflexion due to poor abdominal tone in the late third trimester. Most often seen in grand multiparas, this may result in abnormal fetal presentation or lack of engagement. Uterine prolapse however, also usually seen in a multipara, may occur during any trimester. Treatment requires bed rest with a slight Trendelenburg position to avoid premature labor and rupture of membranes. Cesarean section may be necessary. More severe than prolapse is uterine inversion, which may occur immediately following delivery. In this case, the uterus turns inside out and protrudes through the cervix and outside the vagina. This condition can be acute, subacute, or chronic. It happens most often to multiparas with a lax uterus, from fundal pressure following delivery, and from excessive umbilical cord traction.

Myoma uteri is a benign tumor of the uterine muscle, occurring in some 40% to 50% of women, as determined by autopsy. These tumors may enlarge during the first 12 weeks of pregnancy, but are usually stable after that time. There is a slight chance of late abor-

**Table 10-4. Effects of Gastrointestinal Diseases on Pregnancy[2,3,4]**

| Disease | Symptoms | Effects on Mother | Effects on Fetus |
| --- | --- | --- | --- |
| *Nausea and vomiting* (after first missed period, may last up to 12 wk) | May be related to elevated levels of steroid hormones and hCG | Usually none | Usually none |
| *Hyperemesis gravidarum* (protracted nausea and vomiting occurring throughout pregnancy, any time of day in 3.5/1000 pregnancies) | Weight loss, electrolyte imbalance, dehydration, ketonemia, possible renal or hepatic damage, bleeding from strained throat muscles; increased gastric acid causing gum recession | Endurance may be decreased; nutritional deficiency | No increase in congential malformations or abortion |
| *Appendicitis* (occurs 1/1500 deliveries) | Pain in right lower quadrant in early pregnancy, in right upper quadrant in third trimester; mortality 2% overall; 7% in third trimester and in general population 1.8%; increased morbidity due to delayed diagnosis from pregnancy masking signs and symptoms | Possibility of appendix rupture with infection if removed near term; retention sutures used so mothers can push during delivery and not disturb wound | Mortality 97%; increased with generalized peritonitis |
| *Reflux esophagitis* (heartburn complicates up to 25% of pregnancies; associated with reflux secondary to progesterone and relaxation of lower esophageal sphincter) | Substantial burning, worse after eating and lying down or bending over; usually appears at end of second month; most severe at 32 wk gestation | No known complications | No known complications |
| *Intestinal obstruction* (uncommon in pregnancy; can be caused by adhesions) | Abdominal pain, steady or colicky; vomiting, nausea, abdominal distention, constipation | Surgical intervention needed if stomach decompression not successful; possible hypoxia or hypertension during surgery | Negative effects from complications of surgery |

## Table 10-4. Continued

| Disease | Symptoms | Effects on Mother | Effects on Fetus |
|---|---|---|---|
| *Peptic ulcer disease* (pregnancy has beneficial effect on the disease; 45% of patients symptom-free in pregnancy; pregnancy may protect against development of duodenal ulcers; prostaglandins assert protective effect on gastric mucosa) | Upper gastrointestinal bleeding, usually worse when the stomach is empty; relieved by food or antacids | High incidence ulcer recurrence during lactation; breast-feeding usually not recommended | |
| *Inflammatory bowel disease* (chronic relapsing and remission disease little affected by pregnancy; includes ulcerative colitis and Crohn's disease) | Decreased fertility rate; weight loss, abdominal pain, diarrhea, fever | Relapse common in pregnancy | No increase in prenatal mortality, anomalies or abortion |
| *Pancreatitis* (related to gallstone in 2/3 of cases) | 24–48 attack of right upper quadrant and abdominal pain, nausea and vomiting, pain radiating to back | 37% mortality | Perinatal mortality 37.9% |
| *Cholecystitis* (gall bladder emptying time may be slowed) | Pain in the mid-epigastrum, right scapular and shoulder pain, nausea vomiting, right upper quadrant pain, jaundice | Surgical treatment, if medical therapy doesn't respond in 4 days | Negative effects only from complications of surgery |
| *Intrahepatic cholestasis* (estrogen-related defect in hepatic bile excretion) | Develops late in pregnancy with itching of hands and feet as early as the 6th wk; jaundice if severe | No serious maternal effects; symptoms resolve within few wk of delivery | Perinatal mortality is 4 × that of controls; fetal distress present in 40%; increase of preterm labor, stillbirths, meconium staining |
| *Acute fatty liver of pregnancy* (rare, lethal disorder of unknown etiology; occurs between 30 and 38 wk of pregnancy; more common in twin and male births and in primigravidas) | Repeated vomiting, abdominal pain, nausea, jaundice; in severe cases, hepatic encephalopathy, renal failure, and hemorrhage; may not occur in subsequent pregnancies | Prognosis for the fetus and mother 75%–80% mortality | Early delivery when lung maturity reached may reduce infant mortality |

**Table 10-4. Continued**

| Disease | Symptoms | Effects on Mother | Effects on Fetus |
|---|---|---|---|
| *Chronic liver disease* | Treated with prednisone and azathioprine | No affect on maternal survival nor number of occurrences of hepatitis | Increased incidence of fetal morbidity and mortality |
| *Cirrhosis* (rare disease in pregnancy; complications in estrogen metabolism may result in infertility) | Increased portal pressure due to increased blood volume; esophageal varices due to added weight of gravid uterus on vena cava | Possible fatal hemorrhage, deteriorated liver function; complications from bleeding or esophageal varices, postpartum hemorrhage | Perinatal mortality increased |
| *Hepatic tumors of pregnancy* (adenoma; associated with prior contraceptive steroid use) | Highly vascular tumors enlarged in response to estrogen, may rupture and hemorrhage | Successful pregnancy possible but contraindicated in patients with an unresected adenoma | |

tion, premature birth, or fetal death in utero. Symptoms include pain in the right lower quadrant on the side of the myoma. Ultrasound confirms diagnosis and placement to determine if the myoma overlies the placenta. If they do overlap, there is a 75% complication rate and a two-fold increase in limb anomalies. Cesarean section may be indicated.

Ovarian tumors may occur in the first trimester, and 35% of

**Table 10-5. Effects of Dermatologic Diseases on Pregnancy**

| Disease | Symptoms | Fetal/Maternal Complications |
|---|---|---|
| *Pruritus gravidarum* (affects 20% of pregnant women; associated with cholestasis) | Severe generalized itching in third trimester | None; disappears after delivery |
| *Pruritic urticarial papules* (rash of symmetric, itching papules) | Rash in third trimester in primigravidas | None; disappears after delivery |
| *Herpes gestationis* (unrelated to herpes virus; may recur with subsequent pregnancy, menstruation, or from progesterone medications; usually occurs in second or third trimester) | Malaise, chills, fever, headache, nausea, abdominal and trunk lesions, progressing to extremities; polymorphous, blister-like eruptions | Resolves 3 mo after delivery; fetus small for gestational age; occasionally transient blueness noted in newborn mother |
| *Impetigo herpetiformis* (rare, pustular eruptions; onset third trimester) | Rash in axillae and inguinal folds; may become widespread; malaise, chills, vomiting, diarrhea, sometimes tetany | Remission postpartum; may recur in subsequent pregnancies; treated with corticosteroids; may result in still-birth or placental insufficiency |

women will spontaneously abort. This type of tumor is best removed between 16-18 weeks of gestation to decrease the chance of spontaneous abortion. Malignant ovarian tumors occur once in every 9000 to 25,000 deliveries.

One to 1.5 million women were exposed to diethylstilbestrol (DES) between 1940 and 1970. Exposure in utero has increased the incidence of spontaneous abortion in the first and second trimesters, related to incompetent cervix in the daughters of DES-exposed women. Other anomalies in the female reproductive tract have been linked to DES exposure as well. Thirty-five percent have intrauterine defects, irregular margins, T-shaped uteri, and narrow cavities; 35% have increased incidence of clear cell adenocarcinoma of the vagina; and 24% have cervical structural changes. There appears to be a 20-fold increase in ectopic pregnancies.

DES is also believed responsible for 90% of Mullerian duct anomalies, including divided uteri, two uteri and two vaginas, and an unfused or bifurcated uterus in the vagina. Problems arise with pregnancy. Multiple anomalies of urinary and reproductive tract are the most complex: (1) persistent cloacae when the urorectal septum fails to form, (2) exstrophy of the bladder, and (3) anomalies of the external genitalia due to defective closure of the abdominal wall.

Pelvic infections are yet another reproductive tract dysfunction that the practitioner needs to be aware of when treating patients. These diseases and their effects on the pregnancy are summarized in Table 10-6.

## Neurologic Diseases and Disorders

Neurologic diseases and disorders may be divided into three major categories: (1) disorders of the peripheral nervous system (see Table 10-7), (2) disorders of the central nervous system (see Table 10-8), and (3) neuromuscular diseases (see Table 10-9). Obstetric palsies occur once in every 2600 deliveries. The nerves most commonly injured during delivery include: the obturator (L3-4), caused by compression by the fetal head antepartum or during delivery and resulting in weakness of the thigh abductors with minimal sensory deficit over the medial aspect of the thigh; the femoral (L2-3), caused by psoas muscle hemorrhage, pelvic trauma, or compression in the pelvic cavity and resulting in weakness of the quadriceps or psoas muscles with minimal sensory loss in the anteromedial thigh; and the peroneal nerve (L4-5), caused by compression by stirrups and resulting in weakness of toe extensors and foot eversion with sensory loss over the anterolateral leg and dorsal foot. In all of the above cases, physical therapy is indicated to increase strength and mobility and to instruct in the use of assistive devices or orthoses.

In addition to injuries during delivery, peripheral nerves may

**Table 10-6. Effects of Pelvic Infections on Pregnancy**

| Disease | Symptoms | Effects on Mother | Effects on Fetus |
|---|---|---|---|
| *Syhphilis* (bacterial; transmitted through sexual contact; 25,000 cases/yr in U.S.) | Primary oral and anal cankers extra-genitally; secondary symptoms of skin rashes on palms, soles and perigeni-tally; general ade-nopathy and low-grade fever | Morbidity same as in nonpregnant women | Risk of infection 80%–95% if mother untreated; 25% of fetal death *in utero*; 25%–30% fetal death shortly after birth; syphilitic symptoms in 40% of survivors after third week of life |
| *Gonorrhea* (bacte-rial; asymptomatic in 80%; affects ure-thra, cervix, fallopian tubes, Bartholin's gland) | Pain and tenderness in the pelvic region; cervical discharge; fever and painful urination | Affected in the last 20 wk of gestation of puerperium; in-creased chance of gonococcal arthritis; abortion possible from premature membrane rupture | Neonatal gonorrhea higher *in utero* and during delivery; infections, including conjunctivitis, otitis externa; vulvova-ginitis |
| *Chlamydia* (in-creased incidence of intracellular bacte-ria) | Same as for gonor-rhea | Morbidity and mor-tality same as in nonpregnant women | Transplacental infection occurs; 40%–50% will have inclusion conjunctivi-tis |
| *Trichomoniasis vaginitis* (50% asymptomatic; venereally transmit-ted) | Itching, painful urination | Discomfort | Drugs to be avoided in early pregnancy |
| *Candidiasis vaginitis* (causes more than 90% of vaginal yeast infections) | Itching, burning, red vulva; cottage cheese-type dis-charge; frothy, yellow-green dis-charge | Risk for developing candida vulvova-ginitis; discomfort | Drug not to be used during the first 20 wk |
| *Gardnerella vaginitis* (bacteria may be sexually transmitted) | Slight yellow-gray discharge | Discomfort | Drugs to be avoided in early pregnancy |

become irritated during pregnancy from mechanical disturbance or compression from increased fluid volume (see Table 10-6).

Some studies show a three-fold increase during pregnancy of Bell's palsy, although this disorder is not associated with parity or preeclampsia. Pregnancy does not alter the prognosis for multiple sclerosis patients, but the frequency of exacerbation is most pro-foundly decreased in the third trimester.[1]

## *Musculoskeletal Disorders*

Disorders of the musculoskeletal system are of major interest to physical therapists. Here, our skills are utilized most appropriately in diagnosis and treatment. The multiple musculoskeletal pains of pregnancy in the back, arms, and legs are so commonplace that

**Table 10-7. Effects of Peripheral Nerve Disorders on Pregnancy**

| Disorder | Symptoms | Effects on Mother | Effects on Fetus |
|---|---|---|---|
| *Carpal tunnel syndrome* (occurs in 1%–10% of pregnancies; compression of the median nerve or retinaculum; symptoms appear in third trimester and may persist up to 12 wk postpartum)[9] | Pain and paresthesia along median nerve distribution; pain worse at night, weakness, thenar atrophy; sensory loss | Impaired hand strength requires decrease in activities requiring heavy use of hands; possible steroid injections may require surgical decompression after pregnancy | None |
| *Guillain-Barre syndrome* (acute polyradiculoneuritis; rare during pregnancy; usually follows a viral illness; accompanied by ascending paralysis in cranial nerves; tendon reflexes absent) | Paresthesias and muscle pain; all muscles possibly involved; may be respiratory depression | Onset during third trimester, may increase chance of premature labor; assistance possibly needed during second stage of labor due to weakness of the voluntary abdominal muscles; uterine musculature normal; physical therapy treatment for rehabilitation imperative in recovery phase; recovery rate high with appropriate support and therapies | Possible risk of premature labor during third trimester |
| *Radiculopathy* (involves intervertebral disk bulge, herniation, or nerve root lesion) | Severe back pain with radiating pain into leg; paresthesias, sensory loss, reflex impairment, or weakness in distribution of nerve root lesion. | Extreme discomfort; conservative treatment usually attempted first, involving rest, physical therapy, and support | None |
| *Sciatic neuritis* (pain and tenderness over the sciatic and femoral nerve distributions from relaxation of the sacroiliac joints, subsequent rotation of the pelvis or trauma to the nerves) | Irritation along sciatic nerve and, occasionally, femoral nerve | Discomfort, difficulty in getting around; physical therapy needed to instruct on comfort positions, orthoses use, activities of daily living | None |
| *Polyneuritis* (related to thiamine deficiency from hyperemesis gravidarum; degenerative nerve changes) | Diminished sensation, paralysis, muscular atrophy; may involve single nerve or more | Discomfort depends on degree of disorder; decreased muscular coordination, strength; possibly fatal | Varies according to degree of disease |

**Table 10-7. Continued**

| Disease | Symptoms | Effects on Mother | Effects on Fetus |
|---|---|---|---|
| *Myralgia paresthetica* (common disorder in pregnancy from compression of lateral femoral cutaneous nerve at inguinal ligament or where anterior branch enters tensor fasciae latae; often apears in third trimester | Pain, numbness, and tingling in middle third of lateral thigh; no motor dysfunction; pain may be excerbated by standing or walking, relieved by sitting or supine | Discomfort, restriction in activities; benefits from instruction in posture correction and modification of activities; resolves after delivery | None |

concern and treatment may be overlooked. Simple, conservative, noninvasive measures minimize and eliminate these pains. Etiology is the focus of this chapter. Evaluation and treatment methods for these disorders will be examined in the next chapter.

Low back pain may be caused by sacroiliac pain, ruptured disk, symphysial separation, and dislocation of the coccyx. Muscular pain often occurs in the second and third trimester of pregnancy due to the increased weight of the uterus and the body's center of gravity shifting forward with resulting increased lumbar lordosis, a weakening of abdominal muscles, and relaxation of the sacroiliac ligaments. Excessive stress is placed on the facet joints and posterior ligaments of the lumbar spine. Pregnant women complain of pain in the lower lumbar area, usually aggravated by standing, walking, and lifting and relieved by recumbent or side-lying positions.[10] This lower lumbar pain occurs frequently and is the major cause of back pain in pregnancy. Relaxation of the symphysis pubis and dislocation of the coccyx may also be responsible for referred low back pain.

Cervical spine irritation may result from increased weight gain in the breast tissue, adding strain to the brachial plexus, and causing a change in posture in the neck and upper back positions. The shoulders become naturally rounded and the neck follows. The neck lordosis increases as the eyes look to the horizon. Over time, it may lead to irritation of the cervical nerve roots.

Leg cramps occur in 15% to 30% of all pregnant women usually in the second half of pregnancy,[5] and are painful, tetany-like contractions of the gastrocsoleus groups or occasionally of the thigh muscles. They occur most frequently when women are sleeping and may be strong enough to awaken them. The cramps may last from several seconds to several minutes. The etiology is unknown, but a deficit of calcium or magnesium has been proposed as the cause. Stretching of

## Table 10-8. Effects of Central Nervous System Disorders on Pregnancy

| Disease | Symptoms | Effects on Mother | Effects on Fetus |
|---|---|---|---|
| *Aneurysm* (rupture usually in the angle of bifurcation of vessels in the circle of Willis) | Sudden extreme headache, neck rigidity, nausea and vomiting, hemiplegia, seizures; usually occurs late second or third trimester; rare in delivery or in puerperium | Delivery usually augmented with epidural anesthesia with assisted second stage delivery; morbidity and mortality rate is 47%–70% in patients managed conservatively with bed rest compared to 8% mortality after neurosurgery; possible hemiplegia; physical therapy indicated | Fetal distress and premature labor if hypotension results during neurosurgical procedures |
| *Arteriovenous malformations* (AVM) (commonly located in the frontoparietal or temporoparietal region; more common in multiparas; may bleed in first or early second trimester | Severe headache, seizures present in 30%; focal neurological deficits in 20%; hydrocephalus possible | High morbidity and mortality for mother; Cesarean section at 38 wk offers protection; Valsalva maneuver contraindicated; low forceps delivery with augmentation | Fetal complications as high as 49% |
| *Intercerebral hemorrhage* (primary form is rare in pregnancy; may occur from eclampsia, hypertension, or bleeding from AVM) | Acute onset of headache and alterations in consciousness; other symptoms dependent on location and size of hemorrhage; focal seizures possible | Possibility of hydration, steroid inbalance, ventilatory failure | Unknown |
| *Cerebral artery occulsions* (preeclampsia possible predisposing factor; increased risk of carotid artery stroke in pregnancy) | Signs and symptoms dependent on location and magnitude of infarct; hemiplegia; hemisensory imbalance, visual defects, speech disturbances and headache; seizures | Vaginal delivery favored over Cesarean due to possibility of further infarct brought on by hypotension from hemorrhage or anesthesia; physical therapy crucial | Unknown |
| *Cerebral venous thrombosis* (can occur 1–4 wk after delivery; rare in pregnancy) | Headache usually precedes onset of seizures; recurrence of seizures, implying spreading of the thrombus; fever | Morbidity 30%–50%; survivors less disabled than those who have arterial stroke | No effect |
| *Pituitary tumors* (may increase during pregnancy; may prevent ovulation) | Decreasing vision and visual field deficits form pressure on optic chiasm | Surgery or radiotherapy indicated for rapidly failing vision; remission usually after delivery | None |

**Table 10-8. Continued**

| Disease | Symptoms | Effects on Mother | Effects on Fetus |
| --- | --- | --- | --- |
| *Meningiomas* (may increase in size during pregnancy; astrocytomas and spinal angiomas) | Signs and symptoms dependent on size and location of tumor; headaches, visual field defects; focal neurologic deficits possible and progressive | Anesthesia needed in labor to decrease intracranial pressure from Valsalva maneuver | Unknown |
| *Choriocarcinoma* (occurs after molar pregnancy abortion or sometimes after normal pregnancy) | Usually symptoms appear and progress in the second half of pregnancies; decrease after delivery, but reappear in future pregnancies; metastases, seizures, intracerebral hemorrage, subdural hematoma, subarachnoid hemorrhage | Neurosurgery, if indicated carried out in any stage of pregnancy; therapeutic abortion option for maligant brain tumors; regional anesthesia important to decrease the possibility of intracranial pressure from Valsalva maneuver | Unknown |
| *Epilepsy* (affects 0.3%–0.5% of pregnancies; increased seizure frequency in 37%, decreased in 13%) | Frequency of seizures returns to pregestational level after pregnancy | Risk of seizures if not taking medication or not being properly monitored; after birth, anticonvulsant drugs transported in breast milk, breastfeeding contraindicated | Defects of coagulation rates noted in newborns of mothers who take anticonvulsants; may have hemorrhages shortly after or during birth; congenital malformations in 4%–5% of children with mothers who do not take antiepileptic drugs and 6%–11% in children whose mothers do take anti-epileptic drugs; most common malformations—midline closure-orofacial clefts and cardiac septal defects; 2% increase of seizure activity in children born to mothers having seizure disorders |

**Table 10-8. Continued**

| Disease | Symptoms | Effects on Mother | Effects on Fetus |
|---|---|---|---|
| *Migraine* (recurrent vascular-type headaches that last hours to days; 30% of women with migraines asymptomatic during pregnancy; 50%, fewer or less severe migraines; 20%, worsen or fail to improve) | Usually throbbing, severe headache, may cause photophobia, vomiting, nausea, hemianopsia, or neurologic disturbance | Traditional migraine medicines not suggested during pregnancy; biofeedback and other noninvasive physical measures may be indicated | None |
| *Pseudotremor cerebri* (benign, intracranial hypertension that mimics tumor; spontaneous recovery; may occur 12–20 wk gestation; symptoms stop in 1–2 wk, but intracranial pressure remains elevated; remission after delivery; recurs in 5%–10% subsequent pregnancies) | Headaches; blurred or double vision in 10% of patients; tinnitus, nausea, vomiting, papillar edema, or swelling of optic nerve; present bilaterally, with weakness of the the abducens nerve | Frequent ophthalmologic examinations necessary | None |
| *Wernicke's encephalopathy* (caused by severe cases of hyperemesis gravidarum, leading to thiamine deficiency) | Ataxia, global confusion, horizontal and vertical nystagmus, ophthalomoplegia; Korsakoff's psychosis possible if untreated | Treatment with thiamine and other B vitamins and fluids; disease may be fatal | Possibly fatal if untreated in mother |

the gastrocnemius-soleus group, along with the strengthening of the anterior tibialis, may lead to a reduction in these cramps.

Transient osteoporosis is a rare complication of pregnancy ( 100 cases described up until 1984). It usually does not develop until the last trimester. Vague pains in the pelvis, hip, thigh, and groin may be mistaken for pelvic instability or simple muscular fatigue. There may be unilateral pain in the hip and groin with radiation to the knee. If untreated, this disorder can precipitate complete stress fracture of the femoral neck. It has been proposed that this is a variant of Sudeck's atrophy or reflex sympathetic dystrophy. Symptoms appear gradually. Low back pain is rarely present, and the symptoms usually become so intense that the woman is unable to bear full weight. These women should avoid full weightbearing and use crutches to decrease the stress on the proximal femur. If a stress fracture does occur, surgical treatment may be necessary, and degenerative change in the hip joint may occur in the future. Hip and

**Table 10-9. Effects of Neuromuscular Diseases on Pregnancy**

| Disease | Symptoms | Effects on Mother | Effects on Fetus |
| --- | --- | --- | --- |
| *Chorea gravidarum* (rare disease of pregnancy; form of Sydenham's chorea, may first appear during pregnancy, usually in first or second trimester; goes into remission before delivery) | Nonrhythmic movements that are rapid, jerky, involuntary of extremities, face or trunk; usually aggravated by emotional stress; symptoms decrease during sleep | Maternal mortality greatly decreased since 1930s | Fetal mortality greatly decreased since 1930s |
| *Myasthenia gravis* (autoimmune disease characterized by high titers of IgG antibodies against acetylcholine receptors in striated muscle; remission in 30% during pregnancy; 30-40% have exacerbation, especially in puerperium) | Weakness of muscles innervated by the cranial nerves; visual symptoms, difficulty with speech and swallowing | Uterine smooth muscle unaffected | 12%–20% of offspring develop neonatal myasthenia gravis, mild to severe muscle weakness; symptoms possible first day, persist 2–4 wk |
| *Myotonic dystrophy* (autosomal dominant inherited disease) | Progressive muscular dystrophy with weakness in limbs, cataracts, myotonia, wasting of the muscles of the neck and limbs, baldness, testicular atrophy, mental retardation, arrhythmias | Spontaneous abortion, premature delivery; involved uterine muscle possibly unable to retain fetus | High rate of fetal loss; increased incidence of hydramnios; weakness; diplegia; foot deformity; arthrygrypolis multiplex congenita; hypotonia; difficulty in swallowing, sucking, and breathing[2,3,4] |

groin pain decrease significantly a few months after delivery. Gradually, the proximal femur reconstitutes itself. Four to 6 months after delivery, most women will be asymptomatic and x-rays will appear normal.

Pregnancy has a beneficial effect on symptoms of rheumatoid arthritis. Two thirds of pregnant women with rheumatoid arthritis notice a substantial decrease in pain, swelling, and redness, usually immediately after conception, and continuing until 6 weeks postpartum. Elevated maternal cortisone levels and a generalized suppression of immune response in pregnancy may account for this remission. There is a mild anemia that accompanies this disease that may be exacerbated by the physiologic anemia of pregnancy. If there is deformity of the pelvis or hips, vaginal delivery may be impaired or impossible. The rheumatoid factor does not cross the placenta, and there are no specific effects of the disease on the fetus. Physical therapy and occupational therapy measures are helpful in evaluating function, strength, and range of motion of the involved joints.

Supportive measures would be splinting, strengthening, and restoration of function coupled with protected daily living activities postpartum. Consideration must also be given to increased maternal activities involving care of the infant.

Systemic lupus erythematosus occurs in 1 of every 1660 pregnancies. Clinically, arthralgia or arthritis affects 90% of women with the disease; dermatologic involvement, 70% to 80%; renal disease, 46%; hematologic abnormalities, 50%; and, cardiovascular disease, 30% to 50%. The disease is characterized by periods of exacerbation and remission. Maternal complications involve the cardiac and renal systems, spontaneous abortion, premature labor, fetal growth retardation, and stillbirths. Stillbirths are common in these patients. Pregnancy should be considered only after the patient has a complete understanding of the severity of the disease. There should be a coordinated approach between the obstetrician, rheumatologist, and patient.

Scleroderma can cause excessive fibrosis and vascular changes of the skin, gastrointestinal tract, heart, lung, and kidneys. There is a poor prognosis for the pregnancy if there is severe organ involvement. Labor is not affected by scleroderma, and healing from an episiotomy or Cesarean section is normal. There are no known effects on the newborn and no evidence that scleroderma is transmitted to the fetus. Corticosteroids can be of benefit, and treatment of the disease includes strengthening and range of motion exercises for involved joints and muscles.

Osteogenesis imperfecta is an inherited disorder characterized by bone frailty, blue sclerae, and osteosclerotic deafness. The condition results from hypoplasia of the bone mesenchyme. Usually, patients with this condition have a complicated pregnancy. Previous fractures may have distorted the pelvis, making a vaginal delivery impossible. Weight gain during pregnancy may put additional stress on the pregnant woman's fragile bones, increasing the likelihood of fracture. Uterine labor contractions can be strong enough to cause fractures, if the fetus also has osteogenesis imperfecta, making Cesarean section the preferred method of delivery.

There has been no reported increase in the degree of spinal curvature during pregnancy, despite the additional mechanical stresses and influence of relaxin. Deformities and curves may cause greater discomfort during pregnancy and labor, but there seems to be no increase in progression of the curve as compared to before pregnancy. A daily regimen of stretching and strengthening exercises is believed to be the key to avoiding discomfort in the low back area.

Spinal cord-injured patients are able to carry the fetus to term.

The major problem is that these women are unable to sense the onset of labor. They can have normal contractions but will not feel them. Because of this, second stage may begin before they are able to contact their birth attendant, and they may deliver outside the hospital. During labor and delivery, these patients may suffer from autonomic hyperreflexia. The patient's autonomic nervous system may be stimulated and cause sudden cardiac irregularities, severe hypertension, anxiety, and sweating. These symptoms resolve spontaneously after delivery but should be closely monitored. To avoid this occurrence outside of the hospital or birth facility, due dates should be used to keep a close watch on pregnant women with spinal cord injuries.

Because automobile accidents occur with the same frequency whether a woman is pregnant or not, clients should be advised to wear seatbelts to prevent high-impact skeletal fractures. The lap belt should be worn against the iliac spine, below the enlarged uterus, with the chest strap going across the chest in the normal fashion. If fractures do occur, however, pregnant women have only the traditional treatment options. Surgical fixation may be chosen more often as the stabilization because of the added weight and physical stresses of pregnancy, and, because prolonged skeletal traction for femoral shaft fracture near a pregnant woman's due date would restrict a vaginal delivery. There is also the risk of thrombophlebitis during long periods of bed rest if skeletal traction is considered. If surgery is the answer, procedures are better tolerated by women in their second trimester. X-rays may be taken, if necessary, with careful shielding of the fetus.

Prior pelvic fractures may predispose a pregnant woman to cephalopelvic disproportion, especially as a result of central fracture, dislocation of the hip with residual medial protrusion of the acetabulum and femoral head, and Malgaigne-type fracture dislocations, (ilium on the injured side is displaced in a cephalad direction). Pelvimetry and clinical exam allow the physician to measure the birth canal and predict whether the fetal head will be able to pass. Many women are able to have a normal vaginal delivery following a previous pelvic fracture.

## *Self-Assessment Review*

1. Gestational diabetes is defined as _____.
2. Name two reasons why there is an increased possibility of back pain in pregnancy: _____, _____
3. Pregnant women should not wear seat belts as the belt may exert excessive pressure on the fetus during an accident. True False

4. _____ is a benign tumor consisting of muscle tissue.
5. Preeclampsia is characterized by _____, _____, and _____.
6. Eclampsia, if untreated, will lead to _____.
7. Hyperemesis gravidarum is marked by severe and protracted _____.
8. Asthma (acute or chronic) is a disease characterized by _____, _____, and _____.
9. With an acute viral upper respiratory infection (URI), treatment methods do not include _____.
10. A pregnant woman with a prior pelvic fracture may still be able to deliver _____.
11. Cervical spine irritation may occur in pregnancy due to _____, with resulting _____.

## *References*

1. Spellacy WN: Management of High Risk Pregnancy. Baltimore, University Park Press, 1976.
2. Danforth DN: Obstetrics and Gynecology (5th ed). Philadelphia, JB Lippincott, 1986.
3. Wilson RJ, Carrington ER, Ledger WJ: Obstetrics and Gynecology. St. Louis, CV Mosby, 1983.
4. Niswander KR: Manual of Obstetrics: Diagnosis and Therapy (3rd ed). Boston, Little, Brown & Co, 1987.
5. Queenan JT, Hubbens JC: Protocols for High Risk Pregnancies (2nd ed). Oradell, New Jersey, Medical Economics Books, 1987.
6. Dox T, Melloni BJ, Eisner GM: Melloni's Illustrated Medical Dictionary. Baltimore, Williams & Wilkins, 1979.
7. Queenan JT, et al: Management of High Risk Pregnancy (2nd ed). Oradell, New Jersey, Medical Economics Books, 1985.
8. Bannister R: Brain's Clinical Neurology (4th ed). London, Oxford University Press, 1973.
9. Howell JW, Roseman GF: The evaluation and treatment of carpal tunnel syndrome in pregnancy. Bull Sect Obstet Gynecol 11(2):10-11, 1987.
10. Heckman J: Managing musculoskeletal problems in pregnant patients. Musculoskeletal Medicine 7:14-24, 1984 (Part 1), 8:35-40, 1984 (Part 2).

# Putting It Into Practice

# ELEVEN

# Evaluation and Treatment of the Obstetric Client

Certain restrictions apply when planning an evaluation and designing treatment programs for obstetric clients. These restrictions may inhibit standard physical therapy procedures; therefore, accommodation must be made. Restrictions include avoiding positions that involve abdominal compression in mid to late pregnancy; avoiding the supine position for longer than 3 minutes after the fourth month of pregnancy; avoiding positions in which the buttocks are higher than the chest; avoiding positions or exercises that strain the pelvic floor and abdominal muscles; avoiding exercises that encourage vigorous stretching of hip adductors; avoiding exercises that involve rapid or uncontrolled bouncing or swinging movements[1]; avoiding the use of deep heat modalities or electrical stimulation[2]; and supporting side-lying positions at the waist and under the abdomen.

Perhaps the best place to start is by taking the history. A questionnaire, filled out by the patient before the first meeting, gives the patient time to monitor transient aches and pains, as well as to reduce anxiety about the visit (see Figure 11-1).

Figure 11-1: Patient Questionnaire

Name _____ Home phone _____ Business phone _____

Address _____

Date of birth _____ Occupation _____

Responsibilities at home _____

_____

Level of activity: Sedentary _____ Light _____ Heavy _____ Very heavy _____

Height _____ Weight _____ Due date _____ Doctor _____

Number of pregnancies _____ Number of deliveries _____

Problem _____

_____

_____

Do you have any history of the same problem? _____

How/when did it happen? _____

_____

Describe the pain _____

1) Where felt _____

2) When does it start in the day? _____

3) When does it stop? _____

4) What makes it better? _____

5) What makes it worse? _____

6) Do you sleep through the night without interruption from this pain? _____

7) What percentage of the waking day is it felt? _____

8) How many days a week is it felt? _____

9) What intensity is this pain on a scale from 0 to 10 (0 is none, 10 is the worst)? _____

10) Does this pain prevent you from doing activities of daily living, working, recreation or assuming sexual positions?

_____

_____

11) What self-help measures have you tried? Did they help?

_____

_____

## *Musculoskeletal Evaluation*

### Posture

During the course of pregnancy, the posture changes greatly due to possible hormonal action of relaxin on the ligaments, which allows more spinal movement in all directions; increased breast and uterine weight anteriorly; and forward and upward shift of the center of gravity.[3] The spine will adjust to the added weight and change in center of gravity by increasing the cervical and lumbar curves. As the cervical curve increases, and because of the increased weight of the breasts, the shoulders arch forward. Because the optical righting reflex acts to keep the eyes looking at a horizontal plane, muscles in the posterior neck must work harder to prevent the head from falling forward as the shoulders become rounded. In addition to these spinal changes, the pregnant woman will lean back slightly to allow the weight to shift backwards towards the heels, counteracting the forward influence of the enlarging uterus. If she shifts her weight back, and at the same time relaxes her abdominal muscles, she will tend to walk with a waddling gait and may develop back pain (see Figure 11-2). The key features of this kyphotic, lordotic posture, as

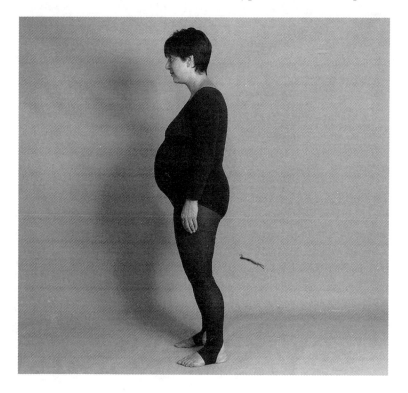

Figure 11-2: Incorrect posture.

described by Kendall, are weakness in the anterior neck, upper back, and lower abdominal muscles; and often shortness in the hip flexors, pectorals, and low back muscles.

When the body is in good alignment, with the buttocks tucked under, the abdominal muscles support the fundus anteriorly, and the uterine weight rests in the pelvic basin.[4] A plumb line, on side view, will bisect the lobe of the ear, the shoulder joint, the bodies of the lumbar vertebrae, the trunk, the greater trochanter of the femur (anteriorly to the midline of the knee), and slightly through the anterior malleolus at the calcaneocuboid joint[5] (see Figure 11-3). Muscle shortness or weakness may cause faulty alignment, and give rise to stretch weakness or adaptive shortening of muscles.[5]

Stretch weakness, from muscles assuming and remaining in a lengthened position beyond neutral, may occur in women with the typical pregnant posture, particularly in the middle and lower trapezius muscle groups, as well as in the lower abdominals. Adaptive shortening of the muscle occurs when it is unable to lengthen in response to relaxation of the antagonist group or to the force of gravity. Consequently, without an outside pull or force, the shortened muscles tend to remain in a shortened position and this is

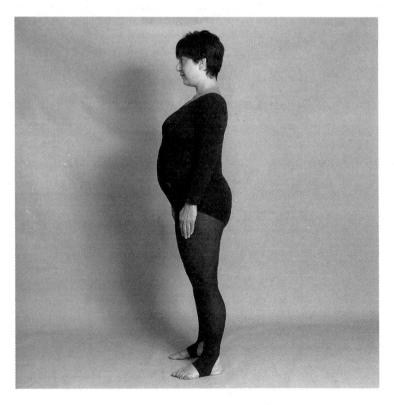

Figure 11-3: Correct posture.

associated with muscle strength.[5] Shortened muscles in the pregnant woman tend to include the low back, anterior shoulder group, and hip flexors. Not all postures will be typical, however, and careful observation of the body will pick up any deviations from the ideal posture. A Polaroid picture taken from a lateral and anterior point of view may help in treatment design. An extra picture, taken with a plumb line superimposed on it, may help the patient understand her posture deviations and actively change them. A program can then be designed to correct stretch weakness and adaptive shortening. Postural defects may be further intensified during recreation, work, and home activities, and attention should be given to an assessment of posture in these positions as well.

Many of the same excellent evaluation tests used on other patients are indicated for pregnant women: observation; palpation; range of motion; and strength, neurologic, coordination, gait, activities of daily living, and functional assessment. Methods of standard evaluations and treatments not included here can be found in *Physical Examination of the Spine and Extremities* by Hoppenfeld; and *Evaluation, Treatment and Prevention of Musculoskeletal Disorders* by Saunders, both excellent references. A musculoskeletal evaluation is included here, however, to highlight a way to evaluate the obstetric client by limiting the number of changes in body position, while at the same time observing pregnancy-related restrictions (see Figure 11-4).

### Muscle testing

Because the mother should avoid the supine position for lengthy periods, as well as avoid positions that compress the abdomen in late pregnancy, some changes are necessary for manual muscle testing positions. Although many of these adaptations do not test the specific muscle in the ideal position against gravity, the therapist is nevertheless able to check for functional strength and substitution. Technically, muscles tested in a nongravity position should not attain a grade better than 2 + out of 5 +, but it is believed the experienced practitioner can palpate the strength through these adapted positions. Examination notes should indicate these modifications. An isokinetic testing device may be used as an alternative for some of the positions.

Suggested alternate positions include stabilizing against the wall, a corner, or a backless stationary stool. If frequent positions requiring the supine position are needed, the therapist can direct the patient to turn to left side lying between tests. However, the pregnant woman with musculoskeletal pain is often extremely uncomfortable during evaluation, and testing positions should be organized in the therapist's mind.

Figure 11-4: Musculoskeletal Evaluation of the Obstetric Client

1. **Standing**
   A. Gait
      Head _____
      Arms _____
      Trunk _____
      Pelvis _____
      Legs _____
      Feet _____
   B. Posture

   | Viewed from | Side | Front | Back |
   |---|---|---|---|
   | 1. Head | | | |
   | 2. Shoulders | | | |
   | 3. Mid/upper back | | | |
   | 4. Abdomen | | | |
   | 5. Low back | | | |
   | 6. Pelvis/hips | | | |
   | 7. Knees | | | |
   | 8. Ankles | | | |

   C. Spinal Movements

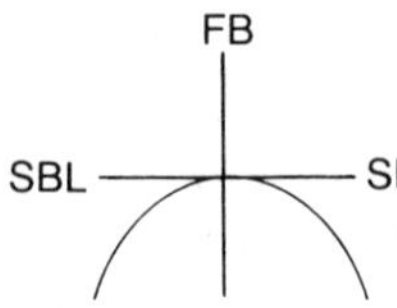

   FB

   SBL ——┼—— SBR

   Normal = N
   Pain = X
   Restricted = 1
   Hypermobile = 2

   D. Pelvis
      Level of PSIS and sacral base-
      Active movement of SI joint (Forward bending—landmarks PSISs)-
2. **Sitting**
   A. Neurologic-Strength

| | Upper Extremities | | | | Lower Extremities | |
|---|---|---|---|---|---|---|
| | | Right | Left | | | Right | Left |
| C1-2 | Chin in | | | L1, 2 | Psoas | |
| C1-2 | Chin up | | | L-3 | Quads | |
| C-3 | Lat Neck | | | L-4 | Tib ant | |
| C-4 | Shoulder shrug | | | L-5 | Ext. H.L. | |
| C-5 | Biceps | | | S-1 | Flex H.L. | |
| C-6 | Wrist extensors | | | S-2 | Hams | |
| C-7 | Triceps | | | | | |
| C-8 | Thumb extensors | | | Reflexes | | |
| T-1 | Intrinsics | | | L-4 | Knee | |
| | | | | S-1 | Ankle | |
| | | | | UMN Babinski | | |

   Reflexes
   C-5, 6  Biceps _____
   C-5, 6  Braco. Rad _____
   C-7     Triceps _____

   0 = absent
   1 + diminished
   2 + normal
   3 + increased
   4 + clonus

   B. Trunk motions
   C. Neck
      Range of motion
      Neck strength
      Neck palpation (vertebrae, muscles)

Figure 11-4: Continued

---

   D. Shoulder/arm:
   Muscle
   Tendon
   Thoracic outlet
   Carpal Tunnel
   Sensation
3. **Supine**—(No longer than three minutes before moving to left sidelying)
   A. Sacroiliac joints
     **Spring**
       Anterior ligaments
       Anterior rotation of ilium or sacrum
       Posterior rotation of ilium or sacrum
   B. Hamstring length
   C. Rectus diastasis
   D. Hip flexor tightness
   E. Leg lengths
4. **Side Lying** (with support at waist and under abdomen)
   A. Sacroliac—(test other side as well)
     Spring test-posterior ligaments
   B. Spinal palpation
     (thoracic, low back, sacrum)
   C. Leg (other side as well)
     Hip flexors
     Quad length
     TFL length
**Impression**
**Plan**
**Goals**

---

Suggested adaptations required for Kendall's standard muscle testing positions include the following:
- Pronator teres and pronator quadratus, supinator and biceps: sitting, arm fixed against a wall;
- Triceps: back lying with arm horizontally adducted;
- Latissimus dorsi: sitting with arm in extension or side lying with the trunk stabilized;
- Teres major: sitting, therapist stabilizes the anterior shoulder;
- Medial and lateral rotators: sitting, therapist stabilizes shoulder and elbow at 90 degrees of flexion;
- Trapezius: standing facing the wall, arm not being tested is bent at the elbow with forehead resting on it;
- Hamstrings: standing with the pelvis in neutral position and one knee flexed; semitendinosus and semimembranosus: internal rotation of the flexed knee; biceps femoris: lateral rotation of the flexed knee
- Gluteus maximus: standing on one leg (can be stabilized in cor-

ner), therapist pushes the bent leg forward from the posterior position;

- Quadratus lumborum: standing against the wall stabilizing the leg and abducting the desired leg;
- Abdominal muscles: test for rectus diastasis before doing a full abdominal test in standard positions;
- Back extensors: sitting on a fixed stool;
- Neck extensors: sitting

### Sample notes for a patient with problem back pain relating to posture

1. Observation: the patient stands with a forward head, rounded upper back, increased lordosis, pelvis is tilted anteriorly, with a protruding abdomen
2. Muscle testing: weak upper back and abdominal muscles
3. Muscle tightness: pectorals, low back muscles, and hip flexors

Goals:

1. Restore full range of motion
2. Increase strength and endurance in weak, target muscles
3. Teach correct posture through serial photographs
4. Increase general fitness level
5. Adapt job, home, and recreational activities to promote proper posture
6. Use upper back support to assist in stretching of pectorals and decrease strain on middle and lower trapezius

Exercises:

1. Stretching:

   a. Head retraction: retract head and swallow; hand pushes in on chin
   b. Wall exercise: stand with back resting on wall, feet 12″ from wall; bend knees, pelvic tilt, keep shoulders and head back, pull chin in and swallow; hold arms out straight, drag arms up wall (palm-up), hold 10 seconds; when arms start to pull away from wall, stop, lower with control, stand up against wall with aligned posture; rest, repeat
   c. Low back stretches: side lying, towel roll under waist, pull single knee to chest; back lying, pull single knee to chest; hands and knees, perform modified buddha and cat exercise (see Chapter 13), long leg stretch with roll underneath knee; slight forward bending to feel stretch in low back and hamstring muscles
   d. Iliopsoas stretch: lying near the edge of the bed, pull both knees to chest and hold one knee as other knee drops over

side of bed and hold 30 seconds, switch to other side (not longer than 3 minutes on back)

e. Pectoral stretch: stand facing into corner, press arms against wall, hold 30 seconds.

2. Strengthening:
   a. Isometric head extensors: later incorporate strengthening of neck rotators, lateral, and forward flexors
   b. Trapezius muscle group: standard exercises
   c. Abdominal muscles: perform modified curl-ups, leg slides, and active standing abdominal contraction, continuing with wall exercises from a sit-to-stand position (assess rectus muscles).

## *Treatment of Selected Musculoskeletal Conditions*

### Sacroiliac joint pain

During pregnancy, the SI joints may become a source of pain. This may occur within the first 3 months, possibly related to the circulation of relaxin and the major physiologic and musculoskeletal changes occurring in the woman's body. In addition, some women find that the SI joint becomes symptomatic premenstrually, as well as, postpartum. Joint movement at the SI has been well-documented.[6-13]

The action of the major muscles around the SI joint will greatly influence rotation. Trained and experience therapists can use mobilization and muscle energy techniques to correct anterior and posterior innominate rotation. Therapists with little training in manual therapy methods should not attempt these techniques on pregnant women, because considerable finesse is required to avoid injuring ligamentous and connective tissue support as well as the joints of the pelvic ring. Indeed, there are many experienced obstetric physical therapists who will not apply these techniques for fear of further injuring the client. Careful assessment of ligamentous stability should be made before carrying out even the most gentle mobilization.

Evaluation of the SI joint includes ligament testing, sacral movement, leg lengths, palpation, and pelvic alignment. After the malposition of the innominate is determined, treatment may involve application of local heat, rest, muscle correction, mobilization, fitting of an orthosis, and a home program to remedy dysfunction. An SI support belt (see Figures 11-5A and 11-5B) can be applied to assist in maintaining a corrected position. Pregnant clients should also be instructed to avoid widely abducted legs when walking on uneven terrain, doing frog kicks, as in swimming, in certain sexual positions,

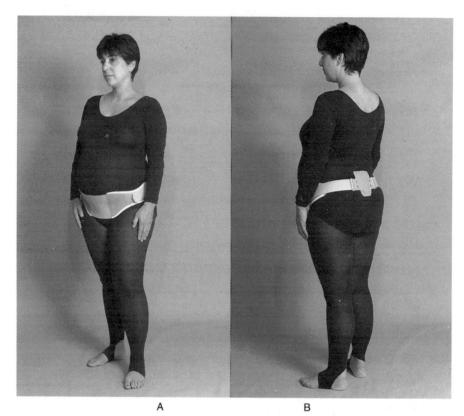

A                                    B

Figure 11-5, A and B: Sacroiliac belt. IEM Orthopedics (See appendix)

climbing stairs more than one step at a time, and swinging one leg out of bed when getting up.

## Posterior innominate

The patient with posterior innominate usually demonstrates unilateral buttock pain and well-localized pain over the PSIS on the involved side. Some or all of the following signs will be positive: in standing, the PSIS is lower on the side of the involvement with the same side iliac crest and the ASIS higher; in supine, the ASIS on the involved side is higher than on the noninvolved side; in supine-to-sit test, the leg on the involved side will appear longer (patient may need support to sit up and lay back); on side or back bending, pain often increases toward involved side; on forward bending, the PSIS on the involved side will elevate higher than on the noninvolved side; and, on spring test over the sacrum, results will be positive.

The patient with posterior innominate requires an anterior torsion force for correction. For self-correction of a posterior innominate, the gluteus maximus is contracted. If the physical therapist feels a need to assist correction, he or she must use *extreme caution* in attempting to correct the rotation. The practitioner should be extremely familiar with applying these techniques to a variety of non-pregnant women before attempting to work with an unstable pelvis under a lax situation. It is important to know that the symphysis pubis can separate in pregnancy and actually rupture with excessive force.

*Muscular correction of posterior innominate*

Patient: Lies supine with involved leg over side of table.

Therapist: Stands on patient's affected side, stabilizing pelvis on opposite side of body; places one hand on the distal thigh with the hip extended and the knee flexed.

Action: Therapist asks patient to flex the hip against therapist's resistance isometrically and hold for 5 seconds. As the patient relaxes, the therapist gently pushes the hip further into extension by taking up the slack, monitoring the ASIS so that it does not move. Repeats 3 times (reexamines after procedure). Repeats, if necessary (see Figure 11-6).

Mobilization for the posterior innominate can be done with the pregnant patient by modifying a technique usually done in prone position.

*Mobilization correction of posterior innominate*

Patient: Lies on side with the affected side up and supported at

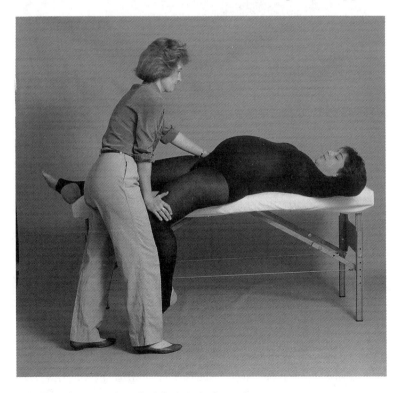

Figure 11-6: Muscular correction of a left posterior innominate.

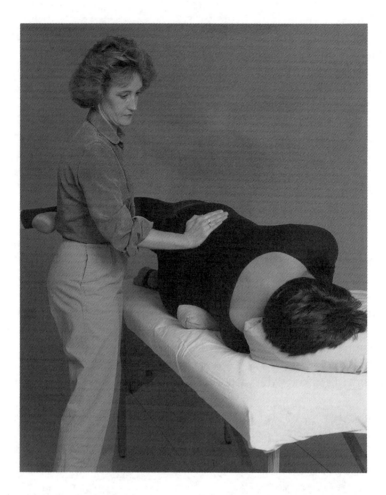

Figure 11-7: Mobilization correction of a left posterior innominate.

the waist and under the abdomen. The unaffected leg is flexed forward to stabilize the lumbar spine in flexion and to hold the ilium posteriorly.

Therapist: Stands behind the patient and grasps the thigh above the knee. The hip is abducted 15 to 20 degrees and extended.

Action: Therapist places opposite hand lateral to the PSIS over the ilium and gently thrusts anteriorly, laterally, and superiorly. Repeats 3 times and reexamines after procedure (see Figure 11-7).

A home program for a patient with posterior innominate should include, in addition to practice in body mechanics and positioning, the following exercises:

1.    Push-pull isometric exercise for posterior innominate:
    a.  Sitting or supine, the patient's hand is on top of the involved thigh, which isometrically flexes against the hand. On the non-involved side, the opposite hand is pushing up from behind

the thigh, while the hip attempts to extend posteriorly (see Figure 11-8 and 11-9).

b. Gluteal stretch: Supine; on involved side, hip is slightly abducted, and patient brings hip and knee into flexion to stretch the buttock muscles (see Figure 11-17).

### Anterior innominate

The patient with anterior innominate requires a posterior torsion force for correction. This patient usually has localized pain similar to that of the patient with posterior innominate, but less severe leg pain. Cervical pain may be associated with this disorder. Some or all of the following signs will be positive: in standing, the PSIS will be lower on the involved side; in supine, the ASIS will be lower on the involved side as compared with the noninvolved side; in the supine-to-sit test, the involved side will appear shorter; on forward bending, there will be pain on the involved side, and the PSIS on the involved side will be higher than on the noninvolved side.[13]

*Muscular correction of anterior innominate*

For self-correction of an anterior innominate, the iliacus is contracted. Other muscle correction may be attempted as follows:

Patient: Lies supine with hip and knee flexed on involved side.

Therapist: Stands on involved side; places most caudal hand under the patient's ischial tuberosity, other hand over ASIS; leans over,

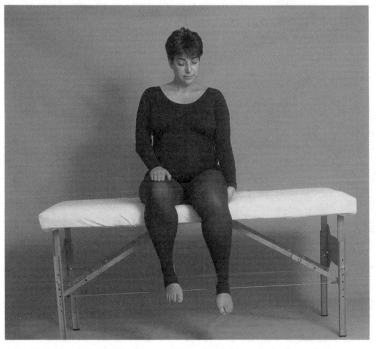

Figure 11-8: Home exercise sitting for correction of a right posterior innominate.

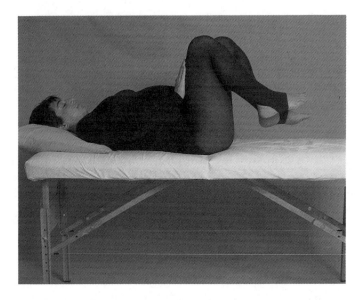

Figure 11-9: Home exercise supine for correction of a right posterior innominate.

takes up slack, and moves patient's hip and knee into further flexion.

Action: Therapist asks patient to extend the hip isometrically against the therapist's chest, hold for 5 seconds, then relaxes, and therapist takes up further slack. Concurrently, the posterior rotation is produced by downward pressure on the ASIS, as well as an upward pull on the ischial tuberosity (see Figure 11-11). Repeats 3 times (reexamines after each).

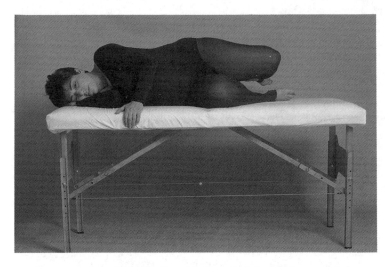

Figure 11-10: Home exercise sidelying for correction of a left posterior innominate.

*Mobilization of anterior innominate*

Mobilization for anterior innominate correction can be performed in different ways. Special caution should be used if the technique is performed as in the first technique listed below:

Patient (*supine position 1*): lies supine with trunk laterally flexed away from involved side, places hands behind the head, fingers interlocking.

Contraindications: If a patient is uncomfortable and unable to tolerate the position, or if there is evidence of lumbar disc disease, try mobilization in a side-lying position or in supine position 2.

Therapist: Stands on the noninvolved side; places one hand on the involved ilium, preventing it from coming up; weaves other hand under the opposite elbow, through the space made by both the patient's elbows and places flat palm on the treatment table. Position allows firm control of the upper torso with one hand, while the ilium is stabilized with the other.

Action: As therapist's arm weaves through the spaces created by

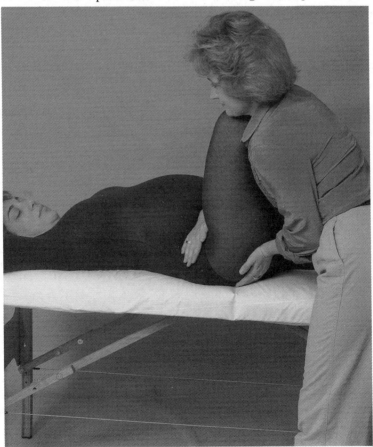

Figure 11-11: Muscular correction of a right anterior innominate.

toward the therapist. (Because the opposite hand keeps the ilium on the table, rotation should be performed slowly to avoid pain. Some patients may be unable to rotate completely.) As therapist rotates the upper trunk, the opposite hand gently thrusts on the anterior superior iliac spine in a posterior lateral superior direction (see Figure 11-12).

Patient (*supine position 2*): Lies supine with leg and knee flexed on involved side.

Therapist: Same position but turns to face patient's opposite shoulder.

Action: Therapist applies pressure posteriorly on the ASIS, while pulling forward on the ischial tuberosity with the opposite hand, and repeats in an oscillating fashion 6 to 8 times (reexamines after each—see Figure 11-13).

Patient (*sidelying*): Lies on side with the affected side up, supports under the waist and abdomen, lower hip and knee are flexed; upper leg flexed and wrapped around therapist's waist.

Therapist: Faces patient so that patient's upper leg is ahead of the therapist who places caudal hand over ASIS and other hand over ischial tuberosity.

Action: Therapist gently thrusts both hands together into poste-

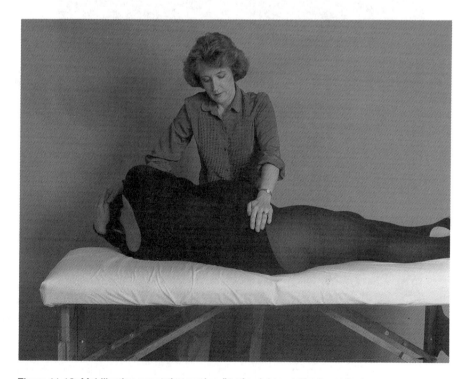

Figure 11-12: Mobilization correction supine #1 of a right anterior innominate.

the patient interlocking her fingers behind her head, patient rotates rior rotation; repeats in an oscillating fashion 6 to 8 times and reexamines after each (see Figure 11-14).

A home program for the patient with anterior innominate should include, in addition to practice in body mechanics and positioning, the following exercises:

1.   Push-pull isometric exercises for anterior innominate:
     a.   Patient sits with knees bent, one hand placed under the thigh of the involved side, against which the hip extends isometrically; the opposite hand is placed on top of the noninvolved thigh, against which the hip attempts to flex isometrically 5 seconds. Both push and pull holds are performed simultaneously. The patient breathes easily, relaxes, and repeats 3 times (see Figure 11-15).
     b.   Patient is supine with knees bent, hand under the thigh on the involved side, thigh pushes down and is held isometrically; at the same time, the other hand is on top of the noninvolved thigh, and the thigh pushes into flexion; contraction is held isometrically (see Figure 11-16).

2.   Iliacus stretch:
     Patient lies on noninvolved side with knee flexed and hip extended on the involved side. Patient holds onto table to stabilize pelvis and actively extends the hip, stretching the iliacus (see Figure 11-10). If the patient is able to maintain pelvic alignment post-exercise, then pelvic tilt and curl-up exercises (check recti) are added.

## Low back

Pregnant clients frequently complain of low back and sciatic pain, which may be caused by the many physical changes of pregnancy: added weight, poor muscle tone, increased lordosis, changes in the center of gravity, and loose pelvic ligaments. Through evaluation, the source of pain must be determined to be muscular or discogenic in origin. Uninterrupted pregnancies may predispose women to herniated disks later in life.[14]

Pregnant women with herniated disks are at a disadvantage, because both evaluation and medications are limited. Evaluations must be performed through clinical exam only, because many imaging techniques and myelograms are contraindicated during pregnancy. Many analgesics and anti-inflammatory medications would be ruled out as well. The patient should be instructed to monitor radicular signs and adjust activity to avoid reproduction of symptoms.

Evaluation of patients with herniated disks would be the same as for nonpregnant patients, and treatment would include:

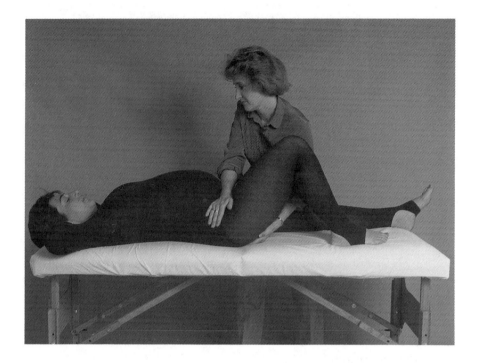

Figure 11-13: Mobilization correction supine #2 of a right anterior innominate.

1.  Frequent rest periods in side-lying positions with support at the waist, under the abdomen, and between the thighs
2.  Cold compresses applied to the low back, 10 minutes at a time, frequently throughout the day with 1 hour between applications
3.  Massage of the low back area in side-lying position
4.  Exercises, including:
    a.  Hands and knees position with head up, maintaining a slight, extended position in the back
    b.  Hands and knees position, performing contralateral arm and leg lifts
    c.  Standing position with hands on hips, slight lumbar extension
    d.  Supine position, leg slides maintaining pelvic tilt and lowering legs with control
    e.  Standing position, contracting abdominal muscles
5.  Body mechanics and back care—avoiding bending or lifting; avoiding sitting as much as possible; taking meals standing up; coughing or sneezing in extension with both hands supporting the small of the back; avoiding constipation
6.  Posture—maintaining correct posture through strengthening

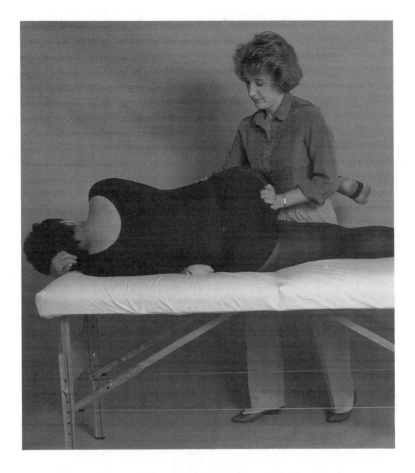

Figure 11-14: Mobilization correction sidelying of a right anterior innominate.

of the upper back, stretching tight muscles, and exercising with the wall exercise (see this chapter—Posture)

7.  Use of mid and low back supports (see Figures 11-18, 11-19, 11-20)

In the case of a low back strain, treatment consists of

1.  Rest in a side-lying supportive position with pillow between knees, under abdomen, and towel roll at waist
2.  Heat applied for short periods in the side-lying position with strap above and below the abdomen to hold it in place
3.  Massage of entire back in sidelying position
4.  Exercises
    a.  Alternate knee-to-chest movement, maintaining pelvic tilt, slightly abducting hip to avoid hitting abdomen
    b.  Pelvic tilt, both knees to chest
    c.  Hands and knees position, performing cat exercise (see Chapter 13)

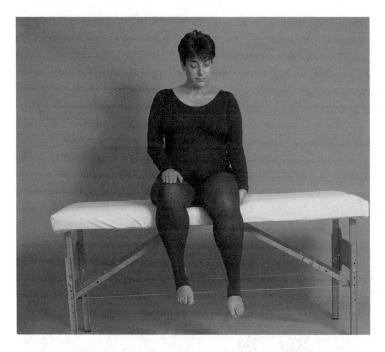

Figure 11-15: Home exercise sitting for correction of a left anterior innominate.

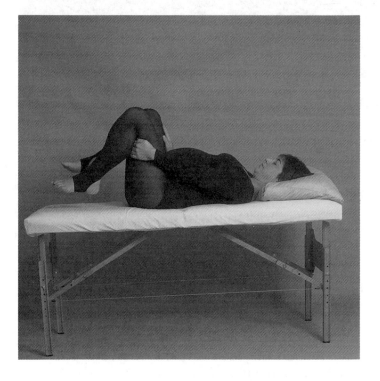

Figure 11-16: Home exercise supine for correction of a left anterior innominate.

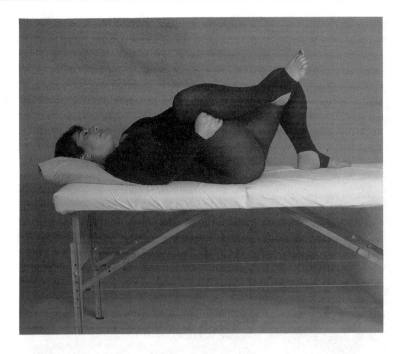

Figure 11-17: Gluteal stretch. Home exercise for correction of a right posterior innominate.

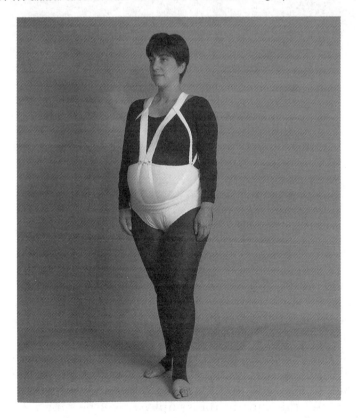

Figure 11-18: Low back support. The Baby Hugger from Trennaventions (See appendix.)

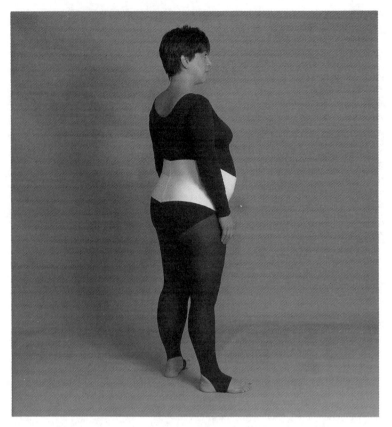

Figure 11-19: Low back support. The Dale active lumbosacral support phase IV from Life Lines Medical, Inc. (See appendix.)

   d. Modified buddha position (see Chapter 13)
   e. Contralateral arm and leg lifts
   f. Ipsilateral arm and leg lifts
   g. Sitting side bends
   h. Knee rock: on back, knees bent, drop knees easily side-to-side, head turns in opposite direction
   i. Posture correction, strengthening upper back, stretching tight muscles; wall exercise (see this chapter—Posture)

### Symphysis pubis

The symphysis pubis may separate a small amount during delivery. With a large baby, or a forceful extraction, more serious injury can result. On examination, the physical therapist may find the following symptoms: Pain: The patient will describe severe pain in the symphysis pubis and SI joints. The urine may be bloody from injury to the bladder neck and urethra. Palpation: The symphysis pubis will be tender, and the ends of the symphysis will be separated. Movement: The bones are usually mobile, and a shift of several centi-

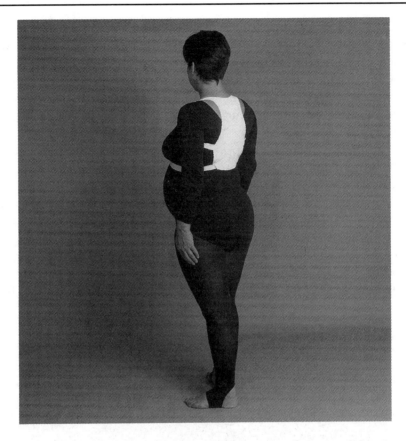

Figure 11-20: Mid back support. From Educational Opportunities. (See appendix.)

meters may be felt when the patient shifts weight from one foot to the other.[15]

Treatment may consist of application of heat or cold, a tight binder to immobilize the symphysis pubis, and instruction on performing activities of daily living so the patient's legs are not widely abducted beyond a comfortable resting position. If separation is severe and causes great pain, the patient may require instruction in the use of an assistive device for ambulation.

## Piriformis

The piriformis may shorten or spasm in pregnancy due to the postural changes and waddling gait. The patient may complain of persistent, severe, radiating low back pain extending from the sacrum to the hip joint over the gluteal region and posterior portion of the upper leg (sciatic nerve distribution).[16] Evaluation may be performed by placing the patient supine with the legs extended. The hip on the involved side will show an increase in external rotation due to the shortened position of the piriformis. On palpation, the buttock on the involved side may be very tender, and the leg on the involved side may appear shorter from contracture of the piriformis. In quad-ruped position, the sacral base on the involved side may appear to lie anteriorly in relation to the PSIS.[15]

Treatment may consist of heat application in a side-lying position with the affected side up and support at the waist, abdomen, and between the knees. The therapist may attempt to relieve the tight-ness in the piriformis by applying pressure with the elbow to the affected piriformis near its insertion, while adducting and internally rotating the hip of the affected side, gently stretching along the course of the muscle for 10 seconds and repeating 3 times (see Figure 11-21). The patient should experience immediate relief. Deep friction massage to the piriformis muscle may also help, and the physical therapist can instruct the patient's partner on how to apply pressure to the piriformis. The patient may also apply pressure herself by leaning into a tennis ball up against a wall, or by side lying

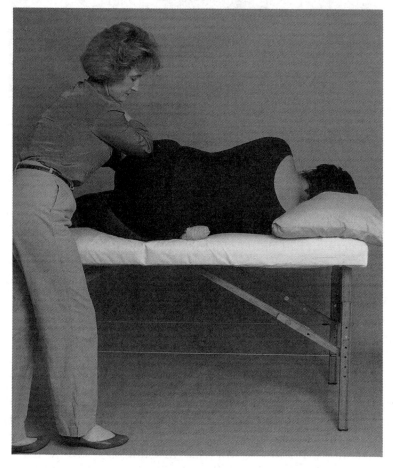

Figure 11-21: Piriformis stretch.

with support, while adducting and internally rotating the hip of the affected side.

## Coccyx

Normally, the coccyx extends in sitting and flexes in standing. Injury to the sacrococcygeal joint may occur during pregnancy or during childbirth. After childbirth, in fact, the coccyx may become subluxed, heal in extension, and become hypomobile.[12] Consequently, the soft tissue over the distal end of the coccyx is quite painful. The physical therapist may assist the woman by placing her in a supported side-lying position, inserting a gloved, lubricated index finger into the rectum (patient relaxes sphincter to allow insertion), and placing the thumb externally over the coccyx. An anterior/posterior glide movement and longitudinal traction may be applied to mobilize the joint (see Figure 11-22). Additionally, the patient may be instructed to apply ice externally over the coccygeal area for short periods throughout the day and to use a coccyx pillow for sitting.

## Neck and upper back strain

Due to changes in posture that often accompany pregnancy, pain may occur in the lateral aspects of the neck and upper back. The trapezius and upper and mid-cervical muscles may frequently be tender or in spasm with trigger points. Lateral flexion and rotation movements are restricted, and neck flexion and extension may be painful at the end of the range. In addition to standard treatment for neck muscle strain,[17] exercises should include pectoralis stretch, head retraction and swallow, upper back stretch at the wall, self-massage, side-bending mobilization using the lateral aspect of the hand as a fulcrum, stretching the levator scapulae, and deep cervical muscle isometrics.[11] Posture correction, relaxation exercises, and upper back supports may also be important. (see Figure 11-20)

## Temporomandibular joint

The temporomandibular joint may be affected in pregnancy, because the laxity of ligaments may allow hypermobility. Usually this is due to an underlying condition that is brought about with the added laxity, allowing the joint to ride over the displaced disk. Problems may also develop from excessive facial muscle tension thrusting the jaw forward during pushing in delivery.[18]

By minimizing the stress on the jaw, the problem may not arise. The patient usually experiences pain in the face and neck muscles and on opening the mouth, and clicking may be felt in the affected joint. There is usually tenderness over the joint and in the upper cervical facial muscles (masseter, temporalis, and pterygoid). Treat-

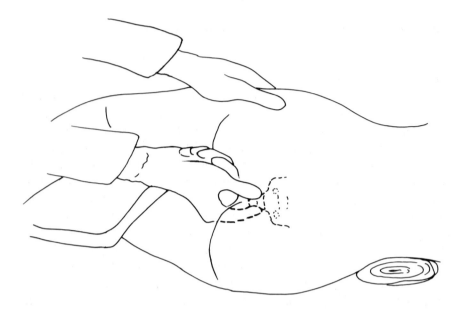

Figure 11-22: Coccyx mobili:

ment consists of applying heat to the joint followed by mobilization techniques for anterior and lateral glide, plus the Rocobado exercise series to reeducate muscle and jaw movements.

## Carpal tunnel syndrome

Carpal tunnel syndrome arises from compression of the median nerve at the wrist (see Chapter 10). Women will complain of pain over the median nerve distribution, paresthesia, numbness, clumsiness, and atrophy in the hands. Nocturnal awakening may occur secondary to pain or paresthesia. Phalen's test will be positive, (*i.e.*, signs will be reproduced by holding wrist firmly in flexion for a minute).[11,12,19] Tinel's sign will also be positive (percussion over the median nerve at the wrist will reproduce tingling in the cutaneous distribution of the median nerve).[11,12,19] Treatment consists of immobilization at the wrist in neutral position with the fingers free to permit activities of daily living.[19] Sometimes only nighttime wearing is required, or alternate splint-wearing time may be needed if both hands are involved. Usually, symptoms resolve postpartum; however, mothers who breast-feed tend to have a longer recovery.[19]

## Thoracic outlet

Symptoms of thoracic outlet syndrome may occur secondary to head and neck postural changes, causing compression of the neurovascular bundle at the cervicothoracic dorsal outlet. This bundle is comprised of brachial plexus nerve fibers and the subclavian artery and vein, usually involving C8 to T1 nerve roots. In the case of scalenus anticus and cervical rib syndrome, Adson's test is positive. The patient is instructed to take a deep breath, extending the neck fully, turning the chin towards the side being examined. In a positive test, the radial pulse disappears, and pain and other symptoms are reproduced. Treatment consists of exercises to stretch the upper trapezius and levator scapular muscles to bring the shoulder complex upward and backward.[12] If costoclavicular syndrome exists, the subclavian artery and brachial plexus are entrapped as they pass between the clavicle and the first rib. To test for this syndrome, the patient takes a deep breath and holds it while retracting and depressing the shoulder. Again, the radial pulse disappears, and symptoms are reproduced in the arm.[12] Treatment consists of mobilization of the clavicle at the sternoclavicular joint and posture exercises to elevate the shoulder girdle. In the hyperabduction syndrome, the subclavian vessel and brachial plexus are entrapped beneath the pectoralis minor tendon and under the coracoid process. To test for this syndrome, the arm is held in a hyperabducted position with the radial pulse diminished and symptoms reproduced. Patients usually complain of pain after sleeping with the arm overhead. Treatment consists of posture correction and stretching of the pectoral muscles.

### Muscle, tendon injuries
Because the use of deep heat modalities and electrical stimulation is contraindicated during pregnancy, the treatment of tendon injuries is limited to superficial heat; transverse friction massage across the tendon, muscle, or ligament to break down adhesions;[10] and the tendon injury program proposed by Curwin and Sandish:[11]

1.  Warm up the part involved
2.  Stretch the part 30 seconds, 3 times
3.  Perform eccentric contraction slowly on days 1 and 2, at moderate speed on days 3 through 5, and quickly on days 5 through 7; thereafter, resistance is increased; the patient should be able to do 3 sets of 10 repetitions each at a particular weight, the third set slightly straining the muscle;[20]
4.  Stretch the involved part (tendon or muscle) using contract/relax techniques, and
5.  Apply ice over the part for 10 minutes

The program is repeated twice daily, increasing weights so that the third set is always a slight strain to the muscle involved. Ace wraps and supports may be helpful, as well.

## Self-Assessment Review

1. When evaluating an obstetric client, two positions that should be avoided are _____ and _____.

2. List three reasons why posture changes occur during pregnancy.

3. The difference between adaptive shortening and stretch weakness is _____.

4. List three reasons why muscle testing positions may have to be changed for the obstetric client _____, _____, _____.

5. The posterior innominate position will require stretching of the _____.

6. List four activities patients with SI joint problems should avoid:

7. List three or more treatment suggestions for low back pain in the obstetric client:

8. The symphysis pubis may be injured or ruptured during _____.

9. A presenting sign of possible piriformis muscle tightness is an _____ position of the hip.

10. During childbirth, the coccyx may become _____.

11. The temporomandibular joint may be painful after delivery because _____.

12. Primary treatment of carpal tunnel syndrome is _____.

13. Tendon and muscle injuries may be treated in pregnancy by _____, _____, _____.

## References

1. Perinatal Exercise Guidelines. Alexandria, Bull Sect Obstet Gynecol, APTA, 1986.
2. Griffin JE, Karselis TC: Physical Agents for Physical Therapists. Springfield, Illinois, Charles C Thomas, 1982.
3. Fries EC, Hellebrandt FA: The influence of pregnancy on the location of the center of gravity: Postural stability and body alignment. Am J Obstet Gynecol 46:374, 1943.
4. Hassid P: Textbook For Childbirth Educators. New York, Harper & Row, 1978.
5. Kendall FP, McCreary EK: Muscle Testing and Function (3rd ed). Baltimore, Williams & Wilkins, 1983.
6. Grieve E: Lumbo-pelvic rhythm and mechanical dysfunction of the sacroiliac joint. Physiotherapy 67(6):171-173, 1981.

7. Golighty R: Pelvic arthropathy in pregnancy and the puerperium. Physiotherapy 58(7):216-220, 1982.

8. Grieve GP: The sacro-iliac joint. Physiotherapy 52(12):384-387, 1976.

9. Kim LYS: Pelvic torsion a common cause of low back pain. Ortho Rev 13(4):61-66, 1984.

10. Cyriax J, Cyriax P: Illustrated Manual of Orthopedic Medicine. London, Butterworth's, 1983.

11. Hoppenfeld S: Physical Examination of the Spine and Extremities. New York, Appleton-Century-Crofts, 1976.

12. Saunders HD: Evaluation, Treatment and Prevention of Musculoskeletal Disorders. Minneapolis, Viking Press, 1985.

13. Erhard R, Bowling R: The recognition and management of the pelvic component of low back and sciatic pain. Bull Sect Orthoped, APTA 2(3):4-15, 1977.

14. Fast A: Low back disorders. Arch Phys Med Rehab 69:880-891, 1988.

15. Wilson JR, Carrington ER: Obstetrics and Gynecology. St. Louis, CV Mosby, 1983.

16. Retzloff EW, et al: Piriformis. JAOA 73(6):799-807, 1974.

17. Travell JG, Simons DG: Myofascial Pain and Dysfunction. Baltimore, Williams & Wilkins, 1983.

18. Iglarsh ZA: Telephone interview with R Gourley, March 1989.

19. Howell JW, Roseman GF: The evaluation and treatment of carpal tunnel syndrome in pregnancy. Bull Sect Obstet Gynecol, APTA 11(2):10-11, 1987.

20. Curwin S, Sandish W: Tendinitis: Its Etiology and Treatment. Lexington, MA, DC Heath & Co, 1984.

# TWELVE

# Evaluation and Treatment of the Gynecologic Patient

One of the most important, if not *the* most important, aspects of physical therapy evaluation and treatment of the gynecologic patient, is taking the history. Although a careful history is valuable when dealing with any patient, the gynecologic patient may tell the physical therapist, who takes the time to listen, things about her condition that she has not told her physician. For instance, a busy physician, nurse, or even physical therapist can miss the relationship between symptoms and the menstrual cycle, and therefore miss possible conditions of dysmenorrhea or premenstrual syndrome. Certain types of incontinence can sometimes be determined only through careful history-taking. In the latter case, the description of the patient may even decide whether the patient can be helped with physical therapy. However, because little documentation exists on the benefits of physical therapy treatment of gynecologic problems, and because the next step for many patients is surgery, it's probably worth it to the patient to attempt a trial whether the problem is muscular or neurologic. More important, the methods the physical therapist can employ to treat gynecologic disorders keep expanding; currently the most common include exercise instruction, relaxation training, biofeedback, transcutaneous electrical nerve stimulation (TENS), and electrical stimulation.

## *The History*

Most practitioners find they develop their own system of patient interviewing, similar to developing a standard routine to conduct an evaluation. A sample history and evaluation, which for some patients or physical therapists may serve as the entire assessment, is described in Table 12-1. In this particular evaluation, no internal assessment of pelvic floor strength is included. This is an area still under debate by physical therapists—should an internal exam be conducted? Some believe the physical therapist is not thoroughly trained to perform an internal pelvic exam. Others believe this is essential to proper management of a gynecologic problem. The answer probably lies somewhere in the middle, in other words, a complete internal exam should be performed by a gynecologist or urolo-

**Table 12-1. Incontinence Evaluation**

1. Is there past or current history of urinary tract disease, infection, injury?
2. Is there past or current history of muscular paralysis or disease; diabetes; surgery on the spine, bladder, pelvis or brain; hysterectomy?
3. Was urethral dilatation performed in past? Why?
4. As a child, was there difficulty holding urine or bed wetting?
5. As an adolescent or adult, was or is there difficulty holding urine or bed wetting?
6. When urinating, is the amount small, medium, or large?
7. Is there difficulty stopping the flow or is there dribbling?
8. Does urine flow uncontrollably when associated with any of the following: coughing, sneezing, vomiting, standing, sitting, laying down, walking, running, straining, changing position, during intercourse, laughing, lifting, pushing? Does urine loss occur at the same time or shortly afterward?
9. Did the problem start after pregnancy, during pregnancy, after vaginal or abdominal surgery, after Cesarean surgery?
10. Is there ever a need for protection? When? What is used?
11. Are medications used; including over-the-counter or recreational drugs?
12. Is the patient aware of urine leaking? Does it leak prior to reaching the toilet?
13. Is there a strong urge to urinate? Can the urge be controlled?
14. Does the patient awaken at night with a strong urge to urinate? Is the bladder full?
15. Is there pain on urination?
16. Is there any difficulty passing urine or starting the flow?
17. Have other family members had trouble with incontinence or bed wetting in the past or do they now? Age of onset? Any pelvic surgery?

Orthopedic Evaluation (strength and range of motion):   Hips   Back
   Pelvis   Knees   Ankles   Feet
Neurologic Evaluation:   Sensory   DTR
Urinary Tract/GYN exam:   Prolapse   Menstrual   Uropressures
Psychologic:
Comments:

Summary:

gist prior to physical therapy; if not to rule out serious pathology, then to rule out communicable disease. The physical therapist can assess the strength and tone of the pelvic floor by palpating on the perineum or by inserting sterile, gloved, and lubricated fingers no more than an inch or two into the patient's vagina. If a biofeedback device is used, such as a perineometer, which measures the strength of contraction of the pubococcygeal muscle, the patient can insert it herself with verbal instruction. This also applies to electrical stimulation units. Again, each of these instruments must be sterilized before and after use with each patient.

The questions in the sample history and evaluation are directed at different types of incontinence problems to assist the clinician in assessing whether the problem is neurologic, muscular, or both. Psychologic factors may also enter into the ultimate diagnosis and treatment. To use this evaluation effectively, then, the practitioner must have a basic understanding of the anatomy and physiology of the urinary system. This system is extremely complex, and only an introduction to this topic is included in this chapter.

## *Bladder*

The urinary bladder has an outer longitudinal, middle circular, and inner longitudinal layer that gives rise to the urethral musculature and the trigonal musculature. The trigone is the area in which the muscle tissue changes from the tubular structure of the urethra to the flat, thin sheet of the bladder. The detrusor contraction, or the contraction of muscles that causes a pushing down of the bladder contents, is the sum of many decussating forces. The bladder outlet is surrounded by deep trigonal muscles and middle circular layers. At the outlet, there is also a band of muscular tissue called the sling of Heiss that is further supported by the pubourethral ligament. This ligament has three divisions; posterior, lateral, and anterior (see Figure 12-1). Through these divisions, the ligament joins with the

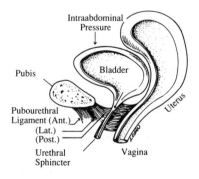

Figure 12-1: Pressures on and support of the bladder

urethra, the levator ani muscles, and the urogenital diaphragm to maintain the relationship of the urethra within the abdomen. Aging, injury, or childbirth are believed to alter the integrity of this ligament; when combined with pelvic floor weakness, the bladder rotates posteriorly and the urethra falls from its position in the "abdominal pressure zone."[1]

This abdominal pressure zone actually refers to the pressures on the urinary bladder imposed by normal intraabdominal pressure. Within the bladder (intravesical pressure), the pressure force is the sum of this intraabdominal pressure plus the detrusor contractions. Intraabdominal pressure is sometimes estimated by balloon catheter measured via the rectum. This pressure can be increased voluntarily when a person strains, coughs, or performs the Valsalva maneuver. Urologists have devised ways to measure the detrusor contraction pressure by subtracting intravesical pressure from the intraabdominal pressure measured rectally. With all these pressures acting on the bladder, how does the bladder hold urine? Fortunately, the bladder connects to a urinary sphincter before leading to the urethra. Maintaining urine in the bladder depends simply on the pressure in the urethra being greater than the pressure in the bladder. To urinate, a person must relax the urethra to reduce the intraurethral pressure. Detrusor contractions follow to expel urine. Flow, normally at a rate of 20 to 30 ml/sec[2] at midflow (maximal), stops when the bladder is empty. The rate can be increased by increasing intraabdominal pressure.

## *Incontinence*

But what happens when the person is unable to relax the urethra, detrusor contractions are weak, or the intraabdominal pressure is reduced because of poor position of the bladder? Frequently, incontinence is the result. Because of the complexity of the urinary system, however, multiple factors can lead to incontinence; these include relaxation of pelvic structures (urethrocele, cystocele, enterocele, rectocele, prolapses, and vaginal outlet), fistulas (urethrovaginal, vesicovaginal, uterovaginal, rectovaginal—see Figure 12-2), and neurologic dysfunction.

Relaxed ligamentous and fascial structures, similar to those mentioned with the sling of Heiss, contribute to "-celes" from the Greek word for hernia.[3] The urethra, bladder, rectum, or posterior vagina may herniate into the vaginal canal. These herniations are described as first degree, second degree, or third degree, third degree being the most severe. The symptoms of each, however, can be quite different. A cystocele may cause no incontinence, in fact, no symptoms at all until the posterior urethrovesical angle becomes so acute that the

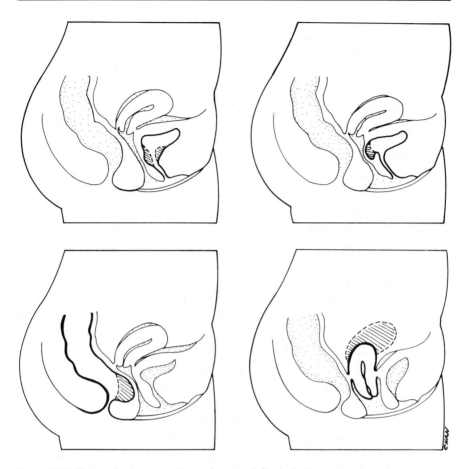

Figure 12-2: Types of pelvic relaxations—from top left, clockwise; cystocele, enterocele, prolapse, rectocele.

patient has difficulty initiating voiding, or retains urine, leading to urinary tract infection. In the patient with an urethrocele, on the other hand, the posterior urethrovesical angle decreases to the point that incontinence results. Enteroceles produce few symptoms until severe; they may herniate through the vagina. Often accompanying an enterocele is a rectocele. The latter may block bowel movement.

Although there are other causes, fistulas (unnatural openings) usually result from carcinoma or trauma, sometimes as a result of other gynecologic surgery. In the United States, this surgery is commonly abdominal hysterectomy. In a severe vesicovaginal fistula, the urinary stream may be continuous through the vagina. Less severe fistulas of this type may cause intermittent watery vaginal discharge. The treatment for large fistulas is almost always surgery.

Four neurologic pathways have been identified in the control of micturition: cerebral-brain stem (loop I), brain stem-sacral (loop II), vesical-sacral-sphincter (loop III), and cerebral-sacral (loop IV).[4] Voluntary control is mediated by loops I and IV, the former over the micturition reflex, and the latter over the striated external urethral sphincter. The fourth mediates voluntary control. The second and third loops regulate detrusor contractions to empty the bladder and coordinate the efforts between the detrusor and the urethra.

In addition to these links to the cerebrum and brain stem, there are four reflexes that assist in continence and storage of urine, two that assist in initiation of flow, five that coordinate the actual flow, and one that stops the flow and reestablishes storage mode. With 12 reflexes (see Table 12-2), it is a wonder that this system works so well in so many people for as long as it does.[5]

Physical examination by a urologist or gynecologic urologist includes checks for hernias, prolapse, pelvic relaxation, fistulae, or diverticula. Tests that may easily be performed by the physical therapist include neuromotor evaluation of sensory and motor function of the lower extremities and of the voluntary sphincters. Standard tests for lower extremity sensation via dermal distribution should be performed, as well as tests of motor strength for lumbar and sacral nerves: knee flexion (L5, S1), knee extension (L3, L4), hip extension (L4, L5), hip flexion (L2, L3), foot eversion (L4), foot inversion (L5, S1), ankle dorsiflexion (L4, L5), and ankle plantarflexion (S1, S2). Deep tendon reflexes should also be evaluated at the knee and ankle, as well femoral, popliteal, and pedal pulses. It is believed that control over the external voluntary anal sphincter links to control of the pelvic floor musculature. The anal sphincter integrity is assessed by stroking skin lateral to the anus; a tap, or squeeze, of the clitoris, or stroking urethral mucosa elicit the bulbocavernosus reflex (con-

**Table 12-2. Spinal Cord Reflexes Associated with Micturition**

*Storage of Urine*
Sympathetic detrusor inhibiting reflex
Sympathetic sphincter constrictor reflex
Perineodetrusor inhibitory reflex
Urethrosphincteric guarding reflex

*Initiation of Flow*
Perineobulbar detrusor facilitative reflex
Detrusodetrusor facilitative reflex

*Control the Flow*
Detrusourethral inhibitory reflex
Detrusosphincteric inhibitory reflex
Urethrodetrusor facilitative reflex
Urethrodetrusor facilitative reflex II
Urethrosphincteric inhibitory reflex

*Stop the Flow*
Perineobulbar detrusor inhibitory reflex

traction of the bulbocavernosus and ischiocavernosus muscles); and a cough or deep inspiration increase intraabdominal pressure and verify integrity of abdominal muscles (T6-L1) and periurethral striated sphincter contraction (see Table 12-3). Should these responses not occur, the problem may be related to central or peripheral nerve dysfunction and referral to a neurologist is warranted.[5]

Urinary incontinence is classified by international standards. Although stress incontinence is a term bandied about, it can result from many disorders. "The term stress incontinence,' on its own, only designates the symptom and the sign, but is not the diagnosis."[6] Types of urinary incontinence include genuine stress, urge, reflex, overflow, and enuresis.

Genuine stress incontinence is pressure-related. One exceeds the other. As a symptom, stress incontinence occurs when exercising; as a sign, it occurs as intraabdominal pressure increases. Genuine stress incontinence should be differentiated from an unstable bladder, in which physical stress results in a delayed loss of urine as detrusor contractions occur that the patient cannot control. A patient may have both types of incontinence problems, however. Two studies suggest that almost half of all pregnant women experience genuine stress incontinence, and about 10% to 20% may have episodes of urge incontinence by the third trimester.[7] Urge incontinence is loss of urine with a strong urge to urinate. It may have a motor component (uninhibited detrusor activity) or sensory component. Although treatment of this type usually focuses on the bladder, recent studies suggest unstable urethra may be a factor with or without unstable bladder.[8] Reflex incontinence, again, may occur without a sensation to urinate and is related to neurologic dysfunction. Overflow incontinence is self-explanatory; it is caused by a bladder that does not respond to stretch feedback. Enuresis is any involuntary loss, particularly bothersome as nocturnal enuresis during sleep.

Other noninvasive tests for types of incontinence, excluding flow studies (urodynamics), include stress tests, voiding diaries, and pad tests. The stress, or cough, test requires the patient to cough while standing. Small amounts of urinary leakage when coughing suggest genuine stress incontinence. If leakage is considerable, or occurs after the cough, an unstable bladder (patient cannot control detrusor contractions) may be responsible. The patient who keeps a voiding diary records times during the day when incontinence occurs, amount of fluid intake and urinary output, as well as whether an urge is associated with leakage. One-hour and 12-hour pad tests may be conducted to assess the effect of normal activities on continence.

**Table 12-3. Tests of Neurological and Vascular Integrity**

*Sensory*
Dermatomal distribution T6-S2

*Motor*
Hip flexion/extension
Knee flexion/extension
Ankle dorsiflexion/plantarflexion
Foot inversion/eversion

*Vascular*
Femoral
Popliteal
Pedal

*Reflexes*
Knee
Ankle
Anal sphincter
Bulbocavernosus
Periurethral striated sphincter

The pads are weighed to determine volume of urine output over time.[9]

Methods of physical therapy management for genuine stress incontinence include pelvic floor (Kegel) exercise instruction, dietary counseling to avoid diuretic substances (such as caffeine), biofeedback via perineometer, and possibly electrical stimulation. Instruction in pelvic floor exercise should be offered to any woman who comes in for physical therapy. Dr. Arnold Kegel conducted several studies to assess the efficacy of strengthening pelvic floor musculature to control continence. He and others have reported improvement in three fourths of women included in study samples.[10]

In the Kegel exercise, loop IV is activated to use cortical impulses to contract fast-twitch, striated periurethral sphincter muscles via the pudendal nerve. It is believed that these muscle fibers can hypertrophy with prolonged training, and therefore, most physicians and patients may become impatient with this method. No optimal number of repetitions has been standardized and probably depends on the tissue integrity of each woman, often a factor of age[11] and race.[12] Sometimes treatment may require several months of persistent exercise to achieve hypertrophy, and ergo, continence. This is where perineometers may have value—as not only an assistive device for the woman to become aware of the correct muscle contraction, but also as a biofeedback device.[13] The perineometer is a pneumatic resistance device, measuring contraction in millimeters of mercury (mm Hg), inserted into the vagina. As the patient contracts the pubococcygeal muscle, located one to two inches inside the vagina, the meter reflects pressure change and can provide visual encouragement. There are a few units on the market. The Kegel perineometer no longer is sold, but its prototype lives as a unit sold by Interactive Medical Technologies. A computerized unit with a printout is available through Biotechnologies, but its cost limits its use to those treating many patients of this type.

Yet another form of therapeutic intervention is through functional electrical stimulation. Although electric current was first applied to the pelvic floor and bladder via surgical implants, external units were found to have fewer complications and a higher success rate. Inflatable vaginal cuffs with electrodes, intravaginal electrodes, and intraanal electrodes are available. There are even some that the patient can wear during the day. In either case, stimulation should be intermittent to avoid muscle fatigue. Electrical stimulation has been used successfully in cases of sphincter weakness as well as to promote bladder inhibition. Recommended frequencies are 50 Hz at a pulse of 1 to 2 msec for urethral closure (pudendal nerve) and 10 Hz for 2-msec pulses for bladder inhibition (pudendal nerve to reflex spinal cord inhibition of pelvic nerve to relax detrusor).[14] Voltage may vary from 2 to 12 depending on individual tolerance and comfort. Units worn all day seem effective when cycled 25 seconds every 10 seconds. Several commonly-used electrical stimulation units have vaginal or anal electrodes.

Compliance can be a problem in the treatment of incontinent women, but results can be dramatic. And given the choice of exercise versus drugs or surgery, motivation may be high for some women. If women can be convinced to fit exercise into their daily routine—and the Kegel exercises are some that can be done anywhere, anytime—improvement should be noticeable within a few weeks. Even if the physical therapist has reservations about internal evaluation of muscle strength, instruction can and should be given verbally. The patient can be taught how to feel for the muscle contraction herself; and contractions can be practiced alone or during sexual intercourse—an added benefit for both the woman and her partner. Patients often report increased sexual enjoyment when pelvic floor muscles strengthen. This problem has come out of the closet, and incontinence clinics have opened across the nation. The physical therapist has the responsibility to treat the patient by whatever means are comfortable.

## Pelvic Pain

While the majority of gynecologic patients may present with problems of relaxed pelvic supporting structures, they may occasionally complain of pain during sexual intercourse or while going to the bathroom that is unrelated to infection or identifiable pathology. In some women, particularly those who may have had an episiotomy during delivery, pelvic muscles are tight, or the episiotomy scar is unyielding. Relaxation training, heat, and perineal massage with a lubricant may be of help to these women. Limited experimentation has been conducted with deep heat modalities, TENS, and behavior modification.

TENS is thought to be effective for relief of chronic, noninflammatory type pelvic (or mastectomy) pain from previous gynecologic or oncologic surgery, endometriosis, or dysmenorrhea.[15] Post-hysterectomy TENS and exercise, for pelvic floor musculature (if the vaginal approach was used) or for abdominal muscles and posture (if the abdominal approach was used), can be incorporated into any hospital or clinic setting. TENS and relaxation training could also be offered as alternatives to medications for relief of premenstrual symptoms of low back ache, cramping, or headache. Placement of electrodes depends on symptoms. Likewise, the endorphin-inducing effects produced by an individually-designed exercise program may help in the relief of stress-related physical complaints. Again, history is of great importance to determine the kind of pain and whether it is associated with menstruation.

The practitioner should be aware that gynecologists are, on the whole, unfamiliar with the role of the physical therapist in the treatment of such disorders. Treatment, however, even by a physician is often palliative for problems of chronic pelvic pain. It is up to the physical therapist to market this developing service for gynecologic clients—to help the gynecologist or gynecologic urologist think of physical therapy before prescribing medication or more radical approaches.

## *Self-Assessment Review*

1. Of utmost importance for the physical therapist conducting a gynecologic patient evaluation is _____.
2. Physical therapists have differing opinions on whether to conduct an _____ exam on patients referred for pelvic floor dysfunction or incontinence problems.
3. Patients with incontinence cannot be treated by a physical therapist unless the physical therapist first assesses pubococcygeal muscle strength. T F
4. Even in states with direct access, it's a good idea to recommend patients be examined by a gynecologist or urologist before physical therapy to rule out _____ or _____.
5. Genuine stress urinary incontinence is largely a symptom related to a difference in _____.
6. _____ pelvic support may result in rectocele, cystocele, urethrocele, or enterocele.

7. The physical therapist who examines a patient referred because of genuine stress incontinence should perform a neurologic screening to include:

8. Name and define at least three types of incontinence.

9. Name the four major neurologic loops that control micturition.

10. Name at least one way in which to treat the following: premenstrual syndrome, dysmenorrhea, genuine stress incontinence, post-hysterectomy, post-gynecologic surgery.

## *References*

1. Cutner LP, Ostergard DR: Modified Pereyra procedure: Vaginal approach to retropubic urethropexy. In Ostergard DR (ed): Gynecologic Urology and Urodynamics: Theory and Practice (2nd ed). Baltimore, Williams & Wilkins, 1985.

2. Tanagho EA: Urodynamics: Uroflowmetry and female voiding patterns. In Ostergard DR (ed): Gynecologic Urology and Urodynamics: Theory and Practice (2nd ed). Baltimore, Williams & Wilkins, 1985.

3. Dorland's Illustrated Medical Dictionary (24th ed). Philadelphia, WB Saunders, 1965, p. 268.

4. Burnett LS: Relaxations, malpositions, fistulas, and incontinence. In Jones HW, Wentz AC, Burnett LS (eds): Novak's Textbook of Gynecology (11th ed). Baltimore, Williams & Wilkins, 1988.

5. Ostergard DR: Neurological control of micturition and integral voiding reflexes. In Ostergard DR (ed): Gynecologic Urology and Urodynamics: Theory and Practice (2nd ed). Baltimore, Williams & Wilkins, 1985.

6. Stanton SL: Introduction to preoperative evaluation of the incontinent patient. In Ostergard DR (ed): Gynecologic Urology and Urodynamics: Theory and Practice (2nd ed). Baltimore, Williams & Wilkins, 1985.

7. Francis WJA: Disturbance of bladder function in relation to pregnancy. J Obstet Gynaecol Br Emp 67:353-366, 1960.

8. Ulmsten U, Henriksson L, Iosif S: The unstable female urethra. Am J Obstet Gynecol 144:93-97, 1982.

9. Pierson CA: Pad testing, nursing interventions and urine loss appliances. In Ostergard DR (ed): Gynecologic Urology and Urodynamics: Theory and Practice (2nd ed). Baltimore, Williams & Wilkins, 1985.

10. Jones EG, Kegel AH: Treatment of urinary stress incontinence. Surg Gynecol Obstet 94:179-188, 1952.

11. Faber P, Heidenreich J: Treatment of stress incontinence with estrogen in postmenopausal women. Urol Int 32:221-223, 1977.
12. Zacharin R: A Chinese anatomy: The pelvic supporting tissues in the Chinese and occidental female compared and contrasted. Aust NZ J Obstet Gynaecol 17:1-11, 1977.
13. Burgio KL, Robinson JC, Engel BT: The role of biofeedback in Kegel exercise training for stress urinary incontinence. Am J Obstet Gynecol 154:58-64, 1986.
14. McCarthy TA: Functional electrical stimulation. In Ostergard DR (ed): Gynecologic Urology and Urodynamics: Theory and Practice (2nd ed). Baltimore, Williams & Wilkins, 1985.
15. Mannheimer JS, Whalen EC: The efficacy of transcutaneous electrical nerve stimulation in dysmenorrhea. Clin J Pain 1:75-83, 1985.

# THIRTEEN

# Instructing Educational Classes

Among the many educational classes that the physical therapist can offer to expectant mothers and their partners are classes for early pregnancy; childbirth preparation; breastfeeding; prenatal, postnatal, or post-Cesarean exercise; and infant care. Although much of the background information needed by a physical therapist who wishes to teach these classes can be learned through reading and obstetric observation, experienced instructors usually agree that potential instructors should acquire extra continuing education to teach a specific topic within the general obstetric and gynecology (OB/GYN) specialty.

Although certification is not required to teach or gain access to OB/GYN clients, it is helpful for physical therapists in some locations to become certified as childbirth educators. There are several organizations, listed in the resource guide in the appendix, that conduct programs leading to certification. Some courses are run weekly for a few months. Others are held intermittently on an intensive basis; the participants often completing most of the instruction over a weekend. More recently, home self-study guides have become part of the teacher instruction arsenal. In addition, obstetric experience, a written or oral test, preparation of a class syllabus, and student teaching may be part of the certification requirements. Continuing education or viewings of labors and deliveries to update knowledge may be required by some organizations to maintain certification. The physical therapist that is exploring certification, then, should examine current and future requirements to evaluate which certification process, if any, fits best into plans for practice and marketing.

## *The Physical Therapist as an Instructor*

The teacher must be able to assess the students' needs by observation and nonverbal and verbal communication, as well as streamline information to the needs of a particular group. Courses for single teenage mothers will most likely require a format different from that for married couples, but the basic content must still be presented to both groups. The childbirth educator who implements a plan formulated from an assessment of the goals, needs, and objectives of the group, as well as from their experiences, will probably have a more successful educational program.[1]

Yet, the job does not stop there. Instructor evaluation is a critical component. If the material presented and the manner in which it is presented is not under constant scrutiny, the program will likely become inflexible and static. A teacher who is self-aware will constantly evaluate and be alert to verbal and nonverbal feedback from class participants. However, formal course evaluation is also recommended, not only as a means of self-evaluation, but as a way of gathering feedback for referring physicians, nurses, midwives, childbirth educators and colleagues. (See Table 13-1)

The teacher should be aware of class participants' emotions that become barriers to their learning. Couples may be anxious because

**Table 13-1. Sample Course Evaluation**

---

1. Did this course meet your goals? Explain.

2. Did you find the handouts valuable?

3. Would you recommend this course to others?

4. Was the information presented in a clear, understandable manner?

5. Do you have any suggestions or added comments?

Date:_____

---

of social issues (*e.g.*, an argument before the class or financial problems). Some couples may monopolize a class session by engaging in manipulative games with each other, often using the instructor as a front for their concerns about the birth of the baby, care of the child, or changes that may result in their relationship. It is a challenge for the teacher to uncover these issues, draw people out, and assist couples in learning about the events to come, while at the same time, addressing their underlying concerns.

One theory ascribes that groups of people in a classroom setting learn by passing through various phases. Initially, a tuning-in phase may occur when the students and the teacher make observations about the setting and other couples in the room and are generally mindful of the surroundings. In the following contractual phase, the teacher introduces himself or herself, relates background experience, and explains what is expected from the class. The students complete this phase when they introduce themselves. As class content is introduced, the work period begins. During this phase, reinforcement is necessary to provide feedback to the class. The final phase is the ending, during which some students may feel anxiety about separation from the instructor. The teacher can reduce anxiety by summarizing the information that was covered by giving homework for the week, and by presenting an overview of the next class. These five phases are part of every class, whether the subject is early pregnancy, childbirth preparation, or exercise.[1]

## *Early Pregnancy Classes*

A woman should be encouraged to join early pregnancy classes as soon as she knows she is pregnant; the sooner, the better. The typical class introduces anatomy, physiology, nutrition, body mechanics, muscle strengthening, and an understanding of emotional issues. The three goals of early pregnancy classes are to assist women and their partners (1) to recognize physical and emotional changes that occur during pregnancy; (2) to learn appropriate comfort measures, and (3) to provide a forum for women and their partners to enter the experience together and express their immediate concerns.[2] The classes consist of discussions, audiovisual presentations, handouts, and practical sessions. Using this information, women will be able to make appropriate choices regarding exercise, relaxation, nutrition, body mechanics, and plans for delivery. Usually, women are encouraged to bring a partner, either a spouse, boyfriend, sibling, parent, or friend. It is particularly helpful for the prospective mother to work with the same person she will bring with her for labor and delivery.

Logistically, the early pregnancy class is geared to the woman 1 to

5 months pregnant and her partner. Three weekly 2-hour classes should provide enough time to cover the necessary material, provided the class is limited to 8 to 10 couples. The classroom should be located where the instructor and couples can have some privacy and quiet for teaching and learning relaxation. Bathrooms should be easily accessible.

Tables 13-2 and 13-3 illustrate a sample registration form and class outline for early pregnancy education classes. If word-of-mouth doesn't draw participants, the instructor may need to advertise the class in the local newspaper or send letters to local obstetricians and midwives.

If a promotional letter is mailed, a statement of objectives, course outline, goals, and possibly, handouts, as well as the physical therapist's resume, may help encourage referrals. A follow-up phone call to answer any questions may also prove fruitful. It often takes a while to increase the size of the class, depending on whether it's private-based or hospital-based. Classes taught in a hospital or clinic tend to receive instant approval by both physicians and clients.

A comfortable way to start the class is for the instructor to discuss personal obstetric experience and rationale for attending early preg-

---

**Table 13-2. Sample Class Registration Form**

Class date: _____

Name: _____

Partner: _____

Doctor/midwife: _____

Home phone number: _____

Work phone number: _____

Address: _____

_____

Contacted:_____

Concerns: _____

Notified of:  time/place: _____

            fee: _____

            clothing/pillows/other: _____

Additional Comments:

_____

_____

**Table 13-3. Suggested Outline for an Early Pregnancy Class**

| | |
|---|---|
| Class 1 | Introduction |
| | Relaxation instruction |
| | Immediate concerns of couples |
| | Break |
| | Emotional aspects of pregnancy |
| | Options for delivery |
| Class 2 | Continue options and planning for delivery |
| | Nutrition |
| | Pelvic floor toning |
| | Break |
| | Body mechanics |
| | Pelvic tilt/Positions of comfort |
| | Relaxation |
| Class 3 | Continue relaxation |
| | Fetal and maternal changes |
| | Father's role |
| | Break |
| | Stretching and toning, body mechanics review |
| | Discussion, questions |
| | Course evaluation |

nancy classes. The participants can then introduce themselves, name their physician or midwife, share their due date, and explain why they are attending the class. This goes for both the woman and her partner. It's often fun to tell husbands it's okay to say their wives made them come. This discussion often breaks the ice and facilitates group interaction.

After introductions are made is a good time for the instructor to go over the contents of any handout packet, which can be added to every week. It is probably a good idea to include in the initial packet, or even with paid registration, a bibliography of suggested reading for pregnancy and childbirth, nutrition, breastfeeding, parenting, and postpartum. It is also helpful to give referral numbers, such as the number for the La Leche League, a nursing mothers' support service, or for labor and delivery classes that require early registration. Packets may also include prepared statements available for purchase, such as the "Pregnant Patient's Bill of Rights" and the "Pregnant Patient's Responsibilities" available from the International Childbirth Association (see Appendix).

**Relaxation: Why it is important**

Many physiologic changes of pregnancy cannot be controlled and may affect a woman's psychological state. For instance, she may have physical discomfort, bizarre dreams, concerns over safety of the baby, or anxiety over birth and parenting. These are normal responses to pregnancy, and fathers may experience similar feelings. This increased anxiety can be stress-producing, but even more stress can occur during labor and delivery. The uterine contractions of labor and delivery occur without voluntary control and can be quite painful. This pain can in turn lead to increased muscular tension as a response to pain. To decrease pain associated with increased muscular tension, relaxation is often the key. However, to relax her body, the laboring woman must be able to relax her mind. Education often provides the answers to stress-inducing questions, thereby decreasing anxiety. Through active relaxation exercises, men and women can not only learn to relax tense musculature, but can develop an awareness of tense musculature. The woman who is able to release tense muscles during labor and delivery will avoid working against herself and, theoretically, will experience less discomfort.

The man or woman who practices relaxation techniques will experience an increased awareness and ability to selectively let go. Relaxation can be helpful in other situations to increase energy and decrease stress, and would certainly be useful to remember when meeting the demands of parenting. Relaxation instruction can take several forms, but only two will be discussed for use in early pregnancy: (1) passive—a meditation-type relaxation in which a person temporarily withdraws from the surrounding environment as a way of breaking from the stress in a state of restful alertness; and (2) active—an conscious recognition and release of tension, which deals with stress by helping the person focus calmly. In the latter type, the person is actively involved in the environment and has an awareness and ability to selectively relax without undue tension and muscle energy expenditure.

In the initial early pregnancy class, the instructor might explain the reasons for relaxation and diaphragmatic breathing and begin relaxation techniques. An effective way to begin relaxation instruction is to first teach class members comfort positions. Both may participate in the exercise. Some women may be comfortable lying on their sides, propped on pillows brought from home, or some may prefer to semi-recline, perhaps against the body of their partner. Playing a tape of music or environmental sounds may be helpful to decrease stress. Jacksonian-type relaxation, in which various body parts are contracted and let go, coupled with deep breathing techniques, can be introduced as a way to bring about total body relaxation. A sample progression would be contractions of the muscles of the forehead, face, jaw, tongue (pushed against the roof of the mouth), shoulders, biceps, fists, abdomen, buttocks, quadriceps, heels (pushing into the ground) and feet (dorsiflexing). A sample command would be, "Tighten the forehead and hold—2,3,4—feel the tension in your forehead ... take a deep breath in through your nose, and as you blow out through your mouth, let the tension go ... and, relax...." This sequence should be repeated for each selected body part. It is important to emphasize the letting go of muscular tension, rather than simply relaxing. To work at relaxation too hard may defeat its purpose.

The second class in relaxation repeats the first class; however, the partners end their relaxation early for instruction in working with the mothers to check for areas of tension and tightness. This will require specific instruction to focus on tension areas like the forehead, jaw, shoulders, arms, and legs. Mothers can be encouraged to find a focal point as a stimulus for conscious relaxation with their eyes open. The teacher assists each partner in checking for the mother's relaxation.

In the third class, relaxation cards, with a body part written on each, may be handed out to the women indicating the part to keep tense. The partners then lead the women through a relaxation session that encourages concentration on a visual focal point. The partners are then asked to find where the area of tension is located on the mother, and the instructor verifies this.

### Emotional aspects and changes

A discussion of emotional influences during pregnancy may be facilitated with a flip chart, the instructor listing changes that may have been experienced by the mothers or noted by their support person. After 15 to 20 changes have been listed, the instructor can step back and ask the class to look at the overwhelming number of changes that can occur in such a short time. Such a list may help couples understand that many of their changes are normal and are experienced by others. Many pregnant women have new outlooks on life, changing interests, and different feelings about themselves and their bodies. They may laugh, cry, or become upset easily. They may be more self-confident or more insecure. Some women are unsure whether they really want to change their life are unsure of their capacity to care for a newborn, and wonder how this child will affect their relationships. Others worry if they will be able to adjust financially if one parent has to stop working. They may also be concerned about the baby's well-being, as well as the progress of labor and delivery. All these factors can cause deep-seated stress in a relationship. The partners need to be aware of these changes; they can help each other by listening when feelings are expressed.

Sexual interest changes in both men and women during pregnancy. In the first trimester, there may be a decrease in interest, if the mother experiences nausea and fatigue. Her partner may believe he will hurt the baby. However, this imagined harm is virtually impossible with the protection afforded by the amniotic fluid and membranes surrounding the fetus as well as by the mucus plug at the opening of the cervix. The muscular abdominal wall and bony pelvis additionally serve to protect the fetus. In the second trimester, there may be renewed sexual interest, but in the third, the mother may be less interested because of discomfort, fatigue, and difficulty in the mechanics. Position changes may be a solution. It is important to realize that these changes may be a variation from what the couple is used to; a discussion of concerns and feelings for each other may help ease tension.

Another well-received educational tool is a slide/tape show of an uncomplicated vaginal delivery. Couples may find it reassuring to watch another couple go through a delivery. A show such as this may also be a good introduction to a discussion of delivery options, many of which will be unfamiliar to most of the couples. For instance, couples these days need to consider whether they prefer hospital labor and delivery rooms, hospital birthing rooms, birthing centers, or home deliveries. Once this matter is settled, it becomes easier to think about the things or people they wish to take with them to increase their comfort during labor and delivery. There might be a favorite object, music, focal point, or backup support person. Whatever they decide, the mothers and their partners should write down questions about their concerns for labor and delivery to facilitate communication at their next health check. Homework for the week includes practice of relaxation daily for 15 to 20 minutes, to talk over their expectations and list what is important to each for labor and delivery.

## Weight gain and nutrition

The discussion of nutrition and weight gain is particularly appropriate for early pregnancy classes. As stated in Chapter 4, most physicians no longer put mothers on restricted weight gain.[3]

It is important to point out that it is never too late to start eating right. There are four major reasons for proper nutrition: (1) to monitor proper weight gain (should gain at least 22 pounds); (2) to ingest adequate high-quality protein to meet the needs of the mother and fetus; (3) to ingest adequate caloric intake to metabolize the protein for use by the body; and (4) to assess the selection of a balanced and varied diet that includes items from all basic food groups. On an allowance of 2000 calories/day, 40% should be from high-quality protein, such as meat, fish, poultry, or eggs; 30% from fats or oils; and 30% from fruits, vegetables, cereals, and breads.

The five food groups are (1) dairy products, (2) protein, (3) vegetables and fruit, (4) breads and cereals, and (5) fats. Dairy products supply calcium, protein, and riboflavin. Mothers need about 4 or more servings a day, 6 or more when lactating. An example of a serving would be 1 ounce of cheese, 1 cup of milk, 1/2 cup of cottage cheese, 1/2 cup of ice cream, or 3/4 cup of plain yogurt.[45] (See Table 13-4 for handout on calcium-rich foods.)

Protein sources supply iron and B vitamins. These include lean meats, poultry, eggs, peanut butter, dried beans, lentils, and tofu. Generally, during pregnancy, 75 to 100 gm of protein are needed as compared to the 45 to 50 gm needed when nonpregnant. Calories may vary between different meat sources. For example, an ounce of beef has 65 calories, whereas an ounce of fish, delivering the same amount of protein, has 35.

Vegetables and fruits provide Vitamins A and C and roughage. A pregnant woman needs 4 or 5 servings per day of dark green and yellow vegetables and citrus fruits and juices. Raw fruits and vegetables retain more vitamins. The longer a fruit or vegetable has been cooked, the more the vitamins and roughage have been removed.[45]

Complex carbohydrates, grown from the ground as opposed to man-made refined carbohydrates, stripped of vitamins and minerals, are utilized better by the body and require the body to use less B vitamins to synthesize their products. Breads and cereals supply B vitamins, carbohydrates and iron. Four servings a day of whole grain products (corn, barley, oats, rice, wheat, or millet) are recommended.

A suggested serving of fats is 2 tablespoons per day to aid the function of the hormones of the adrenal cortex, and to be available to the valuable bacteria in the intestinal tract. Unsaturated fats, found in vegetable oil such as safflower, sesame, and canola oils are suggested. Hydrogenated, partially hydrogenated, processed cheeses, solid cooking fats, fried animal fats, and coconut or palm oils should be avoided. Also recommended are unrefined or cold pressed oils that need to be refrigerated, because they do not have preservatives.

Because the daily caloric requirement is already increased, pregnant woman cannot afford to indulge in nutritionally-poor, highly-refined sweets and starches. It must be emphasized that they should get the most from what they eat. All these foods work in combination, so women need to be taught not to eat all their protein at one meal, or all fats at another. Certain foods must be eaten together to get the most out of each calorie. Because the smooth muscle in the colon slows down in pregnancy, women should consume more bulk, water, and raw bran products in their diet. This may also help them avoid hemorrhoids, which may result from the increased vascularity, pressure of the fetus, and constipation caused by ingestion of prenatal vitamins.[45]

So much iron is needed during pregnancy that the National Research Council has advised that supplements be given to expectant

**Table 13-4. Calcium Content of Selected Foods***

| Average Portion | Calcium (mg) |
| --- | --- |
| Milk, whole fresh | 1 cup 288 |
| Milk, nonfat | 1 cup 298 |
| Buttermilk, whole | 1 cup 293 |
| Buttermilk, skim | 1 cup 296 |
| Yogurt, plain whole | 1 cup 271 |
| Yogurt, plain skim | 1 cup 293 |
| Cheese spread | 1 ounce 158 |
| Cheese, American | 1 ounce 195 |
| Cheese, Swiss | 1 ounce 248 |
| Cream cheese | 1 ounce  17 |
| Cottage cheese, creamed | 1 cup 211 |
| Cheese, cheddar | 1 ounce 211 |
| Ice cream | ⅔ cup 131 |
| Ice milk | ⅔ cup 140 |
| Nonfat dry powdered milk | 1 cup (dry) 220 |
| Sardines, canned | 3½ ounces 409 |
| Shrimp, canned | 3½ ounces 115 |
| Bread: whole wheat | 2 slices  57 |
| white | 2 slices  48 |
| cracked wheat | 2 slices  50 |
| rye | 2 slices  46 |
| Beans, common white | ½ cups  57 |
| Beans, common red | ½ cups  44 |
| Beans, lima | ½ cups  54 |
| Beans, snap, yellow | ½ cups  57 |
| Collards, cooked | ½ cups 215 |
| Kale, cooked | ½ cups 214 |
| Lettuce, iceberg | 4 ounces  78 |
| Onion, raw | 1 large 180 |
| Parsnips, cooked | ½ cups  52 |
| Okra, cooked | ½ cups 105 |
| Sweet potato (with skin) | ½ cups  46 |
| Broccoli, cooked | ½ cup 101 |
| Molasses, light | 2 T  50 |
| medium | 2 T  87 |
| blackstrap | 2 T 205 |
| Figs, dried | 2 ounces  66 |

*United States Department of Agriculture, Composition of Foods, Handbook No. 8, 1975.
Protein sources supply iron and B vitamins.

mothers. The greatest amount of iron is needed during the last three months of pregnancy when the mother is building iron stores that will be transferred to the baby at birth. Additionally, she will need a supply of iron following delivery to replenish the iron in her own blood. It is wise, therefore, to encourage participants in the early pregnancy class to choose iron-rich foods, such as dried fruits, wheat germ, dried beans, and blackstrap molasses. Couples may benefit from a handout with a list of iron rich foods (see Table 13-5).

Although salt restriction was previously prescribed to pregnant women to prevent preeclampsia, the American College of Obstetrics and Gynecology now states that salt restriction in pregnancy is unnecessary.[5] Sodium ingestion is needed to maintain normal salt levels in bone, muscles, and brain to balance the growth of blood

**Table 13-5. Foods High in Iron**
**(more than 1.5 mg of iron per listed serving size)**

| FOOD | SERVING | FOOD | SERVING |
|---|---|---|---|
| Apricots dried | 5 halves | Molasses | 2 T |
| Beans | 1/2 cup | Oysters | 1 ounce |
| Beef, cooked | 2 ounces | Peaches, dried | 3 halves |
| Beet greens, cooked | 1/2 cup | Pork (cooked) | 2 ounces |
| Brazil nuts | 6 medium | Prunes, dried | 4 medium |
| Cereals* | 1 ounce | Prune juice | 1/4 cup |
| Chard, cooked | 1/2 cup | Raisins, dried | 1-1/2 oz |
| Chicken, cooked | 1/2 cup | Sardines | 2 ounces |
| Cider, sweet | 10 ounces | Scallops | 2 ounces |
| Clams | 1 ounce | Shrimp | 2 ounces |
| Corn syrup | 2 T | Spinach, cooked | 1/2 cup |
| Dandelion greens | 1/2 cup | Strawberries | 1 cup |
| Dried beef | 1 ounce | Tomato juice | 3/4 cup |
| Egg, whole | 2 | Tongue, cooked | 2 ounces |
| Ham, cooked | 2 ounces | Tuna | 1/2 cup |
| Heart, cooked | 2 ounces | Turkey, cooked | 1 ounce |
| Instant breakfast | 1 serving | Veal, cooked | 1 ounce |
| Kidney, cooked | 1 ounce | Watermelon | 6″ diameter, 1-1/2 slices |
| Lamb, cooked | 2 ounces | | |
| Liver, cooked | 1 ounce | | |
| Liver sausage | 1 ounce | | |
| Maple syrup | 3 T | | |

*15% NDR of iron or more per serving. United States Department of Agriculture. Composition of Food, Agriculture Handbook No. 8, 1975.

plasma and tissue fluids that are a natural outgrowth of pregnancy. Iodine, a natural mineral sometimes added to common salt, is vital for the proper functioning of the thyroid gland. Therefore, physicians recommend mothers salt to taste, or season as they usually do.[5]

It may be helpful for the class to go through an exercise of filling out a menu sheet for the week to see when and what they eat and if they are getting all the necessary nutrients (see Table 13-6). Partners often wish to fill out a menu sheet as well. Excellent nutrition guides during pregnancy are available and are a welcome addition to class handouts (see resources in the Appendix).

It is important to talk to parents about alcohol, smoking, and caffeine use and abuse. The National Institute on Alcohol Abuse and Alcoholism has said that 3 ounces of absolute alcohol are equivalent

**Table 13-6. Weekly Menu Sheet**

| Day | Breakfast | Snack | Lunch | Snack | Dinner | Snack | Calories (Total) |
|---|---|---|---|---|---|---|---|
| Monday | _____ | ____ | ____ | ____ | ____ | ____ | _____ |
| Tuesday | _____ | ____ | ____ | ____ | ____ | ____ | _____ |
| Wednesday | _____ | ____ | ____ | ____ | ____ | ____ | _____ |
| Thursday | _____ | ____ | ____ | ____ | ____ | ____ | _____ |
| Friday | _____ | ____ | ____ | ____ | ____ | ____ | _____ |
| Saturday | _____ | ____ | ____ | ____ | ____ | ____ | _____ |
| Sunday | _____ | ____ | ____ | ____ | ____ | ____ | _____ |

to 6 average-size drinks. Based on that institute's research, a pregnant woman who drinks 3 ounces of alcohol, clearly risks harm to
her baby.[6] The blood alcohol level will increase in the mother and in
the fetus because of transfer through the placenta. In the first trimester, most of the initial growth and development of fetal organs is
taking place. It is at this time, therefore, when utmost caution should
be used. In some cases, however, the mother may be already addicted
to alcohol or drugs, and there is considerable risk that this addiction
can be transmitted to the unborn child. Newborn addicts must then
cope with withdrawal symptoms in addition to the normal adjustments to the environment at birth.

It is unknown whether there is a safe amount to drink below 3
ounces of absolute alcohol; but risk has been associated with ingestion of 1 to 3 ounces of alcohol, and caution should be advised.[6]
Newborns with fetal alcohol syndrome[6,7] may have low IQs, abnormal facial features, narrow eyes, low nasal bridges, or heart defects.
There is also concern that binge drinking, consuming large quantities on an occasional basis, may also prove harmful to the growing
fetus.

It may be important to point out alternatives to alcohol, whether
they be creative nonalcoholic drinks, or expressive, creative outlets.[8]
The physical therapist with a client suspected of alcohol abuse may
seek help from the local Alcoholics Anonymous Council. Studies
suggest that heavy alcohol drinkers who receive counseling are able
to abstain, or significantly moderate, their consumption before the
third trimester.[9] This reduction of alcohol was associated with a
more normal fetal weight, head circumference, and length.[9]

Smoke also crosses the placenta and can restrict a baby's normal
growth in the uterus. Statistics show a direct correlation between
smoking during pregnancy and an increased incidence of spontaneous abortion and stillbirths. Pregnant women who smoke a pack or
more of cigarettes a day put their fetuses at 50% greater risk of
infant mortality.[8] The American Cancer Institute states that babies of
women who smoke usually average a birth weight of 6 ounces less
than babies of nonsmoking women. Nicotine is believed to restrict
blood vessels and fetal breathing movements, and carbon monoxide
reduces the oxygen available in the fetal circulation.

In addition, vitamin metabolism is also disturbed by smoking. A
1976 study by the U.S. Department of Health, Education and Welfare
found that 7-year-old children of mothers who smoked were shorter
in average stature, tended to have retarded reading ability, and rated
lower in social adjustment than children of mothers who did not
smoke.[8] For mothers who smoke then, the risks include: (1) underde-
veloped and underweight babies at birth, (2) babies more prone to

illness in the first critical weeks of life (related to low birth weight), (3) a greater risk of miscarriage, and (4) babies who have a 20% to 25% greater chance of dying within the first 24 hours after birth.[8]

Caffeine also crosses the placenta, and has been known, when used in excessive amounts, to cause fetal growth retardation and fetal loss. The half-life of caffeine is 2 to 3 times longer in pregnant women than in nonpregnant women. Caffeine may be transported across the placenta and membranes to the fetus and amniotic fluid where concentrations may be greater than those of the mother. Studies suggest that caffeine has the effect of reducing placental blood supply in animals, but the human fetus appears capable of maintaining its umbilical vein blood flow at normal levels.[10]

Caffeine increases catecholamines in the circulation, especially epinephrine. There are known cardiovascular effects, linked to the rise in catecholamine levels; however, further investigation is hampered by the lack of noninvasive methods available in studying human fetal placental blood flow. Physicians, midwives, and maternal health educators may offer guidelines to reduce caffeine intake (see Table 13-7).

## Pelvic floor toning

It is important for the instructor to show a chart to the class when discussing the pelvic floor. Most men and women have never heard of the pelvic floor, and anatomic diagrams that show the layers of

**Table 13-7. Caffeine Content of Various Beverages**

|  | Mg caffeine per 5 oz. cup |
|---|---|
| Coffee instant | 66 |
| percolated | 110 |
| drip | 146 |
| Bagged tea | |
| black, 1-minute brew | 28 |
| black, 5-minute brew | 46 |
| Loose tea | |
| green, Japan, 5-minute | 20 |
| green, 5-minute brew | 35 |
| black, 5-minute brew | 40 |
| Cocoa | |
| 2 heaping tsp. instant | 13 |
|  | Mg caffeine per 12 oz. can |
| Diet Rite | 32 |
| Diet RC | 33 |
| RC cola | 34 |
| Pepsi-Cola | 43 |
| Tab | 49 |
| Diet Dr. Pepper | 54 |
| Mountain Dew | 55 |
| Dr. Pepper | 61 |
| Coca-Cola | 65 |

Adapted from: Harvard Community Health Plan, Boston, Massachusetts muscles suspended like a hammock running anteriorly from the pubis posteriorly to the sacrococcygeal area are helpful. A perineal view will provide an added dimension to the location of the pubococcygeal muscle. The importance for pelvic floor toning should be explained: (1) it supports the uterus and pelvic contents; (2) it may help mother develop an awareness of several degrees of contraction and relaxation, which may be helpful for relaxing the pelvic floor during delivery; (3) a healthy, toned pelvic floor may repair more quickly after delivery; (4) adequate muscle tone and the ability to relax pelvic floor muscles may help avoid episiotomy; and, (5) a toned pelvic floor may cause greater voluntary contractions of the pubococcygeus muscle and possibly stimulate pubococcygeal nerve endings through the vaginal walls, resulting in enhanced sexual satisfaction. During delivery, the passage of the baby's head through the untoned pelvic floor may cause tissue injury.[11] Pelvic floor toning should be a component of any general conditioning program. (See Table 13-8)

### Center of gravity and body mechanics in pregnancy

Instruction in body mechanics includes a chart of the center of gravity showing the nonpregnant state versus the pregnant state, and how the center of gravity is measured through the ear, shoulder, iliac crest, knee, and ankle (refer to chapter 11, Figure 11-3). The additional weight of pregnancy, added breast tissue, and other possible physiologic changes, increase the lumbar lordosis. Postural adaptations may cause a woman to stand with her head forward and shoulders rounded. As a result of poor posture, stress on the brachial plexus may produce some tingling in the hands. Also, at this time, relaxin, progesterone, and estrogen are released and may loosen various ligaments in the body. The pelvic girdle increases in size in preparation for delivery.

It is crucial that the strength in the low back muscles and abdominal muscles be strong to counteract the changes in the center of gravity and accompanying weight gain. The instructor should demonstrate the pelvic tilt both in the supine and hands and knees positions. Participants should be encouraged to avoid positions of discomfort, such as bending straight from the waist, sitting for long periods of time, or holding objects far away from their center of gravity as opposed to close to their body. The instructor should also present comfort positions for resting or sleeping. Finding a comfortable position for a woman in later stages of pregnancy can be quite challenging, but the instructor can encourage left-side lying (to relieve pressure from the fetus on abdominal blood vessels), with a pillow under the abdomen, between the knees, and under the head.

## Table 13-8. Handout for pelvic floor exercises

Exercise #1: The Faucet
(Note: Advise women to completely empty bladder after performing this exercise to avoid urine stasis. Women with incontinence may have difficulty contracting the pelvic floor muscles in this gravity-resisted position.)

| | |
|---|---|
| Position: | Sit on the toilet. Spread legs apart for urination and support feet on a stool if voiding is difficult. |
| Exercise: | As you urinate, stop and start the flow of urine a few times, breaking it off smoothly. Try not to allow any dribbling of urine. Hold tight for 5 seconds before starting urine flow again. |
| Progression: | Let smaller amounts of urine pass each time. Do not worry if this difficult. Try to always end the voiding with an uplifting contraction of the pelvic floor. Do not try this exercise first thing in the morning when your bladder is full, or at night if you are tired or uncomfortable. |

Exercise #2: Contract and Relax

| | |
|---|---|
| Position: | Lie on back or side with legs apart and chest relaxed. |
| Exercise: | Draw pelvic floor upward. Feel the squeeze as the sphincters are tightened, and the inside passage becomes narrow and tense. Focus on the front portion of the pelvic floor where the master sphincter surrounds the vagina and urethra. Initially, hold 2 to 3 seconds and then completely relax. Attempt to relax a little bit more, releasing any residual tension. Repeat 2 or 3 times, relaxing and repeating. Always end with a contraction. |
| Progression: | Try other positions such as sitting, standing, and squatting. Do a total of 50 repetitions a day: 5 repetitions at a time, 10 sessions per day, holding each repetitions for 5 seconds. Relax between each contraction. |

Exercise #3: The Elevator

| | |
|---|---|
| Position: | Assume any position, although lying down is easier at first. |
| Exercise: | Imagine you are in an elevator on the first floor. As you ascend to each floor, draw up the pelvic floor muscles a little bit more. When you reach your limit, do not let go, but descend floor by floor, gradually relaxing the pelvic floor in stages. When you have reached the first floor, think about releasing, and continue to the basement. Do not hold your breath, blow out through pursed lips. Feel the perineal muscles bulge. Complete this exercise by bringing the pelvic floor back up to the ground floor. |

Exercise #4: The Sexercise

| | |
|---|---|
| Position: | Assume any position of coitus with the legs spread apart and relaxed. |
| Exercise: | Grip the penis as firmly as you can with your vagina, holding for 5 seconds before you relax. Try to avoid tensing the buttocks and the abdominal muscles. Repeat a few times until your partner tells you the strength of the contractions has diminished. Rest and repeat in a few minutes. |
| Progression: | Your muscle strength will increase as you learn to make the contractions stronger, more consistent and more numerous. |

[Adapted from E. Noble: Essential Exercises for the Childbearing Year[11]]

The instructor might then talk about additional supports that may be needed in pregnancy—corsets, bras, binders, and support elastic stockings. Sacroiliac corsets may be helpful for women who have chronic sacroiliac irritation, and bras are strongly recommended to support the increased weight of the breast tissue. A well-fitting bra improves posture and may minimize upper back ache. Some women may also find wearing a bra to bed comfortable. Broad, nonelastic straps with stability and support are preferable. Mothers should also be encouraged to buy nursing bras with the best support and fit.

Although it is best to assist venous return from the legs by using the pumping action of the muscles, some women, because of the increased blood volume of pregnancy, find that their legs ache and are susceptible to varicose veins. These women may benefit from elastic stockings (examples listed in the Appendix). They should not be too tight or have bands that interfere with blood circulation.

### Fetal and maternal changes

Fetal and maternal changes can be handled with charts or handouts based on the material presented in Chapters 6 and 7. Additional maternal changes are presented below in Table 13-9. The film "When Life Begins" by McGraw-Hill or a similar one is a good overview of ovulation, fertilization, migration, and implantation of an early embryo. The film also shows the development of the embryo; accompanying changes in the maternal reproductive organs, placenta, and umbilical cord; and the relationship of the fetus to the amniotic sac and fetal membranes. The *in utero* shots are fiberoptic pictures of a live fetus who is later shown being delivered without obstetric intervention.

### Father's role

It is important to talk about a father's role and how it changes over the first, second, and third trimesters, and during labor and delivery. In the first trimester, the father's identity is changing, and he is

**Table 13-9. Maternal Changes in Pregnancy[12]**

| Maternal Changes Month | Physiologic Changes |
|---|---|
| 1. Rise in temperature, vomiting, fatigue, tingling breasts, end of menses | Ovulation, fertilization, implantation of ovum, and thickening of uterine lining due to increased estrogen and progesterone |
| 2. Positive pregnancy test; pressure on bladder with frequency of urination; nausea subsiding; profuse, thick vaginal discharge; breasts enlarge | Mucus plug forming in cervix |
| 3. Colostrum leaking from breasts; nausea subsiding; bladder pressure less | Placenta completely formed and secreting estrogen; uterine cavity filled; uterus rising from pelvic cavity into abdomen |
| 4. Abdominal appearance of pregnancy | Blood volume increasing; fundus half way between symphysis and umbilicus |
| 5. Quickening–fetal movement | Placenta covers half of uterine wall |
| 6. Stretch marks; linea nigra appears; possible chloasma (around eyes); period of greatest weight gain starts | Height of fundus at umbilicus; period of lowest hemoglobin |
| 7. Braxton Hicks contractions palpable, intermittent uterine contractions | Blood volume highest |
| 8. 2–3 pound weight gain, Braxton Hicks contractions stronger; stretch marks more pronounced; backache | Longitudinal stretching of uterus |
| 9. Umbilicus protrudes; shortness of breath, varicosities, ankle swelling; descent of head; lightening (primip), baby drops; easier breathing; urinary frequency | Fundus just under diaphragm (before lightening); lightening more common in primiparas; can occur in multiparas; may drop just before birth |

exploring new roles. He is becoming involved in the pregnancy and is preparing for the labor and delivery process. He may have unresolved feelings about having a child or may need to reevaluate what it will be like to be a father again, if he has other children. This may be a time when he reassesses his job, whether or not it is secure; if he has enough salary; and if he has enough life and health insurance. Often, financial matters are the focus.

The father may notice emotional changes in the mother and can be very supportive at this time by helping with diet, exercises, and emotional issues, and by offering love and companionship. In the second trimester, the movement of the baby at 16 to 20 weeks confirms the pregnancy for the father. The mother may not have physically changed much up to this point, but now she is definitely showing signs of pregnancy. This milestone may plunge the father into thoughts about fatherhood, and he may spend time feeling for movements of the baby and listening to hear its heartbeat. The couple may experience sexual freedom and feel generally good about their relationship. At this time, women may look to their partners for help, when ordinarily they would have accomplished tasks independently. A woman may also express unusual anxiety about her partner's safety. It is necessary for the father to recognize these signs and to participate in his own way. He is definitely needed and can be a very positive support.

In the third trimester, the father has worked through some of the psychological issues raised by the pregnancy. For example, the changing environment, his role, financial issues, and his changing relationship to his wife have been confronted and handled. He has seen how he has been needed, and, hopefully, he becomes involved by attending early pregnancy and then childbirth preparation classes. If so, he has helped with practicing relaxation, breathing, and exercise techniques, and pregnancy has become a time of real sharing. The reality of the baby increases, and the father may find himself dreaming of his new child in a real situation with himself.

During labor and delivery, fathers are allowed to be more involved than they were in the past. There have been stories of men in the late 1960s who would handcuff themselves to their wives as they were wheeled to the delivery room so that they could participate in the birth! Although some cultures used to believe a man would die if he saw his wife in labor, that mystique is changing as fathers see they do have a role as comforter, supporter, and motivator in labor and delivery. Fathers today are sometimes allowed to cut the umbilical cord postdelivery and, often, to be in the delivery room if their wives undergo Cesarean sections. It is a very special time for fathers to see the baby they helped create emerge into the world. It is rare for a man to return to a nonparticipatory role once he has experienced such direct involvement through pregnancy classes, labor, and delivery.

## Stretching and toning

The rationale for exercise needs to be made clear so that the couple will understand the advantages of muscle strengthening, breathing, and relaxation, as well as how the exercised muscles are relevant to childbirth. Rationale includes relief of low back pain and preparation for labor and delivery by increasing strength, stamina, endurance, and tolerance for the physical and mental stress. Exercise also produces a psychological boost, and posture may be improved. If the mother exercises throughout pregnancy, postpartum recovery may be easier and faster. Exercise gives the body strength, muscle tone, and flexibility. It also helps develop new powers of concentration and relaxation.

The instructor can safely recommend that 15 to 20 minutes a day be devoted to light exercise during pregnancy. Each woman must perform at her exercise level and should be challenged to perform additional exercises in a gradually increasing manner. Keeping these factors in mind, it is better to design a simple program that has some flexibility and variability in it to decrease the possibility of boredom and increase the chances of compliance.[12-16]

Several cautionary notes must be added here. Prenatal and postnatal patients must get clearance from their physicians before participating in an exercise program. They must be screened for conditions that would limit their medical, cardiovascular, musculoskeletal, or pregnancy-related complications.

Early pregnancy is a good time to teach how to check for diastasis recti abdominis (as described in Chapter 9). If there is a rectus separation, exercise can be modified to maintain tone and to discourage further separation. The patient can be instructed to lie supine (less than 3 minutes) with hands crossed over the lower abdomen in a corset-type of arrangement, breathe in, then breathe out as she raises her head up, and simultaneously approximate the abdominal muscles with her hands. This can be done several times throughout the day.

Exercises for the prenatal period may be individually tailored by the therapist, working with each woman independently to meet unique needs. There are numerous exercises that are appropriate for this population, but there are guidelines that are important to understand before designing an exercise program. General guidelines for clients include: (1) Exercise regularly and do not attempt to make up for lost time by pushing too hard. Exercise sessions should be no more than 2-1/2 days apart. (2) Finish eating at least 1-1/2 hours before working out to avoid gastrointestinal discomfort. (3) Do not diet during pregnancy. (4) Stop exercising if any dizziness, pain, or persistent discomfort is experienced. (5) Drink water before and after a workout.

Specific exercise guidelines and contraindications that should be followed by physical therapists include: (1) After 4 months of gestation, avoid exercises requiring women to lie supine for longer than 3 minutes to prevent compression on the inferior vena cava. (2) Avoid exercises that promote straining of the pelvic floor or abdominal muscles. (3) Avoid exercises that excessively stretch hip adductors, which may cause strain and possible trauma to the symphysis pubis. (4) Avoid exercises that involve sharp twists, rapid or uncontrolled swinging or bouncing movements. (5) Avoid exercises that utilize positions in which the buttocks are higher than the head, as in bridging, supine bicycling motions, or modified quadruped position because of potential air embolus introduced through the vagina. (6) Avoid inversion activities. Figure 13-1 illustrates a suggested exercise series for an early pregnancy class.[14,15,17]

Questions will undoubtedly arise regarding the safety of aerobic exercise during pregnancy. Aerobic conditioning in pregnancy still involves strengthening the cardiopulmonary system by making the heart work over a 20 to 30 minute period to create a demand for oxygen met by increased breathing. The types of aerobic conditioning best suited for pregnancy are walking or swimming. A program in which the mother exercises a minimum of 3 times a week, possibly increasing the frequency to 4 to 6 times, should be beneficial.

To have true aerobic conditioning, the heart rate should fall within the target zone. The recommended target zone in pregnancy, and until 12 weeks postpartum, is 60% to 70% of the safe, maximum, attainable heart rate. To determine what that safe heart rate is, the formula is 220 multiplied by 60% to 70% (see Table 13-10).[13] Mothers should be taught how to take an accurate pulse, using the carotid or radial artery.

The aerobic program should start with a 5-minute warm-up to prevent injury and to increase flexibility. Stretches should include hamstrings; quadriceps; gastrocnemius-soleus groups; and arm, neck, and shoulder muscles. The heart rate should range in the target zone a minimum of 12 minutes, but 20 to 30 minutes is better. The aerobic program should end with a 5-minute cool-down phase. After delivery, the mother who wishes to continue with her aerobic walking or swimming program should decrease the total time slightly from the amount she was exercising just prior to delivery, and then slowly increase the challenge of her program.

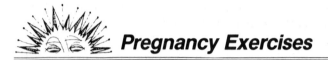

# Pregnancy Exercises

## 1 FULL BODY STRETCH

*Purpose:* To warm up by stretching the entire body.

*Position:* On back, straighten out arms & legs. Point toes and extend fingers, then flex toes toward knees (hold 5 sec.) relax, let arms and legs go limp.

*Amount:* 3x

## 2 HAMSTRING STRETCH

*Purpose:* To stretch the hamstring muscles (back of the thigh) at both ends of the muscle.

*Position:* On back, bend both knees. Bring one knee to chest with hands under knee: (gently hold to chest) extend leg up as high as possible with straight knee and flexed foot. (hold for 10 sec.) lower slowly, switch and repeat.

*Amount:* 3x each leg

## 3 NECK CIRCLES

*Purpose:* To increase flexibility in all neck muscles and relax shoulders.

*Position:* Sit upright with ankles crossed. Gently rotate head in a full circle, breathe gently.

*Amount:* 5x to right, 5x to left

## 4 NECK STRETCH

*Purpose:* To increase flexibility and range of motion in all neck muscles.

*Position:* **A.** Ankles crossed. Look down and place hand on back of head and gently push down until you feel more stretch in the back of the neck. **B.** Turn head to right, with right hand on cheek, push head gently more to the right. Repeat to the left with left hand. **C.** With right hand on top of head, pull head gently so that right ear approaches right shoulder. Switch and repeat.

*Amount:* 3x each exercise in each direction

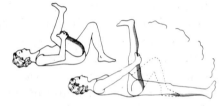

## 5 ABDUCTOR AND LOW BACK STRETCH

*Purpose:* To strengthen thighs and arms.

*Position:* Sit with knees up and ankles crossed, hands under knees. Hands hold and resist downward push of knees (hold 10 sec.) Breathe out as you hold.

*Amount:* Repeat 5x

## 6 FULL BODY TWIST

*Purpose:* To stretch waist, upper body and neck, and increase flexibility throughout the spine.

*Position:* Legs crossed indian-style, place left hand on right knee and twist right. Put right palm on floor behind you next to spine with elbow straight. Inhale slowly, then exhale. Switch and twist to left.

*Amount:* 2x each side

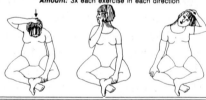

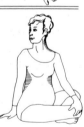

Figure 13-1: Suggested pregnancy exercise regime from Gourley R.

**7** *SHOULDER, ARM AND UPPER BACK STRETCH*

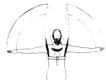

*Purpose:* To increase range of motion and flexibility in shoulders, arms and upper back muscles.

*Position:* Sitting with back against wall, legs out straight. Start with straight arms, palms up at shoulder level. Drag arms slowly up wall maintaining contact with wall. Hold at point where arms want to push away from wall, (hold for 10 sec.), lower slowly. *Amount:* 3x

---

**8** *CAT EXERCISE*

*Purpose:* To relieve back pain and increase flexibility in low back muscles.

*Position:* On hands and knees, arch the back up and drop head down. Reverse the action, to head up and back raised to flat position. *Amount:* 10x

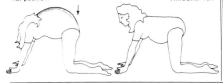

**9**

BUDDHA

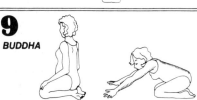

*Purpose:* To stretch upper back, arms, wrists, and low back muscles.

*Position:* Sitting on heels with knees a comfortable distance apart, place hands on thighs. Keeping knees bent slide hands forward (on floor) until arms and back are stretched forward, breathe out, stretch. (hold position, breathing easily, for 10 sec.) *Amount:* 5x

---

**10** SQUATTING

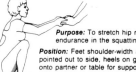

*Purpose:* To stretch hip muscles and increase endurance in the squatting position.

*Position:* Feet shoulder-width apart and knees pointed out to side, heels on ground, squat holding onto partner or table for support, (hold for 10 sec.), stand, repeat. *Amount:* 4x

**11** *HIP STRETCH*

*Purpose:* To stretch front of thigh and increase flexibility in legs.

*Position:* Squat on floor. Place one leg behind and shift weight to bent leg keeping hands on floor. Pull self forward until knee of bent leg is directly over ankle, (hold for 10 sec.). Switch and stretch.

*Amount:* Alternate 3x each leg

---

**12** SIDE BENDS

*Purpose:* To stretch arms and trunk.

*Position:* Feet shoulder width apart. Hold elbow of right arm with left hand. Gently pull right elbow behind head as you bend to the left, (hold 10 sec.). Switch to left. Hold left elbow with right hand.

*Amount:* 3x each side

**13**

CALF STRETCH

*Purpose:* To stretch calf muscles and front of thighs.

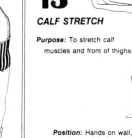

*Position:* Hands on wall, straighten left leg behind. Feet pointing straight forward, lean into wall until stretching is felt in calf muscles (hold 10 sec.). Same position, bend the back knee (hold 10 sec.). Switch and stretch opposite leg. *Amount:* 3x each leg

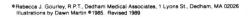

Figure 13-1: Suggested pregnancy exercise regime from Gourley R. (continued)

**Table 13-10. Target Heart Rate Zones for Pregnant Women and New Mothers**

| Age | Beginners (60%-70% of SHR*) | Fit before pregnancy (70%-75% of SHR) |
|-----|-----------------------------|---------------------------------------|
| 20 | 120-140 | 140-150 |
| 21 | 119-139 | 139-149 |
| 22 | 118-138 | 138-148 |
| 23 | 117-137 | 137-147 |
| 24 | 117-137 | 137-147 |
| 25 | 116-136 | 136-146 |
| 26 | 115-135 | 135-145 |
| 27 | 115-135 | 135-145 |
| 28 | 114-134 | 134-144 |
| 29 | 113-133 | 133-143 |
| 30 | 113-133 | 133-143 |
| 31 | 112-132 | 132-142 |
| 32 | 111-131 | 131-141 |
| 33 | 110-130 | 130-140 |
| 34 | 110-130 | 130-140 |
| 35 | 109-129 | 129-139 |
| 36 | 108-128 | 128-138 |
| 37 | 108-128 | 128-138 |
| 38 | 107-127 | 127-137 |
| 39 | 106-126 | 126-136 |
| 40 | 106-126 | 126-136 |
| 41 | 105-125 | 125-135 |
| 42 | 104-124 | 124-134 |

From White R: Fitness in Pregnancy. Seattle, Pennypress, 1984.[13] *SHR = safe, maximal attainable heart rate

## Childbirth Preparation Classes

Classes in psychoprophylaxis describe physical and psychological preparation for labor and delivery. These classes are designed to be held as close to the mother's due date when motivation peaks. The repeated practice of the techniques learned in this class will encourage a conditioned response by the mother and her partner when they need it during labor and delivery. Women are again encouraged to bring their partner or other support person. Labor and delivery is a time when support is most definitely needed. A class is usually 1 1/2 to 3 hours each time, with a break in the middle. Fees for the classes will vary, depending on how the teacher will be reimbursed. A hospital or physician may pay the instructor directly and charges to the client included in the hospital's or doctor's fees. If the instructor is in private practice, fees will probably need to be calculated to cover the length of class, rental of equipment (films, projectors), and space; or the fee charged to students may be a reflection of the resources and customs of the community. Some childbirth classes may be covered by the couples' insurance; however this is unusual. Class size should probably be limited to 8 couples.

Publicizing the classes is often another job of the instructor; if she is in private practice or works for a sponsoring agency, articles written periodically in a local newspaper may help remind the community of available classes. Calling local hospitals and physicians is a must to exchange information between instructor and referral sources. Some hospitals and doctors ask that the instructor show them some of the class handouts and information used. Prepared packs given to these potential referral sources will supplement the initial contact. Offering to stock the hospital or doctor's office with brochures allows them to give out some information about the instructor and classes (objective, content, and logistics). Some instructors keep a running calendar at the doctor's office to post when the next class will start. When starting up a new class, it may be helpful to advertise and show a childbirth film free to the public.

A hospital tour should be arranged or encouraged for the class members. Communication is enhanced for the participants if there are realistic expectations between hospital, doctor, and childbirth educator. At the final class, a course evaluation and scheduled postpartum meeting with all the babies will encourage further group contact and support.

A suggested outline of a 7-class series in childbirth preparation is included and a list of items for couples to bring to the hospital are provided for ideas (see Tables 13-11 and 13-12)

No matter what type of childbirth education is offered, relaxation exercises are the stepping stones to controlled breathing and to a prepared response to the pain of labor (see Figure 13-2). To achieve

**Table 13-11. Suggested Outline for 7-Class Series in Childbirth Preparation**

| | |
|---|---|
| Class 1 | Content<br>Introduce self. Give background information. Have students introduce themselves. Discuss course content and goals, overview of class. Introduce psychoprophylaxis and its relevance to pain, labor, and delivery. Discuss fetal and maternal development. Introduce relaxation. Give overview of labor and delivery, showing charts. Teach pregnancy stretches. |
| Class 2 | Answer questions. Practice relaxation. Show exercises for pelvic floor and abdominal muscles. Discuss body mechanics and positions of comfort. Discuss labor and coaching role. Start basic breathing techniques. |
| Class 3 | Answer questions. Review breathing techniques. Practice breathing techniques. Practice relaxation. Discuss transition and review labor. Discuss variations of normal labor. Review pregnancy stretches. |
| Class 4 | Answer questions. Practice relaxation exercise. Teach expulsion. Discuss second stage of labor. Discuss coach's role. Discuss what to bring to the hospital. |
| Class 5 | Answer questions. Review labor, including hospital procedures. Show film on labor and delivery. Discuss appearance of the newborn. Discuss postpartum period expectations—emotional and physical changes. |
| Class 6 | Answer questions. Review all breathing exercises. Review all relaxation exercises. Show film of postpartum period, adjusting to the newborn. Instruct in postpartum exercises and supplement with handouts. |
| Class 7 | Visit the hospital. View labor and delivery rooms, birthing rooms, and birthing chair, if provided. |

**Table 13-12. What to Bring to the Hospital**

For the Labor Bag: watch with a second hand, lip balm, ice pack, socks, money for phone calls, phone list, powder for abdominal stroking, pen and paper, food for partner, cards, books, magazines, focal point, camera/flash and film, lollipops to decrease nausea, labor guide, tennis ball for counterpressure in case of back labor, paper bag for hyperventilation.

For the Mother: slippers, two to three nursing nightgowns, bathrobe or bed jacket, bras, underpants, sanitary pads, toilet articles, address book and birth announcements, reading material, writing material, loose-fitting going home outfit (probably one worn at 4-5 months of pregnancy)

For Baby: pacifier, undershirt (newborn size), diapers, pins, plastic pants, going home outfit, blanket, sweater, hat, car seat.

a conditioned response, relaxation and breathing start automatically in response to a uterine contraction; however, participants must practice relaxation and breathing exercises daily.

There are two basic breathing techniques taught in preparation for labor and delivery: (1) rhythmic, deep breathing, which is about 8 breaths per minute or 2 per 15-second period, and (2) shallow chest breathing, which is 30 to 40 breaths per minute.[1] The mother uses rhythmic or slow breathing when she can no longer walk or talk through a contraction. She signals the beginning of a contraction with a cleansing breath. She focuses on one spot to enhance concentration, rhythmically and gently inhales through the nose, and exhales through the mouth. After the contraction is over, she gives

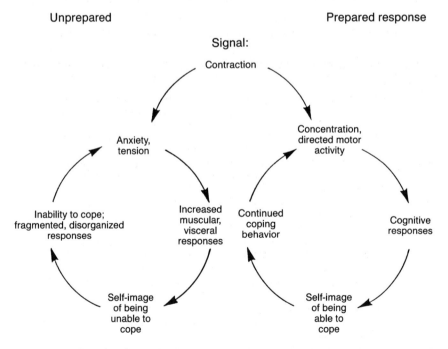

Figure 13-2: Responses in the prepared and unprepared woman. (From Hassid P. Textbook for Childbirth Educators, Hagerstown, Maryland: Harper & Row, 1978)

another cleansing breath (see Figure 13-3A) Coaches are encouraged to breathe along with mother during practice and in late labor.

Shallow chest breathing is used when the rhythmic chest breathing is no longer adequate to cope with the contractions. This technique begins with a cleansing breath, the mother focuses, and con-

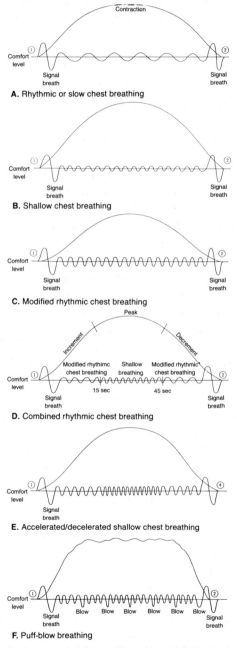

Figure 13-3: Breathing for labor and delivery. (From Hassid P. Textbook for Childbirth Educators, Hagerstown, Maryland: Harper & Row, 1978)

tinues with 30 to 40 breaths per minute. It should be practiced for at least 1 minute and should end with a cleansing breath. These breaths are shallow, brief, held high in the chest, and are very light. There is little chest exertion noted (see Figure 13-3B).

Based on these two breathing methods, other breathing patterns and activities are adapted to suit the needs of the laboring woman. For example: 1) Add abdominal stroking to rhythmic chest breathing to increase concentration and sensory input. 2) Modify rhythmic chest breathing by incorporating variations, such as inhaling for a count of 1, exhaling for a count of 2 to 3 (see Figure 13-3C). 3) In active labor, perform combined rhythmic breathing by starting with a cleansing breath, continuing with modified rhythmic chest breathing, but, during the peak of contraction, use shallow chest breathing, and end with a cleansing breath (see Figure 13-3D). 4) Use accelerated/decelerated shallow chest breathing when labor has been prolonged or during difficult labor. It is more complicated and requires more concentration. After a cleansing breath, start with shallow breathing, 1 every 2 seconds; after 15 seconds, increase to the rate of 1 per second, then at 45 seconds decrease to 1 every 2 seconds, alternating with shallow chest breathing (see Figure 13-3E). 5) Use puff-blow for transition. After a cleansing breath, take a series of three shallow breaths (inhale and exhale) and a blow. By counting these breaths, more concentration is required, which helps pass the transition contractions that may last 90 seconds or more. The coach can also have the mother vary the puff-blow techniques to encourage distraction, (*e.g.,* 3 breaths to 1 blow, 2 breaths to 1 blow, 3 breaths to 1 blow again, and 1 breath to 1 blow—see Figure 13-3F). Add abdominal stroking for greater comfort in transition. 6) Use rapid repeated blows when feeling a premature urge to push (not pictured).

Hyperventilation may result from repeated blowing, prolonged exhalations or breathing at a rapid rate. As the $CO_2$ blood level drops, respiratory alkalosis may occur, and vasoconstriction may cause dizziness or tingling around the mouth and fingers. If the alkalosis state is continued, spasms of the wrist and feet may occur. To relieve symptoms, exhaled $CO_2$ can be reinhaled by placing a paper bag over the mouth or cupping hands over the nose and mouth. To avoid recurrence, instruct the woman to slow down and pay more attention to relaxation.

Preparing a couple for pushing involves using relaxation as well as muscle contraction simultaneously. To practice the technique, mothers should first empty their bladders. Women are then instructed to assume a comfortable position. The most common are sitting or semi-reclining, described as follows:

Position:     Sit with feet touching the floor and hands grasping the

|  | thighs, or recline to about 40 degrees from sitting (three to four pillows behind) with knees pulled up, hands under thighs. |
|---|---|
| Breathing: | Take a deep breath in to lower the diaphragm, lean forward, if sitting; if reclined, pull thighs to chest. Relax jaw and perineum. Direct the push low down in front, increasing the pressure in the abdomen as you bear down, letting breath out. Refuel with 1 to 2 slow deep breaths at the end of the contraction. |

Women who have been experiencing many Braxton Hicks contractions or who have had previous miscarriages should practice only the positions and breathing, and not the actual pushing. Some instructors, in fact, do not allow any women in late pregnancy to practice pushing in class or at home for fear of causing premature labor.

Discussion about drug analgesia and anesthesia should be presented in an overview fashion, so that the couple can make informed choices. It should not be the role of the teacher to discuss every type of analgesia or anesthesia available. The mother is given guidelines so that she will know when to ask for medication. If she is unable to cope with contractions at 4 cm of dilation, she may need intervention because of the many hours left until delivery. She may request medication at 8 cm dilation, but with strong support from her doctor, midwife, and coach, she may be able to get through without medications. The idea of a psychoprophylaxis class is to teach the mothers how to better cope with pain through the many techniques she has learned. These techniques should greatly reduce her need for medication,[18] a factor which can only help both mother and infant.

Mothers and their partners should be introduced to the possibility of a Cesarean section, because these surgeries account for one out of every four births. In a class of eight couples, then, two may have a Cesarean section. The reasons Cesarean sections are performed should be the focus of the instruction. A few reasons for Cesarean birth are cephalopelvic disproportion, placenta previa, abruptio placentae, malposition, malpresentation, fetal distress, toxemia, premature rupture of the membranes without labor, and prolapsed cord. Participants should be encouraged to talk about their fears, and realize that having a section is, indeed, having a baby. Medications, incisions, and postpartum care after Cesarean can also be covered in the class. If the mother is to have a general anesthesia, or if the father is not there, a picture taken at the time of delivery may make the transition from pregnancy to parenting easier.[18] A film about Cesarean delivery can be shown to reduce anxiety and fear (see resource section in Appendix).

Many emotional and physical changes occur during postpartum. Initially, even if the mother is exhausted, she may feel an emotional high. Soon after, however, she may be more concerned about her body image and about how she has managed her labor. These feelings may have an effect on her nurturing abilities. She may feel that she did not live up to her own expectations, and as a result, may have less confidence in herself. The dramatic physical and hormonal fluctuations after birth will have an influence on the mother's well-being as well. Her family, partner's love and support, rest, and exercise will help speed her recovery.

Understanding these changes will enable partners to be supportive, even if the mother has days of emotional lability and strong, uncharacteristic dependency needs. Special time should be set aside for partners to spend together, perhaps necessitating child care arrangements. Even a walk around the block together may become a scheduling hassle. New parents need this time to sort out their new roles and priorities and to maintain mutual support for each other. In childbirth preparation classes, these emotional needs can be brought to the attention of the father. He should be encouraged to schedule time with the mother and to share child care responsibilities so mother can feel she has some time alone as well. Group support can be very important to both the new mother and father. A class roster with home phone numbers can be useful to the class. The instructor may also want to make a follow-up call to each family, postdelivery, before the class gets together after everyone has delivered. Extended families and friends can also be solicited to help with household tasks, so mother can rest and attend to child care.

## *Postpartum*

Physical changes of the mother have been detailed in Chapter 9, but it is important in childbirth preparation classes to remind couples that the uterus may be sensitive after delivery and after fundal massage. In the days that follow delivery, the bleeding will be heavy and gradually diminish, but if a mother physically overexerts herself, she may have a period of red flow, and she should slow down. The perineum will also feel sore from stretching, even if an episiotomy was not done. The mother may find some comfort from applying ice packs to the perineum to decrease swelling. Early pelvic floor exercises should help decrease discomfort while urinating. These exercises can be started immediately upon delivery and should be done every hour after that. This will promote an increase in circulation, which will decrease stiffness and edema. Sitz baths may help reduce perineal pain and promote healing. On the third day postpartum, the abdominals should be checked for diastasis recti abdominis. Gentle abdominal exercises, leg slides, pelvic rocking in sitting and on all fours, and diagonal curl-ups may be started.

Advice should also be given regarding the restoration of normal voiding. The bladder and urethra may undergo trauma. As a result, the mother may have some loss in sensitivity to pressure build-up in the bladder. She should be reminded to frequently empty the bladder, especially during the first week postpartum, when there is considerable natural diuresis. There is also a slowing of intestinal peristalsis after delivery. The abdominal muscles are lax, and the mother may be constipated. If she has not had a bowel movement by the third day after delivery, she may need an enema to stimulate peristalsis. Roughage in the diet, plenty of milk, and mild exercise help relieve constipation. If hemorrhoids develop from pushing efforts, sitz baths, pelvic floor exercises, and avoiding constipation may help relieve the discomfort.

Mothers may look to the childbirth educator for advice on when to return to work after delivery. This choice really rests with the couple and depends on how they plan to raise their child, their lifestyle, and their family situation. They should be encouraged to seek their own answers. Some women arrange day, or live-in care, immediately for their newborn so they can return to work quickly, either because of finances or preference. Other families will pick a number of months for mother or father to stay home with the child or will wait and see, deciding as time passes when to return to work. The mother who wants to continue breastfeeding and working, may express and freeze the milk.

In addition to instruction about the breast anatomy and physiology of lactation, prospective parents should be taught what nursing behaviors to expect from the infant. The baby may be sleepy for the first few days, recovering from labor and delivery, and adapting to the new stimuli outside the womb. It may need to be awakened to nurse. Cool water on the baby's forehead may help awaken the baby enough to suck.[19] Initially, the baby should be fed every 2 to 3 hours, or on demand, whichever comes first.[20]

The mother should build up the sucking time gradually in each breast from 5 to 15 minutes. The feedings may stretch out to every 3 to 4 hours after the first few weeks. An experienced mother or nurse can offer assistance for the first-time mother when nursing is started. The nipple and areola should be held between the second and third fingers of one hand with the opposite hand held behind the baby's head to bring it to the nipple. This way, the nipple and areola can be placed well back into the baby's mouth so that it is sucking on the areola. If the baby needs some encouragement, stroking the cheek next to the nipple will elicit the rooting reflex, and the baby will turn to the nipple and suck. The baby will suck quite naturally; the letdown reflex may come slowly at first, but continued suckling will encourage it.

Sometimes the suction with which a baby holds on may be a problem. It will need to be broken so that the baby can be switched to the other side. A finger placed in the corner of the infant's mouth will relieve the suction. The baby needs to be burped before changing sides and at the end of the feeding to expel swallowed air. The next feeding should start on the breast that was finished last. A safety pin attached to the bra, changed from side to side after each feeding will help the mother remember which side to start on.

Sometimes the baby will strongly prefer one breast over the other. This may mean that the baby has an inborn cerebral dominance, expressed as a preference for a certain head position that he was accustomed to *in utero*[19]. By changing from the standard cradling position, the mother can still have the child nurse from the nonpreferred side. Other possible positions are mother and child side lying, or the football hold, in which the baby is held on the forearm alongside the mother rather than across her (see Figure 13-4). The mother should bring the baby up to her and avoid leaning to the baby when feeding, or upper back pain may result. A pillow placed under the child and behind the mother, so that she can maintain a supported position, will decrease back strain.

### Postnatal Exercise Program

Postnatal exercise contraindications and guidelines are the same as with prenatal exercises, except supine lying and abdominal compression (unless post-Cesarean section) are not restricted. Postdelivery mothers will need to be checked for diastasis recti abdominis. To restore maximal overall strength postnatally, exercises should concentrate on pelvic floor toning, abdominal muscles, posture realignment, strengthening of upper back, upper body, and lower extremities to increase strength and circulation.[21] The challenge to the physical therapist is to create an exercise regime that will meet the needs of the mother, avoid contraindications, and be fun to do. Some programs have been developed using the baby as part of the exercise.[21] Designing two programs that can be alternated every other day helps to prevent boredom. Additionally, music and a class format will assist in motivating the mothers. Table 13-13 is a sample of a postnatal program. It is not meant to be inclusive, and physical therapists should use this only as a guideline for developing a pro-

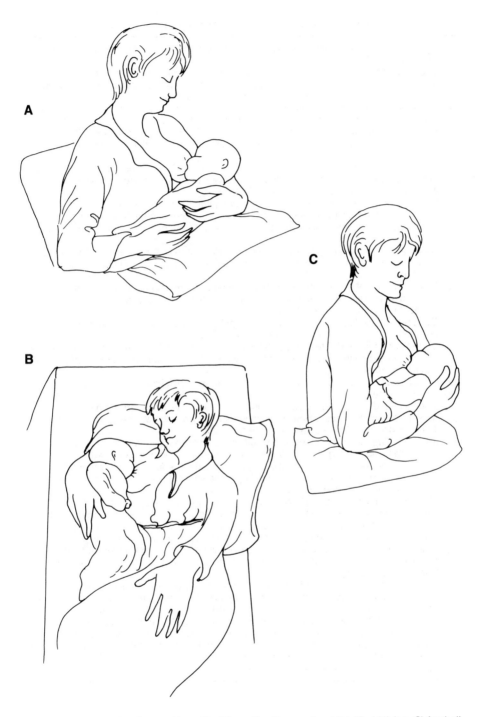

Figure 13-4: Breastfeeding positions A) sitting with pillow under child, B) sidelying, C) football hold.

**Table 13-13. Sample Postnatal Exercise Program**

1. Pelvic floor toning—supine, contract-relax exercises. Hold the contractions for 5 seconds, 10 repetitions.
2. Single straight leg raise—supine, alternate knee bent, raise leg straight up and down, stretching the hamstring in the back of the leg, hold at maximal stretch for 5 seconds, lower with control, switch legs left and right, 10 repetitions each.
3. Pelvic tilt exercise—knees bent, flat on back, hold stomach in, flatten back against the floor simultaneously doing a pelvic floor contraction, 10 repetitions.
4. Knee drop—knees together and bent, flat on back, drop knees side to side, allowing hips to come up, shoulders remain flat, head turns in opposite direction of knees, 10 repetitions.
5. Single knee to chest—on back, knees bent, pelvic tilt, pull knee towards chest, lift head, head returns to flat position, lower leg to knee bent position and alternate with other leg, 10 repetitions each leg in an alternating fashion.
6. Hula—in supine, legs straight, hike hip up straight and down, keeping legs straight, alternate side to side 10 times each side. Use hip muscles. Do not lift up buttock.
7. Gluteal set—in supine position, legs straight, squeeze buttocks and hold 10 seconds, relax, repeat 10 times.
8. Ankle pumps—legs straight, flat on back or sitting, pump ankles up and down together 10 times, then circle both feet together 10 times in one direction, 10 times in the other direction.
9. Leg slides—towel under feet, knees bent, flat on back, maintain a pelvic tilt while sliding legs almost to a fully-extended position and bring them back up to a knee bent position without losing the pelvic tilt, 10 times.
10. Curl-ups—on back, pelvic tilt, arms out straight, knees bent, lift head, chest and shoulders up 45 degrees and down, repeat 20 times. Breathe out as head lifts.
11. Sit-backs—-(avoid if diastasis recti abdominis) in sitting position, knees bent, hands touching knees, lean back at a 45 degree angle and hold 5 seconds, return upright, rest and repeat 10 times.
12. Cat exercise—on hands and knees, drop head down, raise back up, return to neutral, repeat 10 times.
13. Modified buddha—on knees, sit back on heels, lean forward with arms extended and back stretched, drop head. Hold 10 seconds and return to knee sitting position. Repeat 10 times. (Do not raise buttocks above head level.)
14. Knee standing side stretch—on knees, pillow under knees, maintain upright position, bend side to side, trying to touch fingertips to either side. Do not lean forward.
15. Neck stretches—sitting comfortably, stretch neck side to side, holding 5 seconds each way. Also, rotate neck left and right, holding 5 seconds each way, up and down without holding. Repeat the series 5 times.
16. Shoulder series exercises—sitting upright, shrug shoulders up, pull shoulders down, pull shoulders forward, pull shoulders backwards, rotate shoulders forward 5 times, rotate shoulders backward 5 times each, repeat the series 5 times in all.
17. Upper back lifts—prone lying, a) arms out straight overhead, lift head, neck, and chest up and down; b) arms straight out at shoulder level, lift head, neck, chest and arms up and down; c) arms out to sides, elbows bent, lift head, chest, upper back up and down. Repeat series 10 times.
18. Head retraction—sitting, hand on chin, pull chin in and swallow. Repeat 5 times.
19. Posture correction exercise at wall—standing, feet 6 inches from wall, back against wall, bend knees, do a pelvic tilt, shoulders back, arms out at the side, palms up, head back and retracted, drag arms up the wall until there is a stretch in the upper back, hold 5 seconds, stand up slowly, maintaining a pelvic tilt, lower arms, relax and repeat 5 times.
20. Hamstring stretch—long sitting, lean over legs and hold 10 seconds, feel gradual stretch, come up to a long sitting position, repeat 10 times.
21. Pelvic floor exercises—repeat as in Number 1.

gram that best suits the needs of their client and their own teaching style.

## Post-Cesarean Exercise Program

Exercises are the key to successful physical rehabilitation, and breathing exercises should be first on the list. Because general anesthesia is used, the mucus may pool in the lungs. Therefore, the mother should be encouraged to breathe completely, so that the lung is totally ventilated. Additional exercises may be started in the hospital before discharge, focusing on abdominals, pelvic floor, and general conditioning. The following is a sample exercise list for the first week post-Cesarean:

**Day 1**
1. Diaphragmatic breathing—mother splints incision with her hands or a splint pillow whild performing deep breathing.
2. Mid-chest expansion—mother puts hands along the side of the lateral chest wall while directing air into lungs so that ribs expand into her hands.
3. Upper chest expansion—mother places one hand over the sternum, the thumb and fingers are over the clavicle, while she directs the chest expansion into her hand.
4. Huffing—mother splints incision and breathes in through the nose and on exhalation, she repeats a forced "Ahhhh."
5. Pelvic floor exercises.

**Day 2 and 3**
All of the Day 1 exercises should be done plus:
1. Pelvic tilt—side-lying or sitting positions.
2. Leg slides—knees bent lying on back, pull stomach in, flatten back, slide one leg up and down, maintaining pelvic control. Do not extend legs down fully.
3. Hula—lying supine, legs flat; hike hip up and down.

**Day 4 and 5**
If mother is up and about easily, discontinue breathing exercises.
1. Check for diastasis recti abdominis and do corrective exercises, if needed; mother crisscrosses hands across abdomen, approximating the rectus abdominis and lifts head up.
2. Partial lower trunk rotation—on back, knees bent, shoulders flat, knees drop together from side to side, head turns in opposite direction of the knees.

**Day 6**
Do all exercises as previously listed, plus:

1.  Pelvic tilt—on all fours, then gradually add more challenging abdominal exercises, including for the oblique muscles.

The physical therapist can help the post-Cesarean section mother correct her posture. A Polaroid picture of the mother can show her postural problems, and instruction in proper body mechanics can aid her recovery from surgery. The physical therapist may also wish to provide written guidelines for body mechanics to patients:

### Body mechanics guidelines for post-Cesarean patients:

1.  Getting up from a lying down position: Do not sit up straight (jackknife). Go slowly. Roll to the side. Swing legs over the edge. Push with the elbow of the side you were lying on and the other hand.
2.  When sitting, avoid soft chairs. They are hard to get up from and have poor back support. Avoid extremes of rounded or arched back. Use a cushion or roll in the small of the back for support. Sit on a firm straight chair.
3.  Stand with chin in and contract abdominal muscles.
4.  Climb stairs slowly, one at a time, to avoid exhaustion. Propel the body up the stairs, using the thigh and buttock muscles, keeping the weight over the feet.
5.  When bending over, keep a curve in the low back, and one foot in front of the other. Bend the knees and lower the trunk. Legs should take most of the weight, back maintains a vertical position.
6.  To lift, maintain one foot in front of the other, bringing the object close to the body at waist level. Make frequent trips to decrease the weight of heavy loads.
7.  When reaching, use a stool for overhead objects. Do not over-extend when reaching. Put frequently used objects closer to shoulder level.

[Adapted from Frahm J: *Hutzel Hospital Physical Therapy Department Post-Cesarean Section Program.*[22]]

Using these guidelines, the mother is taught to adjust daily activities. Huffing gently will discourage her from holding her breath. Household tasks should be done with the weight evenly distributed over each leg and can incorporate pelvic floor and pelvic tilt exercises. When completing repetitive rotational activities (sweeping, mopping, vacuuming, and raking), she can put one foot in front of the other and lunge forward and back while shifting weight, decreasing the full arc of trunk rotation.

## *Infant Care*

The physical therapist offering full client services may wish to provide a class on basic infant care. The class may include physical and emotional needs of the infant and special care immediately after birth. To describe the physical characteristics of the newborn, audiovisual aids are a must. Many couples have never seen a newborn, and they may have a "Gerber-type" baby in mind. Discussion of the head molding, lanugo, vernix, color of the skin, fontanelles, and enlarged genitals is important. The female infant may have a pink vaginal discharge due to the high hormonal level of the mother. For the same reason, both males and females may have enlarged genitals and breasts with some minor milk secretion. Besides discussing the characteristics of the newborn, the instructor can offer couples the opportunity to diaper, bathe, or dress a newborn doll.

Part of the class should focus on the physical changes and needs of the infant, such as:

1. Umbilical cord care—cord usually falls off in 10 days, if kept dry and clean; alcohol wiping sometime recommended.
2. Diapering—baby needs to be changed frequently after soiling or wetting diapers; first stools are green, tar-like meconium, often present until the third day. As the mother feeds the baby, the movements will change in consistency and color (frequency of movement will differ from baby to baby).
3. Washing—nonirritating soaps should be used for washing the baby's clothes, diapers, and body (baby usually given a sponge bath until the cord falls off).
4. Circumcision—usually, the tip of the penis will be healed within a week after circumcision, although it may be sore for a day or two after the surgery. Parents can learn how to position the baby side lying, using rolled blankets or towels, to help avoid pain caused by pressure on the incision.
5. Suckling— the infant needs to suckle and in spite of nursing, a pacifier may be helpful to satisfy the suckling need and develop the mouth and throat muscles.
6. Stimulation—the infant needs to be held, stroked, talked to, and played with; red, noisy objects are believed to encourage the baby to focus and follow the stimulation.
7. Feeding—usually on demand, but at least every 2 to 3 hours.
8. Sleeping—sleep schedule varies with each baby. It is best to rest when the baby does to conserve energy, especially if the mother is nursing.

Bonding between mother, father, and child takes time. It is important as a childbirth educator to dispel the notion that instant

**Table 13-14. Infant Development**

| Motor Milestones | Gross Motor | Fine Motor |
| --- | --- | --- |
| Birth to 1–2 months | Random, reflexive asymmetrical; prone head raising; prone propping on forearms | Hands fisted, hand to mouth |
| 4–6 months | Symmetrical, good head control; pivots on belly; sitting, independently; rolling supine and prone; on hands and knees | Hands to midline; holds objects placed in hand; prereaching, ulnar reaching and palmar grasp |
| 7–9 months | Trunk rotation; reciprocal crawling, pull to stand | Transfers objects; cup drinking, finger foods, thumb and forefinger grasp |
| 10–12 months | Cruising, walking, lordosis, base of support | Pincer, smooth grasp and release |
| 18 months | Running awkwardly, frequent falls | Uses spoon |

(Adapted from Merril J: University of New England, Pediatric class notes)

parenting happens with delivery of the child. Over time, the family will sort out priorities, and the feeling of being a parent will develop. Physical closeness and caring can encourage the bonding process and should be started as soon as possible. If keeping the baby warm is a concern, a warming light can be placed over the baby, mother, and father immediately after delivery, so the baby and parents will not be separated. Separation during this critical time is discouraged unless medically indicated for the mother or infant. During this bonding period, the infant is encouraged to suckle. (This helps stimulate uterine contractions.) If the mother has not received medication, the infant will be responsive during the first 1 to 2 hours after delivery and may attempt to focus on mother's and father's faces. The baby will then most likely become drowsy and sleep.

Integrating the new baby into the family will involve changes in all relationships, whether it is the first child or the last. Usually, by the end of 6 weeks, the postpartum adjustments have been resolved, and the family has made its adjustments and prioritized family, home, and baby care.[21]

## Infant Development

Parents may express a desire to understand their baby's future motor development, or the physical therapist may want to instruct infant development or infant stimulation classes. In childbirth preparation classes, this topic can be covered through a handout (see Table 13-14) or photographs. Suggested reading lists can also be distributed in any class (see appendix).

## *Self-Assessment Review*

1. Identify two areas of possible concern to prospective parents.
2. What are two types of relaxation and how do they differ?
3. How many calories should be added to a pregnant woman's diet to insure adequate caloric intake, given that she is maintaining a good diet?
4. It is recommended that a pregnant woman gains _____ pounds in the first trimester and _____ pounds per week in the second and third trimester.
5. The center of gravity moves _____ during pregnancy with added weight gain.
6. List six precautions when designing perinatal exercises:
7. Two benefits of early walking and exercise post-Cesarean section are _____ and _____.
8. The two basic types of breathing for labor and delivery are: _____ and _____.
9. Reasons for a partially open glottis during pushing are _____, _____, _____.
10. What exercises should be started first to speed recovery after Cesarean section?
11. How often should a baby be allowed to nurse in the first weeks of life?

## *References*

1. Hassid P: Textbook for Childbirth Educators. Hagerstown, Harper & Row, 1978.

2. Gourley R, Leland P: Early Pregnancy—Promotional Packet, unpublished, 1980.

3. Danforth DN, Scott JR (eds): Obstetrics and Gynecology (1st ed). Philadelphia, JB Lippincott, 1986.

4. BACE: Handbook in Prepared Childbirth. Newtonville, MA, BACE, 1976.

5. Goldbeck N: As You Eat So Your Baby Grows. Woodstock, Ceres Press, 1980.

6. American Council on Alcoholism: Drinking and Pregnancy. Baltimore, MD, American Council on Alcoholism, 1984.

7. U.S. Department of Health, Education & Welfare: Alcohol and Your Unborn Baby. Rockville, MD, No.78-521, 1978.

8. American Cancer Society: Why Start a Life Under a Cloud? Washington, DC, ACS, 1984.

9. Rosett HL, et al: Strategies for prevention of fetal alcohol effects. Obstet Gynecol 57(1):1-7, 1981.

10. Kirkman P, et al: The effect of caffeine on placental and fetal blood flow in human pregnancy. Am J Obstet Gynecol 147(8):939-942, 1983.

11. Noble E: Essential Exercises for the Childbearing Year, (2nd ed). Boston, MA Houghton-Mifflin, 1982.

12. Gourley R: Early Pregnancy Education, class handouts, unpublished, 1981.

13. White R: Fitness in Pregnancy. Seattle, WA, Pennypress, 1984.

14. Perinatal Exercise Guidelines. Alexandria, Virginia. Sect. on Obstet. Gynecol., 1986.

15. O'Connor L: Exercising more ways, enjoying it less. J Obstet Gynecol Phys Ther 13(1):8-9, 1989.

16. Gourley, R: Pregnancy stretches. Dedham, MA, DMA, 1985, rev. 1989.

17. O'Connor L: Proposed guidelines on perinatal exercise for the physical therapist. Bull Sect Obstet Gynecol, APTA 10(1):5-6 1986.

18. Noble E: Rationale for Prenatal and Postpartum Exercise. In Simkin P, Reinke C (eds): Kaleidoscope of Childbearing Preparation, Birth and Nurturing. Seattle, WA, Pennypress, 1978.

19. Brazelton TB: Infants and Mothers. New York, Delta, 1969.

20. Walker M, Driscoll JW: Nursing Mothers Council of BACE: Breastfeeding Your Baby (2nd ed): Wayne, NJ, Avery Publishing, 1981.

21. Fienup-Riordan A: Shape Up with Baby. Seattle, WA, Pennypress, 1980.

22. Frahm J: Post-Cesarean Exercise Program: Detroit, MI, Hutzel Hospital, 1986.

# FOURTEEN

# Getting Started in OB/GYN Physical Therapy

## *Instruction for Physical Therapy Students*

Compared to 10 years ago, the number of physical therapy curricula offering segments in obstetrics and gynecology to students has increased. This increase reflects not only an interest by physical therapists in this field, but also the need among female clients for such a service. Although not documented, many physical therapists became, and still become, interested in this field because of their own or spouse's pregnancies. Prior to the formation of the Section on Obstetrics and Gynecology of the American Physical Therapy Association (APTA), physical therapists interested in this field had no avenues to reach clientele other than through childbirth education, or by referral of a patient who was seen for some disorder and who also happened to be pregnant. Yet, although the field of obstetrics and gynecology is relatively new to the realm of the physical therapist, some physical therapy curricula included this topic at least 15 years ago.

In 1974, Terry Ruby, P.T., now living in Massachusetts, lectured to a class of 40 physical therapy students at the University of California, San Francisco, about the benefits of practice as a childbirth educator. After a brief review of the physical changes of pregnancy, labor, and delivery, Ruby told students how to apply for certification as an instructor in the Lamaze method of childbirth. At that time, childbirth education was the major method of obtaining education in this field and the primary way to obtain access to obstetric clientele. Although that was as much as could be covered in the hour allowed by the curriculum, it was the portal to a new field for several students in that class.

Prior to that time, and since that presentation, therapists who eventually practiced in the field of obstetric and gynecologic physical therapy attempted to pass on this information to other physical therapy students across the nation. However, not every curriculum includes a segment on obstetrics and gynecology.[1] This omission by certain curricula, whether because of insufficient time in the program, or lack of interest or qualified personnel, has caused physical therapists to initiate instruction in this area, either as part of the regular academic staff, or more often as a guest lecturer. In fact, the obstetric physical therapist who is not necessarily a childbirth educator is a relatively new phenomenon.[2] It is no wonder, then, that curricula education in this aspect is not firmly established.

Samples of course content and objectives by two guest lecturers are included below. Each offers a slightly different perspective, and the time allowed for each presentation differs slightly.

## Sample content I:

PHT 412 Clinical Science
OB/GYN Unit General Outline
Ann Dunbar, M.S., P.T., Guest Lecturer

   I.  Introduction: The role of the physical therapist in OB/GYN
  II.  How it all began
      A.  Reproduction; overview of male and female anatomy and physiology
      B.  Conception and implantation
      C.  Very early pregnancy
 III.  Pregnancy
      A.  Anatomy and physiology of pregnancy
          1.  Bodily changes associated with uterine growth
          2.  Changes in bodily systems
      B.  Emotional changes of pregnancy

  C. Physical therapy intervention
   1. Musculoskeletal dysfunction
   2. Exercise
   3. Pelvic floor changes
 IV. Labor and delivery
  A. Theories on initiation of labor
  B. Sources of labor pain
  C. Average labor process
  D. Management of labor pain
   1. Overview of childbirth education
   2. Relaxation
   3. TENS
  E. Complications and variations of labor and delivery Cesarean: postpartum management and rehabilitation
 V. Postpartum
  A. Anatomy and physiology
  B. Psychologic changes
  C. Physical therapy intervention
   1. Exercise
   2. Diastasis recti abdominis
   3. Pelvic floor restoration
   4. Posture and body mechanics
 VI. Women's health care issues: The physical therapist's role
 VII. The physical therapist's role in talking with bereaved parents

OB/GYN Unit Objectives
At the completion of the unit, the student will be able to:
1. Given a list of 10 events leading up to conception and implantation, arrange the items in correct sequence.
2. Define amniotic membrane and placenta including the general location and function of each.
3. List five physiologic changes occurring during pregnancy and a common complaint associated with each.
4. Given a list of 10 physical and emotional characteristics of pregnancy, identify the trimester(s) in which each characteristic occurs.
5. Demonstrate the three principles of body mechanics discussed in class in the following situations: sit to supine and return, lifting, and sitting. Demonstrate a position of good posture and state the rationale for its use.
6. Discuss according to class lecture the possible sources of back pain during pregnancy.
7. Design a small group prenatal exercise program stating the rationale and goal for each exercise.

8. State the rationale for Kegel's exercise.
9. Discuss two sources of labor pain by stating, (a) segmental innervation of the involved tissues, and (b) phase/stage of labor in which each source is more likely to occur.
10. Outline the use of TENS during labor. Discuss the neurophysiologic rationale for its use.
11. State the three stages of labor and the three phases of stage I. Describe each phase and stage including three characteristics of each phase and stage listed.
12. Plan, in outline form, a program for post-Cesarean pain management including TENS and exercise. State the goal and rationale for each exercise.
13. Name two different relaxation techniques used for labor pain management. Discuss the educational process of client instruction for one labor pain management technique, including content, client rehearsal, and terminal behavior.
14. Define the postpartum period as described in class.
15. Given a patient problem, state at least three postpartum changes pertinent to consider in a physical therapy program. State the rational for each choice.
16. Design a small group postpartum exercise program including goals and rationale for each exercise.
17. Demonstrate the assessment technique for diastasis recti abdominis. Describe the physical therapy intervention to assist restoration.
18. List three considerations for communication when working with bereaved parents.

OB/GYN Unit Lab Sessions
1. Relaxation: Jacobsen's method and use of imagery
2. Video of labor and delivery
3. Posture and body mechanics for pregnancy and postpartum, Kegel's exercises, diastasis recti abdominis restoration

OB/GYN Unit Class Assignment
Develop a Class or Home Program
Exercise is applicable for a wide variety of women's health care problems. For this assignment, choose a situation from below (or one of your own with consent of the instructor) and develop an appropriate exercise program. State a general overview of the problem identifying the implications for exercise (*e.g.,* need to increase circulation). List your exercise/patient education program as if written for a patient. Include starting position, action or movement, and purpose for each exercise. Summarize instruction in posture and body mechanics. Include references you use.

Pregnancy: prenatal
Pregnancy: postpartum
Post-Cesarean
Osteoporosis
Low back pain in pregnancy
Urinary incontinence
Dysmenorrhea Exercise for the older woman

## Sample content II:
Teaching OB/GYN Involvement to Physical Therapy Students
Linda M. Pipp, P.T.

I. Historical Perspectives
   A. Other countries
   B. United States
   C. Preventive medicine
   D. Special interest group/physical therapy association
II. Resources
   A. Organizations
   B. Journals
   C. Articles
   D. Books
   E. Meetings
III. Therapeutic exercise vs. active aerobics
   A. Distinction
   B. Combination
IV. Unique variety of disciplines
V. Changes of pregnancy
VI. Core curriculum
   A. Posture
   B. Body mechanics
   C. Circulation
   D. Pelvic floor
   E. Relaxation/comfort
VII. Rationale for prenatal exercises
VIII. Teaching directives
IX. Exercise choices
X. Rational for postnatal exercises
XI. Postnatal program
XII. Postnatal: Cesarean childbirth
XIII. Role of the physical therapist in labor/delivery and instructing in alternate methods of pushing
XIV. TENS
XV. Clinical contact with pregnant women outside of classes
XVI. Diagnostic ultrasound

XVII.   Obstetric terminology, tests, etc.
XVIII.  Role of exercise/activity/sports and effects on baby
  XIX.  Physical therapy in gynecologic problems
        A.  Pelvic floor
        B.  Neuropathies
   XX.  Obstetric controversies in practice

Portions of the above outlines are appropriate for instructing other disciplines about physical therapy services. For instance, obstetricians and obstetric nursing staffs may be interested in physical therapy for patients in need of prenatal, postpartum, or post-Cesarean exercise; for patients who appear to have musculoskeletal pain; for patients with urinary muscular problems; and for obstetric patients using TENS for labor, delivery, or postpartum. They may also be interested in resources and comfort techniques for pregnant clients. In addition, recent interest by physical therapists in high-risk pregnancy has resulted in the development of several hospital-based programs that may be of interest to nurses and obstetricians.

Childbirth educators would probably be interested in TENS for labor and delivery, as well as any pain management techniques that would be available to clients during pregnancy or postpartum, particularly musculoskeletal pain during the last trimester. Childbirth educators also receive questions about prenatal and postpartum exercise that could be referred to a physical therapist with an obstetric background.

## Research Needs

Although the physical therapist has much to offer other health team members, as well as the pregnant woman herself, there is little in the literature to provide supportive documentation of physical therapy techniques for inquiring obstetricians, family practitioners, or other referral sources. Therefore, the need for research in all areas of obstetric and gynecologic physical therapy is critical. In the last few years, physical therapists have become more interested in performing research in this field. Studies have been published in *Physical Therapy*, journal of the American Physical Therapy Association, and in the *Journal of Obstetric and Gynecologic Physical Therapy*, journal of the Section on Obstetrics and Gynecology, APTA. There have been literature reviews and critiques of obstetric material published by physical therapists and non-physical therapists in other physical therapy, childbirth and lay publications. Yet, to date, actual research studies have been limited to studies of TENS use in labor and delivery, and other attempts to apply standard physical therapy modalities to the pregnant patient. These studies, though, help provide entry for physical therapists who need such traditionally-based methods to convince physical therapy directors or hospital administrative personnel that such a service is needed.

Research is needed in every aspect of obstetric and gynecologic physical therapy, and not only in treatment methods, but also in evaluation and incidence of specific disorders. For instance, the number of studies of incidence of low back pain in pregnancy can probably be counted on the fingers of one hand. Likewise for studies of incidence of diastasis recti abdominis, pelvic floor dysfunction, and postural abnormalities during pregnancy. In fact, research is so scant that there is little to support the notion that the lordosis of pregnancy is a normal anatomic and transient change in posture. Physical therapists have yet to learn what amount of lordosis is normal in pregnancy and, indeed, if any residual lordosis is normal for the parous woman. This lack of evidence tends to leave the physical therapist who desires to start a physical therapy program for obstetric or gynecologic clients with only anecdotal support.

Listed below are only a few of the research questions asked by practitioners who have worked with this population and with OB/ GYN health care team members.

1. What is normal posture for the pregnant woman and for women of all ages?
2. Does the lordosis associated with pregnancy contribute to low back pain?
3. What is the incidence and cause of peripheral joint pain, spinal pain, myofascial pain, or neurologic pain in pregnant women? In the general female population at different ages?
4. How do various pain relief methods relate for women in labor?
5. Are relaxation and conservative nonintervention methods for pain management effective for late labor?
6. Left untreated, how often will diastasis recti abdominis cause clinical symptoms that require treatment?
7. Are corrective measures for diastasis recti abdominis effective?
8. Are preexisting musculoskeletal conditions exacerbated by pregnancy?
9. What is the earliest time during pregnancy that related musculoskeletal changes can cause actual disability and loss of work?
10. Are pelvic floor exercises effective for stress incontinence and for mild prolapse/cystocele/rectocele?

## *Marketing Physical Therapy Services*

With the advent of direct access by the consumer to physical therapists in many states, the physical therapist, in private practice and
even in some hospital settings, has had to rely less on physician
referrals and more on creating a market for services. Perhaps that
accounts for the success of certain physical therapy practices in
some areas and not in others. For instance, orthopedic practice has
always had its niche in the rehabilitation of industrially-injured patients. As the cost of rehabilitative services increased, more efficient
methods of rehabilitation were developed to attract clients, for instance, the back school was initiated. Today, back schools are big
business, and orthopedic specialty clinics are the major source of
income for many private practitioners.

The field of obstetric and gynecologic physical therapy has yet to
establish such a lucrative niche. Although this specialty has been
formally organized since 1977, as a freestanding, money-making
proposition, it has a long way to go before it will be fully accepted by
physicians, allied health workers, and pragmatically, by insurance
companies.

Some progress has been made through a variety of marketing
techniques. In the 1970s, the primary marketing techniques were to
offer childbirth education classes, early pregnancy workshops, and
infant care or infant stimulation sessions. Teaching such classes allowed access to pregnant women and women with problems from
previous pregnancies that could be helped with physical therapy.
These classes were often taught through hospitals, clinics, for specific physicians, or privately. Many physical therapists, however,
found that teaching childbirth education did not allow time to properly treat women with problems, nor was there an opportunity to
evaluate or receive financial compensation according to physical
therapy protocol.

In the late 1970s and early 1980s, the interest of the general
population in exercise boosted a similar interest in the pregnant
population. These women sought classes primarily for conditioning,
but physical therapists struggled to retain their professional role
among minimally trained exercise instructors offering classes
through health clubs, adult schools, and city recreation departments.
True, a physical therapist could often win the role of exercise instructor, but again, opportunity for thorough evaluation and treatment, plus professional reimbursement by insurance carriers, was
lacking. More recently, physical therapists have branched into private practice.

Diane Gent, P.T. in Ohio, developed a role for a consultant physical therapist in Cesarean rehabilitation in a major hospital. Elizabeth Noble, P.T., started a private center for childbearing women and their offspring that offers a variety of exercise and educational classes, as well as the option of individual evaluation and treatment. Others have attempted to develop services for obstetric and gynecologic inpatients, such as programs for high-risk patients on bed rest, pain relief for gynecologic cancer patients, and pelvic floor exercise for patients with stress urinary incontinence. Another fairly successful way to convince hospital administration of the value of physical therapy for these clients is by developing TENS programs, either for post-Cesarean procedures or during labor. Unfortunately, since the TENS device is not specifically approved by the FDA for use during pregnancy, legalistic security is not assured in this situation, nor is financial reimbursement.

A small number of physical therapists have attempted to reach obstetric and gynecologic clients by directly working with obstetricians and gynecologic urologists. Jane Frahm, P.T., of Michigan, has received referrals from a gynecologic urologist for treatment of pelvic floor weakness. Debbie Weinstein, P.T., of California, treated patients on referral for an obstetrician until the obstetrician decided he could not assume the liability in his office. There are many other physical therapists who have had some success in this field, but it is still young and growing. It will take many more determined physical therapists to guarantee the role of our profession in this specialty area.

To assist beginning practitioners, examples of promotional material successfully used to initiate a private practice in obstetric and gynecologic physical therapy are included below. It is hoped that, by sharing examples of marketing tools, others may develop their own literature and practices; and in so doing, promote the growth of this field.

**For marketing to physicians or health care providers:**

Linda J. O'Connor, R.P.T.

Registered Physical Therapist

*Physical therapy services for your obstetric and gynecologic patients with complaints of:*

| | |
|---|---|
| *Lower or upper back sprain/strain (acute or chronic)* | Therapeutic exercise to correct posture; training in safe ways to perform activities of daily living; positioning in sitting, lying, standing, walking, lifting, working; application of local superficial heat, massage, orthoses; TENS for GYN patients; screening for disability referral |
| *Joint dysfunctions or aggravation of previous orthopedic problems (pelvic, wrist, shoulder, elbow, hip, knee, ankle, neck, spine, sacroiliac, symphysis pubis; sprains, strains, tendinitis, bursitis)* | Therapeutic exercise to correct dysfunction; training in activities of daily living; gait; positioning for comfort; range of motion; manual muscle testing; heat/cold; massage; orthoses; TENS for GYN; screening for orthopedic referral |
| *Nerve compressions/neuropathy (carpal tunnel, sciatica, paresis, paresthesiae)* | Neuromuscular reeducation; relaxation; orthoses; TENS for GYN; positioning; functional activities; range of motion; manual muscle testing; exercise; screening for neurologic referral |
| *Muscle weakness (abdominal, pelvic floor causing stress incontinence or mild prolapse, general weakness secondary to bed rest for cervical incompetence or premature labor contractions, diastasis recti abdominis)* | Therapeutic exercise to strengthen and promote circulation; manual muscle testing; home visits for gentle exercise and avoidance of Valsalva during movement for bed rest patients |
| *Discomforts of pregnancy and reduced mobility (assorted areas of pain or weakness)* | Relief measures for discomforts; therapeutic exercise; individualized home programs; circulation exercises |
| *Pain post-Cesarean or post operative; dysmenorrhea* | TENS; positioning; therapeutic exercise; activities of daily living; breathing and coughing |

## Abbreviated list for health care workers or hospital/clinic administrations:

Linda J. O'Connor, R.P.T.

Registered Physical Therapist

### Physical Therapy Services for Obstetric and Gynecologic Patients

Evaluation of muscle strength and range of motion

Therapeutic exercise for musculoskeletal and minor neurologic dysfunction

Fitting of orthoses for relief of muscular strain, neuropathies, and varicosities

Gait training with assistive devices for severe pain on ambulation

Preventative instruction for back care and comfort

Posture evaluation and treatment

Assessment and treatment of pelvic floor weakness

Individualized exercise programs for premenstrual syndrome, dysmenorrhea, or osteoporosis

Post-hysterectomy exercise programs to regain muscle strength in pelvic floor or abdominal muscles

Individualized prenatal and postnatal exercise

Application of heat, massage, ice, TENS for pain relief

TENS for chronic gynecologic pain, including dysmenorrhea

Breathing control for patients with cervical incompetence during transfers and activities of daily living

Post-Cesarean TENS and pain relief measures

Post-Cesarean exercise

Relaxation training or breathing control for individual women preparing for labor and delivery

© L. O'Connor, 1988

## For obstetric patients:

Linda J. O'Connor, R.P.T.

Registered Physical Therapist

Some of those aches and pains you have during and after pregnancy may be helped with physical therapy.

*Low or upper back ache:* hot packs; massage; exercises to correct posture; instruction in proper lifting, carrying, and pushing/pulling/reaching techniques; relaxation; and comfortable positioning for bed or work

*Aching muscles, joints, or aggravation of previous orthopedic problems:* evaluation of problem and exercise as appropriate for pelvic joints, wrists, neck, hips, knees, ankles, shoulders, elbows, pelvic floor

*Tingling or falling asleep of arms or legs:* sometimes related to normal swelling of pregnancy and often relieved through positioning and circulation exercises or joint supports

*Muscle weakness and discomforts of pregnancy:* individualized prenatal/postnatal/post-Cesarean home exercise programs to strengthen and promote circulation, breathing and coughing exercises, pelvic floor exercises

*Pain after Cesarean section or after surgery:* instruction in how to change positions with minimal pain and without straining muscles, relief from gas distension, posture exercises, strengthening stomach muscles, TENS for pain relief

*Evaluation and treatment by: Linda O'Connor, R.P.T., A.C.C.E., physical therapist, certified childbirth educator, instructor in childbirth education and obstetrical exercise, member Section on Obstetrics and Gynecology of the American Physical Therapy Association*

*Private insurance billed as a courtesy*

Ask your doctor for a referral to physical therapy

© L. O'Connor, 1987

---

Brochures with drawings and eye-catching graphics are also helpful in marketing to health care workers and patients alike. Although direct access now exists in many states, the promotional material directed at obstetric clients urges patients to ask their doctor for a referral to physical therapy. It is the opinion of the authors that the backing of a physician when treating this patient population is wise. That does not mean, however, that certain problems cannot be treated within the direct access arena; particularly patients referred by midwives or by other patients. The question of employee versus contractor status has come up in obstetric private practice performed in the obstetrician's office. On the basis of having attempted both methods, my recommendation is to remain on contractor status. This conclusion has been drawn because the volume of referrals from an obstetrician or even a group of obstetricians is limited. To make a private practice in this field pay, the practitioner will probably need referrals from several sources. Some physical therapists have contracted with women's hospitals or the obstetric units of major general treatment hospitals. Physical therapists can also offer special aches and pains clinics, back classes for pregnant women, and home programs for patients on bed rest, in addition to early pregnancy or labor preparation classes.

## Certification and Specialization

Another way to market physical therapy services is by teaching classes: childbirth education; early pregnancy education; refresher for labor and delivery; vaginal birth after Cesarean; preparation for Cesarean; or exercise for prenatal, postnatal, post-Cesarean, or postgynecologic surgery. These have been addressed in the previous chapter. Teaching classes such as these can bring you in contact with pregnant women and provide an atmosphere for relaxed questions and answers. Many physical therapy referrals can be drawn from such sessions. In some areas, however, being a physical therapist is not enough to receive referrals from other childbirth educators. There are a few major childbirth education organizations that offer certification as a childbirth educator. This certification is vital to obtain in some cities, because childbirth educators often approach obstetricians via an organization representative to provide a list of qualified teachers. Sometimes, being on that list can mean many referrals as opposed to few, if any.

The three major childbirth organizations in the United States are the American Society for Psychoprophylaxis in Obstetrics (ASPO/ Lamaze), the International Childbirth Education Association (ICEA), and the Academy of Husband-Coached Childbirth (Bradley Method—AAHCC). These certification courses typically involve either home study or a combination of home study and workshops, plus student teaching, observations of labors and deliveries, and perhaps individual design of an entire 6- or 7-week class on preparation for labor and delivery, complete with objectives and teaching materials needed. The entire certification process may take 2 years or more. In addition, the Read Natural Childbirth Method and other local organizations may offer certification courses as well, but these would be specific to an area. Although the training a childbirth educator receives from these organizations is usually valuable, it may not be necessary for the physical therapist wishing to teach the same methods. The physical therapist is trained in the instruction of relaxation methods and the basic understanding of pain mechanisms and relief. It takes only some additional research and reading to understand the techniques used in almost any method of childbirth training. Reading a book, however, cannot substitute for the actual observations of labor and delivery, the assistance provided by a mentor teacher, and the contacts made by attending such courses.

Childbirth educators are responsible for the acceptance of alternative birthing in this country. Prior to the Lamaze movement of the early 1960s, but even in some places today, women had their babies in positions of convenience for obstetricians or other birth attendants (*i.e.*, flat on their backs and medicated for pain control). Thanks to childbirth educators, these other methods have provided women with a variety of options in birthing, including their own selection of position, form of pain relief, and setting in which to deliver. These actions speak for the subtle but forceful impact of these organizations. Their potential as referral sources should not be overlooked.

There are also certification courses in perineometry. This type of course gives the physical therapist a certificate, but the actual instruction may be redundant for the physical therapist who has researched pelvic floor anatomy and function.

Along the same line as certification as a childbirth educator, the Section on Obstetrics and Gynecology, APTA is in the process of developing a specialization in its field according to the guidelines established for other clinical specialties. The process to develop the certification for this clinical specialty is long and convoluted, but it seems destined to occur. Whether certification will help promote the field or encourage referrals is unknown.

## *Internships*

Where then, can physical therapists who do not want to go through the childbirth education certification course and do not want to wait for the clinical specialty process to be completed, gain some practical experience in this field before striking out on their own? Why not an internship?

Physical therapy interns have had successful experiences in this field. And the internship can take many forms— prenatal/postnatal exercise instructor, assisting a private practitioner, designing and implementing an obstetric program for an established clinic or hospital department, or submitting an article to the obstetric literature. Obstetric and gynecologic physical therapy usually takes a lot of conversation: presenting ideas to nursing staff, resident obstetricians, and even anesthesiologists if TENS is part of the proposal. All a student needs to do is to find a practitioner in this field; the best route for that is either through the APTA or through one of the childbirth education associations. One physical therapy intern developed her own internship and combined writing with practice:

### Practicum in obstetric and gynecologic physical therapy
Kate Layne, P.T.; Linda O'Connor, P.T.; Luray Eshelman, P.T.

In the first 2 weeks of the practicum, the student will assist in the preparation of an issue of the *Journal of Obstetric & Gynecologic Physical Therapy*. Assignments include writing an interview article and a review article; learning basic editing techniques and editing submissions from other writers; and understanding how the publication is produced, published, and mailed.

In the second 2 weeks of the practicum, the student will observe and assist in the instruction of obstetric clients in exercise and childbirth preparation techniques. Assignments include developing a slide set on instruction in body mechanics during pregnancy.

Many other possibilities exist for physical therapy students desiring an internship in this field. At this point in the development of the field, however, the specific criteria for this internship are left to the imagination of the student, academic faculty, and clinical faculty.

## *Working within the OB/GYN Team*

As intimated throughout this chapter, developing a successful practice in obstetric and gynecologic physical therapy requires patience, commitment, enthusiasm, and a belief that other members of the OB/GYN health care team are vital to an enjoyable obstetric experience for the patient. Often it is the physical therapist who must play the role of go-between for physicians and nursing staff. In this situation, the physical therapist on staff at that particular facility stands a better chance of selling services than an outside consultant.

The other critical factor is funding for outside services. Many staff physical therapists who attempt to implement obstetric programs become frustrated when work loads increase and obstetric services are pushed to the back burner. Yet the physical therapist who firmly convinces obstetric nurses and obstetricians that these services are indeed desperately needed by some patients will have a better chance of continuing to adequately evaluate and treat expectant women. In other words, the obstetrician or obstetric nurse that suddenly is assured that some of the complaints of their patients can be alleviated, will be a strong supporter for the physical therapist with both department heads and administration.

Outside of the hospital or clinic situation, one of the best advocates for physical therapy services is the private office nurse or nurse-practitioner who also sees the patients. And, even when physical therapy services are available, it usually takes constant appearances and contact with office personnel to remind them that a physical therapist has a lot to offer the female patient.

## *Self-Assessment Review*

1. Physical therapists often become interested in the field of obstetrics and gynecology as a result of their own _____.

2. The obstetric and gynecologic segment of a physical therapy curriculum could include the following topics: (list three) _____, _____, _____.

3. Instruction to other health care workers about services available from physical therapy for pregnant clients could include what topics? (name three) _____, _____, _____.

4. Describe two ways to market physical therapy services for pregnant clients to obstetricians: _____, _____.

5. Describe two ways to market physical therapy services to pregnant clients: _____, _____.

6. At the present time, the three major childbirth education organizations in the United States are _____, and _____.

7. In the future, physical therapists may have the opportunity to be certified by _____.

8. Obtaining an internship in this field depends primarily on _____ and _____.

9. Since physical therapy services for obstetric clients is a relatively new concept, practitioners may become frustrated when _____.

10. One reason physical therapists need to work closely with other obstetric caregivers is _____.

## *References*

1. Hulme JB, Nieman K, Miller K: Obstetrics in the physical therapy curriculum. Phys Ther 65(1):51-53, 1985.
2. Wallis K, Curtis PR, Kondela-Cebulski P: The physical therapist in obstetrics practice: Results of an initial survey of section members. Bull Sect Obstet Gynecol, APTA 11(1):5-8, 1987.

# Conclusion

While many parts of this book have been designed for use as a clinical reference and self-study guide, others are limited in scope to meet the needs of the clinician and student just starting in obstetrics and gynecology. For the continuing student of obstetrics and gynecology, additional questions will eventually come to mind that were not answered in this introductory text. And, as the field of obstetric and gynecologic physical therapy expands, the practitioner will need to know more about the nuances of obstetric patient care. These answers lie within past, present, and future literature directed at obstetric and gynecologic physician specialists. In addition, other unpublished and invaluable information will be gleaned from interactions with the various members of the female patient's health care team.

It is conceivable that as time passes, the OB/GYN physical therapist will become recognized as a specialist in female patient care. Only the professional who is able to interweave all the factors contributing to the current condition of a female patient may effectively and efficiently evaluate and treat that patient. Knowledge of symptomatology related to reproductive dysfunction or the biomechanical results of bearing children can provide answers where there seem to be none. No specialist in another field of physical therapy can boast an awareness of the interactions of every bodily system, from menarche through menopause, when examining a patient, when communicating with physicians, and when servicing the patient as part of the family unit.

With the vast impact of reproductive events on lifestyle, family dynamics, and psychologic well-being, it is no wonder that OB/GYN caregivers are part of a health care team that depends heavily on each and every member. There is no foreseeable reason that the physical therapist cannot play an indispensable role in educating other team members and the patient about maintaining or attaining a state of fitness, comfort, and health prior to, during, and after pregnancy. Because this role is not yet firmly established in the minds of the medical community and the public, in many parts of the country, it is an exciting time for the physical therapist to unveil various aspects of treatment available for these clients. The only limitations are the imagination of OB/GYN practitioners and the strength of belief in the part they play in providing total patient care.

# APPENDIX A:

# Suggested Reading by Topic

## Breastfeeding

Eiger M, Olds, SW: The Complete Book of Breastfeeding. New York, Workman Press, 1972.

La Leche League International, The Womanly Art of Breastfeeding, Franklin, Illinois, La Leche League, 1963.

Walker M, Driscoll JW: Breastfeeding Your Baby (2nd ed). Wayne, New Jersey, Avery Publishing, 1981.

## Musculoskeletal

Cyriax J, Cyriax P: Illustrated Manual of Orthopaedic Medicine. London, Butterworth's, 1983.

Hoppenfeld S: Physical Examination of the Spine and Extremities. New York, Appleton-Century-Crofts, 1976.

Saunders HD: Evaluation, Treatment and Prevention of Musculoskeletal Disorders. Minneapolis, Viking Press, 1985.

Kendall FP, McCreary EK: Muscle Testing and Function (3rd ed). Baltimore, Williams & Wilkins, 1983.

## *High-Risk Pregnancy*

Cherry SH, Berkowitz RL, Case NG (eds): Rovinsky and Guttmacher's Medical, Surgical and Gynecologic Complications of Pregnancy (3rd ed). Baltimore, Williams & Wilkins, 1985.

Queenan, JT (ed): Management of High-Risk Pregnancy (2nd ed). Oradell, New Jersey, Medical Economics Books, 1985.

## *Exercise*

Simkin P, Whalley J, Keppler A: Pregnancy, Childbirth and the Newborn. New York, Meadowbrook, 1984.

Noble E: Essential Exercises for the Childbearing Year (2nd ed). Boston, Houghton-Mifflin, 1982.

Artal R, Wiswell RA (eds): Exercise in Pregnancy. Baltimore, Williams & Wilkins, 1986.

Section on Obstetrics and Gynecology, APTA: Perinatal Exercise Guidelines. Alexandria, Section on Obstetrics and Gynecology of the APTA, 1986.

Section on Obstetrics and Gynecology, APTA: Post-hysterectomy Exercise Program. Alexandria, Section on Obstetrics and Gynecology of the APTA, 1988.

Heardman H: Physiotherapy and Obstetrics in Gynecology. Edinborough, E & S Livingstone, 1951 (out of print).

Bing E: Moving Through Pregnancy. New York, Bantam Books, 1977.

Fitzhugh ML: Preparation for Childbirth. San Rafael, Margaret B Farley, RPT, 1974.

## *Obstetrics and Gynecology*

Danforth DN, Scott JR (eds): Obstetrics and Gynecology (5th ed). Philadelphia, JB Lippincott, 1986.

Rayburn WF, Lavin JP: Obstetrics for the House Officer. Baltimore, Williams & Wilkins 1984.

Niswander KR (ed): Manual of Obstetrics (3rd ed). Boston, Little, Brown & Co, 1987.

## *Labor and Delivery*

Oxorn H, Foote WR: Human Labor and Birth (4th ed). New York, Appleton-Century-Crofts, 1980.

Noble E: Childbirth with Insight. Boston, Houghton-Mifflin, 1983.

### Infant Development and Parenting

Brazelton TB: Infants and Mothers. New York, Dell Publishers, 1969.

Caplan F: The First Twelve Months of Life. New York, Grosset & Dunlap, 1971.

Brazelton TB: Toddlers and Parents. New York, Dell Publishers, 1974.

Gordon T: Parent Effectiveness Training. New York, Peter Wyden, 1970.

### Nutrition

Brewer GS, Brewer T: What Every Pregnant Woman Should Know: The Truth About Diet and Drugs in Pregnancy. Baltimore, Penguin, 1979.

Goldbeck N: As You Eat, So Your Baby Grows. Woodstock, Ceres Press, 1980.

### Childbirth

Kitzinger S: Giving Birth: The Parents Experience of Childbirth. New York, Traplinger, 1971.

### OB/GYN Books by Physical Therapists

Ebner M: Physiotherapy and Obstetrics (3rd ed). London, Livingstone Publishers, 1967 (out of print).

Wilder E (ed): Clinics in Physical Therapy, Vol 20, Obstetric and Gynecologic Physical Therapy. New York, Churchill-Livingstone Publishers, 1988.

Noble E: Essential Exercises for the Childbearing Year: A Guide to Health Before and After Your Baby is Born (2nd ed). Boston, Houghton-Mifflin, 1987.

Noble E: Having Twins-A Guide to Pregnancy, Birth and Early Childhood: Boston, Houghton-Mifflin, 1980.

Noble E: Childbirth With Insight. Boston, Houghton-Mifflin, 1983.

### Other

Gaskin IM: Spiritual Midwifery. Summertown, The Book Publishing Co., 1978.

Ashford JI: The Whole Birth Catalog - A Sourcebook for Choices in Childbirth. Trumansburg, Crossing Press, 1983 (out of print).

---

# Product Information and Resources

## *Maternity Supports and Orthoses*

### Carpal tunnel support
Freedom Long Elastic Wrist Support
AliMed
297 High Street
Dedham, Massachusetts 02026
$17.50
Wrist circumference determines patient's size; custom-made splints for wrists that are difficult to size.

### Mid-back support
Educational Opportunities
9840 Purgatory Road
Eden Prairie, Minnesota 55344
(612) 944-1656

**Low back supports**

1. Baby Hugger
   Trennaventions
   909 4th Avenue, Suite 610
   Seattle, Washington 98104
   $55 wholesale, $70 suggested retail
   Supports low-back, mid-back, and vulvar varicosities by a panty and strap arrangement to lift up the gravid uterus; designed by a physical therapist.

2. Warm 'n Form
   Jerome Medical
   102 Gaither Drive
   Mt. Laurel, New Jersey 08054
   (800) 257-8440
   $46
   Provides back supports that can be used in pregnancy with a custom-molded insert.

3. Mother-to-Be Back and Abdominal Support
   CMO, Inc.
   PO Box 147
   Barberton, Ohio 44203
   (800) 344-0011; in Ohio, (800) 452-0001
   $50 plus shipping
   Abdominal sling with moldable back insert; order by patient's dress size; S(3-9), M(12-14), L(16-18), XL(18 + )

4. Contour-Form Maternity Support
   Contour Form Products
   12 N. Diamond Street
   PO Box 328
   Greenville, Pennsylvania 16125
   $90

5. Life Lines Medical, Inc.
   4 Franklin Street
   Milton, Massachusetts 02186
   (800) 654-6001 Dale Active Lumbosacral Support Phase IV with insert $40; without insert $23

6. Universal Abdominal Binder
   E.M. Adams, Co., Inc.
   121 West Street
   Medfield, Massachusetts 02052
   (800) 225-4788
   $12

7. Glori-Us
   Mary Jane Company
   5510 Cleon Avenue
   North Hollywood, California 91609
   $26
   Abdominal sling with mild support for back pain, vulvar varicosities, round ligaments, or hypermobile pubic symphysis.

## Sacroiliac support
Maternity Lumbopelvic/Sacroiliac Support
IEM Orthopedics
PO Box 592
Ravenna, Ohio 44266
(800) 992-6594
$55
Leather sacral pad and two velcro side straps, available for pregnant and nonpregnant clients; designed by a physical therapist.

## Perineometers
1. Perineometer and vaginal stimulators
   Interactive Medical Technologies
   2646 Palma Drive, Suite 290
   Ventura, California 93003
   (805) 650-6235
   Gynex(TM) perineometer (Kegel prototype), and Restore(TM) vaginal stimulator.

2. Perineal EMG Biofeedback
   Perineometer Research Institute
   242 Old Eagle School Road
   Stratford, Pennsylvania 19087
   (215) 525-8778

## Maternity pillows, wedges
1. Maternity Support Pillow
   Lossing Orthopedic
   777 Harding Street NE
   PO Box 18298
   Minneapolis, Minnesota 55418
   (800) 328-5216
   $39.99 retail, professional price $25

2. Body Therapeutics
   182 South Alvarado Street
   Los Angeles, California 90057
   (213) 413-8007

**Venous supports**

1. Medi
   76 West Seegers Road
   Arlington Heights, Illinois 60005
   (800) 633-6334
   Stockings measured by a Medi dealer or physical therapist; available in beige, black, off-white and gray.

2. USA Sigvaris and Company
   PO Box 570
   32 Park Drive East
   Branford, Connecticut 06405
   Available in four thicknesses; calf, half-thigh length, thigh-length, and maternity stocking.

3. Gottfried Medical
   PO Box 8996
   Toledo, Ohio 43623
   (800) 537-1968

4. Jobst
   PO Box 653
   Toledo, Ohio 43694
   (800) 537-1063

## *Publications for Childbirth Educators*

1. American Baby Magazine
   249 West 17th Street
   New York, New York 10011

2. American Journal of Obstetrics and Gynecology
   CV Mosby Company
   1830 West Line Drive
   St. Louis, Missouri 63146

3. Birth: Issues in Perinatal Care and Education
   Blackwell Scientific Publications, Inc.
   52 Beacon Street
   Boston, Massachusetts 02108

4. Journal of Obstetric and Gynecologic Physical Therapy Section on Obstetrics and Gynecology of the American Physical Therapy Association
   PO Box 327
   Alexandria, Virginia 22313

5. Childbirth Educator
   249 West 17th Street
   New York, New York 10011

6. Lamaze Parents Magazine
   1840 Wilson Boulevard, Suite 204
   Arlington, Virginia 22201

7. Obstetrics and Gynecology
   Elsevier Science Publishing Company, Inc.
   52 Vanderbilt Avenue
   New York, New York 10017

## *Maternal-Child Health Organizations*

1. American Academy of Husband Coach Childbirth (AAHCC)
   The Bradley Method
   PO Box 5224
   Sherman Oaks, California 91413
   (800) 423-2397 outside CA, or (818) 788-6662

2. American College of Nurse-Midwives (ACNM)
   1522 K Street NW, Suite 1120
   Washington, DC 20005
   (202) 347-5445
   Gives listing of nurse-midwives and nurse-midwifery training
   programs.

3. American College of Obstetricians and Gynecologists (ACOG)
   600 Maryland Ave SW
   Suite 300E
   Washington, DC 20024
   (202) 638-5577
   Offers professional and public educational materials concerning pregnancy and childbirth.

4. American Physical Therapy Association, Section on OB/GYN
   1111 North Fairfax Street
   Alexandria, Virginia 22314
   (703) 684-2782; (800) 999-2782
   Publishes a quarterly journal and provides seminars for physical
   therapists and childbirth educators.

5. American Society for Psychoprophylaxis in Obstetrics
   (ASPO/Lamaze)
   1840 Wilson Boulevard, Suite 204
   Arlington, Virginia 22201
   (800) 368-4404 or (703) 524-7802

Offers certification in Lamaze method of childbirth preparation, publishes the Lamaze Parents Magazine and provides information about pregnancy and childbirth-related topics.

6. Birthworks
   PO Box 152
   Syracuse, New York 13210
   (609) 953-0371
   Offers a holistic approach to childbirth and provides information from a holistic standpoint.

7. Council of Childbirth Education Specialists, Inc.
   8 Sylvan Glen
   East Lyme, Connecticut 06333
   (203) 739-8912
   Childbirth organization offering certification to nurses, physical therapists; offers introductory and advanced seminars.

8. Read Natural Childbirth Foundation
   13301 Elseo Drive, Suite 102
   Greenbrae, California 94904
   Offers preparation in the Grantley Dick-Read method of prepared childbirth.

9. International Childbirth Education Association (ICEA)
   PO Box 20048
   Minneapolis, Minnesota 55420
   (612) 854-8660
   Certifies childbirth educators, has mail-order book store and offers information about pregnancy and childbirth education.

10. La Leche League International
    9616 Minneapolis Avenue
    PO Box 1209
    Franklin Park, Illinois 60131
    (212) 455-7730
    Headquarters for the 3000 groups throughout the world offering support for breastfeeding, through individual counseling and education.

11. Nurses Association of the American College of Obstetrics and Gynecologists
    (NAACOG)
    600 Maryland Avenue SW, Suite 200
    East Washington, DC 20024
    (202) 638-5577
    Organization for nurses specializing in obstetric, gynecologic, and neonatal nursing, with many publications related to preg-

nancy and childbirth; continuing education programs and current maternal and child health information.

12. National Clearinghouse for Alcohol Information
    U.S. Department of Health Services
    PO Box 2345, Department AFTE-FAS
    Rockville, Maryland 20852
    (301) 468-2600
    Offers information on effects of alcohol.

13. National Institutes of Health
    U.S. Department of Health and Human Services
    Building 31, Room 7A-32
    Bethesda, Maryland 20205
    (301) 496-4000
    Offers all NIH publications and information on antenatal diagnosis, Cesarean birth, toxoplasmosis, and ultrasound imaging.

14. U.S. Department of Agriculture
    WIC Supplemental Food Section
    1103 North B Street, Suite E
    Sacramento, California 95814
    (916) 322-5277
    Offers information on nutrition for pregnant nursing women.

## *Audiovisual Aids for Patient Education*

1. ASPO/Lamaze
   1840 Wilson Boulevard, Suite 204
   Arlington, Virginia 22201
   (800) 368-4404

2. BABES (Bay Area Birth Education Service)
   c/o Childbirth Graphics, distributor
   1210 Culver Road
   Rochester, New York 14609-5454
   (716) 482-7940

3. Childbirth Graphics
   PO Box 17025
   Irondequoit Post Office
   Rochester, New York 14617
   (716) 266-6769

4. International Childbirth Educators Association, Inc. (ICEA)
   PO Box 20048
   Minneapolis, Minnesota 55420-0048
   (612) 854-8660 or (800) 624-4934

5. Pennypress
   1100 23rd Avenue East
   Seattle, Washington 98112
   (206) 325-1419

6. Feeling Fine Programs, Inc.
   3575 Cahuenga Boulevard West, Suite 425
   Los Angeles, California 90068
   (800) 443-4040, in California, (800) 531-1212
   Distributes videos produced by American College of Obstetricians Gynecologists.

7. Milner-Fenwick Inc.
   2125 Greenspring Drive
   Timonium, Maryland 21093

8. Ross Laboratories
   A Division of Abbott Laboratories
   625 Cleveland Avenue
   Columbia, Ohio 43216
   (614) 227-3333

9. Barlas/Walker Associates
   15 La Costa Drive
   Natick, Massachusetts 01760
   (617) 893-3553
   Slide set of labor and birth produced by a physical therapist.

10. Polymorph Films, Inc.
    118 South Street
    Boston, Massachusetts 02111
    (617) 542-2004

11. Suzanne Arms Productions
    151 Lytton Avenue
    Palo Alto, California 94301

## *Publications for Patient Education*

1. "Back Care During Pregnancy and Beyond"
   Physical Therapy Services
   8710 Choctaw Road
   Bon Air, Virginia 23235

2. "Shape Up for Pregnancy"
   Kathy Tooman, PT
   2602 St. Mary's Drive
   Midland, Michigan 48640

3. "Exercise During Pregnancy"
   David J. Milano, PT
   BHCPT
   P.O. Box 1272
   Burlington, NJ 08016

4. "Better Baby Series"
   Pennypress
   1100 23rd Avenue East
   Seattle, Washington 98112
   (206) 325-1419
   Pamphlets available for childbirth classes relating to Cesarean births, obstetrical tests and technology, teenage childbirth, siblings at birth, exercise and nutrition.

5. "Ultrasound Exam in Obstetrics and Gynecology" and "X-rays, Pregnancy and You"
   The American College of Obstetricians and Gynecologists
   600 Maryland Ave SW, Suite 300E
   Washington, DC 20024
   (202) 638-5577

6. "Pregnant Patient's Bill of Rights" and "Pregnant Patient's Responsibilities"
   ICEA
   PO Box 20048
   Minneapolis, Minnesota 55420
   (612) 854-8660

7. "For the Expectant Father"
   Maternity Center Association
   48 E 92nd Street
   New York, New York 10018
   (212) 369-7300

8. "As You Eat, So Your Baby Grows: A Guide to Nutrition in Pregnancy"
   Ceres Press
   Box 87, Department D
   Woodstock, New York 12498

9. "Alcohol in Your Unborn Baby"
   U.S. Department of Health, Education and Welfare
   National Institute on Alcohol Abuse and Alcoholism
   5600 Fisher's Lane
   Rockville, Maryland 20857-78521

# ANSWERS TO SELF-ASSESSMENT REVIEWS

## Chapter Three

(1) Relaxin; (2) pelvic; (3) thoracic kyphosis; (4) stretches, weakens; (5) psoas; (6) rib cage; (7) heart; (8) inferior vena cava, aorta; (9) ossification; (10) ischial spines, pubic arch, sacral promontory, ischial tuberosities; (11) abdominopelvic, sacrococcygeal, sacroischial, pubic, sacroilial; (12) rotatory; (13) assist the examiner to determine inlet and outlet size; (14) pelvic diaphragm; (15) pelvic, urogenital.

## Chapter Four

(1) Breathing deeply; (2) increases slightly; (3) contraindicated; (4) reduced cardiac output in the supine position, due to compression by the expanding uterus; (5) 39°C, teratogenic, neurotubal; (6) decrease; (7) increased blood pressure and tachycardia; (8) smooth; (9) ovaries, relaxin; (10) pigmentation, eyes and cheekbones; (11) 14; (12) amenorrhea; (13) decrease in support of the uterus, bladder and rectum.

## Chapter Five

(1) Hormone; (2) autocrine, paracrine; (3) androgens, progestins, estrogens; (4) three; (5) follicular granulosa, corpus luteum; (6) corpus luteum; (7) releasing and interfering; (8) follicular, ovulation, luteal; (9) absence of flow; (10) painful flow, heat, exercise, TENS.

## Chapter Six

(1) Upper third; (2) transportation; (3) false; (4) smoking (or others in text); (5) cocaine (or others in text); (6) true; (7) false; (8) carbohydrates, proteins, fats; (9) Apgar; (10) Brazelton scale.

## Chapter Seven

(1) Breast tenderness, weight gain, nausea, frequent urination; (2) upward, abdomen, bladder; (3) lightening, engagement; (4) Braxton Hicks contractions; (5) lie, position, presentation, station; (6) regular contractions, bloody show, rupture of membranes; (7) Stage I, labor or cervical effacement and dilation; Stage II, delivery of the fetus; Stage III, delivery of the placenta; Stage IV, postpartum; Phases— Early or latent (effacement and 0-3 cm dilation), Active (4-7 cm dilation), Late or transition (7-10 cm); (8) poor cervical dilation, poor fetal descent, placental anomalies; (9) medications/anesthetics, childbirth education, TENS; (10) carefully document cases and submit for publication.

## Chapter Eight

(1) Disproportionate ratio between the child's head and the mother's pelvis; the head is not able to pass through the pelvis; (2) into the anal sphincter; (3) bulging of the bladder into the vagina after damage to the supporting structures of the bladder; (4) maternal position, full bladder, pelvic floor fatigue; (5) urethrovesical junction and urethra; (6) other than the head; (7) the infant's head is delivered, but the shoulders are too wide for the pelvic inlet; (8) vaginal birth after Cesarean, uterine rupture; (9) labor cannot be induced as necessary, labor is unsafe for mother and fetus, fetal or maternal dystocia, an emergency demands fetal delivery; (10) 37 or 38 weeks.

## Chapter Nine

(1) Decrease and return to normal size, decrease in weight, and shed endometrium; (2) lochia; (3) diaphoresis; (4) 2 to 3 weeks; (5) push with legs and buttocks while contracting the pelvic floor and bracing abdominal muscles; (6) pelvic floor toning and gentle abdominal exercises; (7) oxytocin and prolactin; (8) letdown reflex; (9) pelvic floor, abdominal muscles, back muscles, buttock muscles, and deep hip muscles; (10) myocardial disease, congestive heart failure, rheumatic heart disease (class II or above), recent pulmonary embolus,

acute infectious disease, uterine hemorrhage, severe hypotensive disease, diabetes mellitus, radicular arm or leg signs, sacroiliac pain, excessive vaginal bleeding, marked rectus diastasis

## Chapter Ten

(1) Diabetes that first appears during pregnancy; (2) effects of hormones on pelvis and postural positions; (3) False; (4) myoma; (5) hypertension, proteinuria, and edema; (6) seizures; (7) vomiting; (8) bronchospasm, increased airway secretions, hyperactive airways; (9) antihistamines and cough suppressants; (10) vaginally; (11) added breast weight, change in upper back posture.

## Chapter Eleven

(1) Prone lying and supine lying for longer than three minutes; (2) added uterine and breast weight anteriorly, change in center of gravity; (3) adaptive shortening occurs when a muscle is held in a shortened position without appreciable lengthening during relaxation and is associated with muscle strength; stretch weakness defines muscles that remain in a lengthened position; (4) no abdominal compression, avoid a supine position longer than 3 minutes, and side lying should be maintained with trunk and abdomen support; (5) iliacus; (6) walking on uneven terrain, frog kick in swimming, widely abducted legs in sexual positions, taking more than one stair at a time; (7) heat, exercise, lumbar support, posture correction; (8) childbirth; (9) externally rotated; (10) subluxed and extended; (11) mother's head may be thrusted in extension; (12) splinting of the wrist in neutral; (13) heat, friction massage, and a tendon injury program.

## Chapter Twelve

(1) Taking a careful history; (2) internal; (3) false; (4) pathology or communicable disease; (5) pressures; (6) relaxed; (7) sensory and motor tests of lower extremities and sacral nerves, deep tendon reflexes; (8) genuine stress, urge, reflex (see text for definitions); (9) cerebral-brain stem (loop I), brain stem-sacral (loop II), vesical-sacral-sphincter (loop III), and cerebral-sacral (loop IV); (10) exercise, relaxation, TENS (see text).

## Chapter Thirteen

(1) Changing outlooks on life, increased anxiety regarding child raising, concern for the unknown; (2) active relaxation is a conscious recognition of release and tension, passive relaxation occurs when a person withdraws temporarily from the surrounding environment; (3) an additional 300 calories; (4) 2 to 4 pounds, slightly less than 1 pound; (5) forward; (6) after four months' gestation, no exercise in

positions requiring supine position for longer than 3 minutes, no straining of pelvic floor or abdominal muscles, no exercise involving abdominal compression, no vigorous stretching of hip abductors, no sharp twists or uncontrolled swinging or bouncing movements, and no position where the buttocks are higher than the head; (7) incisional healing, correct posture; (8) shallow chest breathing and rhythmic chest breathing; (9) avoids blood pressure fluctuation, maintains pressure of rib cage, abdominal muscles and diaphragm better interact together to push the baby down the birth canal; (10) breathing and pelvic floor exercises; (11) on demand.

## Chapter Fourteen

(1) Pregnancy, birth experience, or spouse's pregnancy; (2), (3), (4), (5) any of the topics or methods listed in the outlines above; (6) ASPO/Lamaze, ICEA, AAHCC; (7) the Section on Obstetrics and Gynecology of the American Physical Therapy Association in conjunction with the clinical specialties certification program of the APTA; (8) finding an OB/GYN practitioner, designing the internship; (9) work loads increase and obstetric services are cut; (10) referral source, support for services, or integrated team approach to patient care.

# GLOSSARY

**abortion** - any loss of pregnancy before the 28th week, either accidentally or intentionally

**abruptio placentae** - premature separation of the placenta from the uterine wall after 20 weeks of gestation

**active labor** - the second phase of the first stage of labor during which the cervix dilates from 4 to 8 cm

**activin** - hormone releasing factor that assists production of FSH at the pituitary

**after pains** - contractions of the uterus after the fetus and placenta are delivered

**afterbirth** - amniotic membranes and placenta, expelled from the uterus during the third stage of labor

**allantois** - the diverticulum from the hindgut of the embryo which appears around the 16th day of development; forming part of the umbilical cord and placenta

**alpha-fetoprotein** · nonhormonal plasma constituent in amniotic fluid used as a determinant of neural tube defects

**amenorrhea** · absence of monthly menstruation

**amniocentesis** · removal of amniotic fluid by a needle through the abdominal wall and uterus to determine the fetal age and genetic characteristics after 4 months' gestation

**amnion** · the innermost thin, tough layer of the sac surrounding the fetus (bag of waters)

**analgesic** · a drug that relieves or reduces pain without causing unconsciousness

**anesthetic** · a drug that produces loss of sensation with or without loss of consciousness

**antenatal** · during pregnancy

**antepartum** · the period from conception to birth (also called prenatal)

**antral** · relating to a body cavity

**Apgar score** · evaluation of the infant's condition in terms of heart rate, respiratory effort, muscle tone, reflex irritability, and skin color at 1 and 5 minutes after birth

**areola** · darkened area around the nipple

**autocrine** · method of intracellular hormonal communication

**back labor** · pain arising from pressure on the lumbar and sacral nerve roots, experienced in some women as the baby's head descends in the birth canal

**bonding** · the crucial attachment that develops between a mother, father, and their new baby after delivery

**Braxton Hicks contractions** · intermittent contractions of the uterus during pregnancy

**Brazelton Neonatal Behavioral Assessment Scale** · scale developed by Dr. T. Berry Brazelton to assess the newborn infant's ability to adapt to itself and the environment

**breech** · describes the position of the fetus in which anything but the head is presented first

**caudal** · a form of regional anesthesia administered below the spinal cord in the canal

**cephalopelvic disproportion** · a condition in which the infant's head is unable to fit through the pelvic outlet and is an indication for Cesarean delivery

**cerclage** · a purse string ring suture placed around an incompetent cervix at the level of the os at 12 to 14 weeks of gestation to prevent premature delivery from an incompetent cervix

**cervix** · the neck of the uterus, which leads into the vagina and thins out and dilates during labor

**Cesarean section** · delivery of a child by abdominal surgery

**chloasma** - mask of pregnancy; pigmentation appearing on forehead and cheeks of some pregnant women

**chloroform** - colorless, heavy liquid-formerly used as a general anesthetic

**cholestasis** - suppression or arrest of bile flow

**chorion** - the outermost membrane that encases the fetus

**chorionic villus biopsy** - biopsy of the chorionic villus that determines chromosomal and metabolic abnormalities of the fetus from 9 to 11 weeks' gestation

**circumcision** - the surgical removal of foreskin from the male infant's penis

**cleansing breath** - the breath taken at the beginning and end of a labor contraction to signal the support person and to begin and end each breathing technique

**climacteric** - major turning point in a female's life from ability to reproduce to a state of nonreproductivity

**clitoris** - small, round-shaped organ at the anterior part of the vulva

**colostrum** - watery-like milk secreted from a woman's breasts during pregnancy and during the first few days postpartum

**contractions** - shortening and tightening of the uterine muscle fibers during and after labor

**corpus luteum** - endocrine body that produces progesterone and develops in the ovary at the site of the ruptured ovarian follicle

**crowning** - indicates the presenting part of the infant visible at the vaginal opening; sometimes refers to the time at which the widest diameter of the presenting part is passing through the vaginal opening

**cryptomenorrhea** - monthly signs of menstruation without blood flow

**cystocele** - downward and forward displacement of the bladder towards the vaginal opening, often related to weakness or traumatized muscles from childbirth

**decidua** - mucus membrane lining the uterus (or endometrium) that changes in preparation for pregnancy and is sloughed off during menstruation and during postpartum

**DES - diethylstilbestrol** - drug given to mothers during the 1950s to prevent miscarriage; caused congenital abnormalities in both male and female offspring

**detrusor muscle** - the muscular component of the bladder wall

**diameter** - measurements of the pelvic inlet and fetal head; (biparietal - the largest transverse diameter of the fetal skull at term)

**dilation (dilatation)** - the stretching and enlarging of the cervical opening to 10 cm to allow birth of the infant

**dipping** - presenting part slightly enters bony pelvis from abdominal cavity

**ductus arteriosus** - the channel between the pulmonary artery and aorta in the fetus, usually closing over soon after birth

**dysmenorrhea** - pain experienced during menstrual periods

**dyspareunia** - painful intercourse

**dystocia** - a difficult childbirth; a fetal dystocia is difficult labor due to abnormalities of the fetus relative to size or position; b) maternal dystocia - difficult labor due to abnormalities of birth canal or uterine inertia

**eclampsia** - an acute disorder related to pregnant and puerperal women, consisting of convulsions and loss of consciousness associated with hypertension, edema and proteinuria

**effacement** - thinning and shortening of the cervix, occurring before or during dilation expressed in percentages of 0% to 100%

**electronic fetal monitoring** - the monitoring of the fetus and uterine contractions through internal and external pressure and sound transducers during labor

**embryo** - baby from conception to 8 weeks gestation

**embryotomy** - extraction of a dead fetus by dismemberment

**endometriosis** - abnormal proliferation of the uterine mucus membrane into the pelvic cavity

**engagement** - signifies that the fetus has firm head-down position within the mother's pelvis, and is no longer floating above the bony pelvis

**enterocele** - herniation of the intestine below the cervix associated with congenital weakness or obstetric trauma

**epidural** - anesthesia injected into the epidural space of the spine which can produce loss of sensation from the abdomen to the toes

**fetal distress** - decrease in fetal heart rate and the possibility of meconium-stained amniotic fluid related to jeopardized fetal oxygen supply

**fetus** - describes the baby from the 8th week after conception until birth

**first stage of labor** - initial part of labor when the cervix effaces and dilates to 10 cm; includes the early, active and transition phases

**fistulas** - abnormal passage between two organs, (e.g., rectovaginal-passage between the rectum and vagina)

**floating** - refers to the fetus floating within the uterus in the abdomen above the bony pelvis

**footling breech** - presentation where a foot is the presenting part

**forceps** - locked tong-like obstetrical instruments used to aid in delivery of the fetal presenting part

**frank breech** · position of the fetus where both legs are flexed against the abdomen and the sacrum is the presenting part

**fundus** · the top upper portion of the uterus

**gestation** · total period of time the baby is carried in the uterus, approximately 40 weeks in humans

**grand multipara** · a woman who has given birth seven or more times

**gravida** · a pregnant woman

**hydatidiform mole** · anomaly of the placenta which forms a nonmalignant mass from cystic swelling of the chorionic villi; no embryo is present

**hysterectomy** · surgical removal of the uterus

**incompetent cervix** · cervix that prematurely dilates as pregnancy progresses

**involution** · the return of the uterus to the nonpregnant size and position

**Kegel exercises** · pelvic floor strengthening exercises developed by Dr. Arnold Kegel

**labia** · the external folds surrounding the vagina and urethra

**labor** · refers to the uterine contractions that produce dilation and effacement of the cervix, assisting in descent of the fetus and delivery through the vaginal opening

**lactiferous** · secreting milk

**lanugo** · fine hair on the body of the fetus after the fourth month in utero

**latent phase** · early phase of the first stage of labor which ends when the cervix is fully effaced and 3 to 4 cm dilated

**letdown reflex** · the involuntary release of milk through the nipples that occurs at the beginning of breastfeeding

**luteinizing hormone (LH)** · a pituitary hormone responsible for developing a corpus luteum

**lie of the fetus** · relationship of the long axis of the fetus to the long axis of the mother

**lightening** · occurs when the fetal head drops into the pelvic inlet, allowing the uterus to descend to a lower level, relieving pressure on the diaphragm and making breathing easier during the last few weeks of pregnancy

**linea nigra** · pigmented line appearing on the abdomen, from the pubis to the umbilicus in pregnant women

**lochia** · discharge of blood, mucus, and tissue from the vagina after delivery, often lasting up to 6 weeks after birth, but usually referring to the bright red discharge of the first 2 weeks postpartum

**malposition** · faulty or abnormal position not favoring normal descent of the presenting part

**malpresentation** - abnormal fetal presenting part

**mechanism of labor** - describes the five positions that the fetal head assumes through the pelvis: descent, flexion, internal rotation, extension, and external restitution

**meconium** - fetal bowel movements

**micturition** - the act of urinating

**midwives** - attendants who assist women during labor and delivery

**molding** - the shaping of the fetal head by the overlapping fetal skull bones to adjust to the size and shape of the birth canal

**mucus plug** - a plug produced by the endocervical glands to seal the cervical canal, which is extruded from the vagina in early labor

**multigravida** - a woman who has been pregnant more than once

**multipara** - a woman who has completed two or more pregnancies to the stage of viability

**multiparity** - refers to a condition of having two or more children

**multiparous** - refers to having given birth to two or more offspring in separate pregnancies

**myoma** - benign tumor consisting of muscle tissue

**myometrium** - fixed, smooth muscle forming the middle layer of the uterine wall

**neonatal period** - represents the first 4 weeks of an infant's life

**occipitofrontal** - a line from the root of the nose to the most prominent portion of the occipital bone of the fetus at term

**occipitomental** - diameter from the chin of the fetus to the most prominent portion of the occipital bone; the correct angle for the application of forceps

**occiput anterior** - fetal occiput to the mother's symphysis pubis

**oligomenorrhea** - longer intervals between menstrual periods from 38 days to 3 months

**oliguria** - low excretion of urine

**oocyte** - a primitive cell in the ovary that after meiosis becomes an ovum

**oxytocin** - hormone stored in the pituitary that causes contraction of the uterus

**papilla** - a nipple-like protrusion from the surface of an organ

**paracervical** - refers to anesthesia injected in one or several locations around the uterine cervix

**paracrine** - method of extracellular hormonal communication

**paracyesis** - pregnancy that develops outside the uterus in the abdominal cavity

**parity** - condition of having produced viable offspring

**parturition** - the act of giving birth, or childbirth

**pelvic contraction** - condition in which one or more diameters of the pelvis is narrower than normal, not allowing for normal progression of labor

**pelvic floor** - sling arrangement of ligaments and muscles that supports the reproductive organs

**pelvimetry** - method of obtaining pelvic measurements by x-ray

**perineometer** - pressure sensitive device inserted vaginally to measure the strength of pelvic floor muscles

**pessary** - a circular ring device used to hold a prolapsing uterus in place when surgical repair is contraindicated

**phases** - three periods of uterine activity during the first stage of labor

**pica** - bizarre appetite

**pitocin** - synthetic oxytocic hormone administered through intravenous drip to induce or augment uterine contractions

**placenta** - organ that develops within the uterus from which the fetus derives its nourishment; also serves as a filtering system

**placenta previa** - condition where the placenta implants in the lower segment of the uterus and partially or completely covers the cervical opening

**premenstrual syndrome (PMS)** - symptoms that occur monthly after ovulation and usually cease at menstruation or shortly thereafter

**podalic version** - manipulation of a breech fetus presentation internally or externally

**polyhydramnios** - excess volume of amniotic fluid greater than 2000 ml

**position** - relationship of the fetus to the mother's pelvis

**postpartum** - period following birth

**precipitate delivery** - unexpected or sudden birth following a very short labor

**preeclampsia** - condition of hypertension, edema and albuminuria noted in late pregnancy, and possibly leading to serious toxemia

**premature rupture of the membranes** - rupture of the amniotic sac before the fetus is at full-term

**presenting part** - the part of the fetus that is first engaged in the pelvis

**primigravida** - a woman who is in her first pregnancy

**progesterone** - a hormone produced by the ovary responsible for changes in preparing the wall of the uterus for implantation

**prolapsed uterus** - uterus that has descended into the vaginal canal due to weakness of the supporting structures

**prostaglandin-synthetase inhibitors** - substances that inhibit the synthesis of prostaglandins

**prostaglandins** - lipid soluble hormone-like acetic compounds occurring in nearly all tissues, used for inducing labor

**pruritus gravidarum** - generalized itching not relieved by medication

**psychoprophylaxis** - psychologic and physical preparation for childbirth as taught in labor and delivery classes

**ptyalism** - increased saliva production, usually returns to normal by the middle of the second trimester

**puerperium** - the time from the end of labor to when the uterus returns to its normal size, approximately 6 weeks

**quickening** - the sensation of fetal movement, usually initially occurring between the 4th and 5th months of pregnancy

**rectocele** - herniation of the rectum with protrusion into the vaginal canal, or prolapse of the rectum into the perineum

**reflex incontinence** - form of incontinence caused by inability to inhibit bladder stimulatory reflexes

**relaxin** - a polypeptide ovarian hormone secreted by the corpus luteum, possibly acts on the ligamentous structures of the body, slackening the ligaments to allow greater opening in the pelvic outlet

**Rh factor** - hereditary blood factor found in red blood cells determined by specialized blood tests; when absent, a person is Rh negative

**ritodrine** - drug given to suppress labor

**round ligament** - pair of ligaments that hold the uterus in place, extending laterally from the fundus between the folds of the broad ligaments to the lateral pelvic wall, terminating in the labia majora

**rupture of the membranes** - refers to the rupture of the amniotic sac prior to delivery

**second stage of labor** - includes the time from 10 cm of dilation until birth of the baby

**shoulder dystocia** - occurs when the presenting part in the pelvic inlet is the fetal shoulder, thereby arresting normal progression of labor

**show** - refers to the blood and mucus plug that is extruded from the vagina in early labor

**speculum** - an instrument used to hold open and dilate the vagina during inspection

**spinal** - an injection of anesthesia into the spinal fluid to produce numbness

**stages** - refers to the three divisions of labor, delivery of the child and delivery of the placenta

**station** - locates the presenting part of the fetus in relation to the mother's ischial spines

**stress incontinence** - occurs when intravesicular pressure exceeds urethral resistance, detrusor activity absent

**stress test** - used at the end of pregnancy to attempt to induce uterine contractions to determine fetal well-being

**striae gravidae** - stretch marks appearing on the distended skin caused by the rupture of elastic fibers due to excessive distention

**suboccipitobregmatic** - diameter of the fetal skull from middle of the large fontanelle to the undersurface of the occipital bone where it joins the neck

**teratogens** - substances which will produce abnormal fetal development if given to the mother in pregnancy through drugs or environmental factors

**terbutaline** - drug given to mothers to stop premature labor

**thalidomide** - drug used as a tranquilizer in the 1950s that in pregnant women produced severe limb abnormalities in offspring

**third stage of labor** - birth of the placenta

**tocolytic** - drug used to arrest labor

**transition** - the last phase of the first stage of labor when the cervix dilates from 0 to 10 cm

**transverse lie** - refers to the fetus in a horizontal position across the mother's pelvis

**trigonal** - relating to a triangular shape

**unripe** - describes a cervix that is not soft and not ready for labor

**urethrocele** - prolapse of the urethra with bulging into the vaginal opening

**urogenital diaphragm** - the perineal membrane, the deep muscle layer of the deep fascial layer which supports the pelvic organs

**uterine dysfunction** - inability of the uterus to contract and relax in a coordinated fashion

**uterus** - the pear-shaped organ in which the fetus grows; also called the womb

**vacuum extractor** - device consisting of a cup, hose, and pump that creates a vacuum against the fetal head and to which traction is then applied to assist in delivery of the fetus through the birth canal

**vagina** - a 5-6 inch long elastic canal from the vulva to the uterus

**Valsalva maneuver** - when intraabdominal pressure is increased by breath holding during exertion

**vulva** - external female genitalia

**Wharton's jelly** - connective tissue with jelly-like material within the umbilical cord that supports the umbilical vessels

**whey proteins** · protein content of mother's milk

**yolk sac** · the highly-vascularized umbilical vesicle surrounding the yolk of the embryo

Definitions adapted from: Dox I, Melloni BJ, Eisner GM: Melloni's Illustrated Medical Dictionary. Baltimore, Williams & Wilkins, 1979; and Thomas CL (ed): Taber's Cyclopedic Medical Dictionary (13th ed). Philadelphia, FA Davis, 1977.

# Index